Deconstructing Toxic Narratives

Lynn R. Webster • Sarah Eichberg

Deconstructing Toxic Narratives

Data, Disparities, and a New Path Forward in the Opioid Crisis

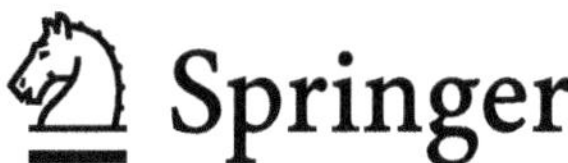

Lynn R. Webster
Lifetree Medical Inc
Salt Lake City, UT, USA

Sarah Eichberg
The Eichberg Group
Dunedin, FL, USA

ISBN 978-3-032-23134-5 ISBN 978-3-032-23135-2 (eBook)
https://doi.org/10.1007/978-3-032-23135-2

This Springer imprint is published by the registered company Springer Nature Switzerland AG
The registered company address is: Gewerbestrasse 11, 6330 Cham, Switzerland

Preface

For much of my professional life, I have lived at the intersection of two often conflicting realities—bearing witness to both the devastation that opioids can cause and the indispensable relief they provide for people living with severe, unrelenting pain. I have seen patients transformed, some shattered, some healed, by these medications. I have also seen the public narrative around opioids shift dramatically over time, often driven less by evidence than by fear, outrage, and misinformation.

This book was born out of frustration: frustration at the pervasive misunderstanding of addiction, the misrepresentation of scientific data, and the oversimplified public discourse that assigned blame without nuance. Early in my career, like many of my peers, I struggled to understand why some individuals misused medications while others did not. We lacked the tools and frameworks to recognize addiction risk or even define addiction itself. At the same time, I heard the desperate cries of patients in pain—patients who were stigmatized, neglected, or abandoned as policy shifted sharply in reaction to rising overdose deaths.

Despite my commitment to science, I came to understand that the opioid crisis was shaped less by data and more by emotional pain: by fear, grief, trauma, and good intentions gone awry. Most people who engaged with the crisis—clinicians, policymakers, advocates, and journalists—did so earnestly. But many were misguided, misinformed, or driven by a need for certainty in the face of overwhelming complexity.

While I initially planned to write a different book on the history of the opioid crisis, I realized I first needed to ask fundamental questions about its underlying dynamics. Several years of research and data analysis convinced me that the content of this book is essential to understanding that history.

My work with the pharmaceutical industry was to seek safer and more effective treatments for pain and addiction with the goal of reducing the need for opioids. This experience provided perspective into how industry operates. It is not an altruistic enterprise. We live in a capitalistic society where incentives for innovation can be a positive force in solving medical problems. However, profit-seeking can unintentionally cause collateral damage. While financial incentives can drive innovation, they become indefensible when the pursuit of profit endangers human lives.

I have always been driven to make a difference, to improve the lives of those I treated and the community at large. When practicing medicine, I feared I would hurt someone. To avoid this and to offer cutting-edge therapies, I felt I had to be on the front line of research. This journey generated clinical questions, with each answer leading to many more unknowns. This book is an extension of my attempt to understand what I did not know and, ultimately, what I believe the larger community should understand as well.

I understand that some readers may question my objectivity or view my perspective as conflicted. I do not dismiss those concerns. Scrutiny of potential bias is valid and necessary in any public health discussion. But it is also important to recognize that engaging with industry has given me unique insights into how treatments are developed, marketed, and regulated. That perspective is not inherently disqualifying; in fact, it can help illuminate aspects of the opioid crisis that are often overlooked. To dismiss a viewpoint solely because of a perceived affiliation is itself a form of bias—one that risks obscuring the complexity of the issues at hand. I ask readers to approach this book with an open mind, evaluating its arguments on the strength of the evidence and reasoning rather than on assumptions about its author.

Though some of my questions have been partially answered through this journey, there are many more that remain unresolved. I would never claim to have all the answers; indeed, the depth of the unknown is vast. But by seeking to understand, by asking difficult questions, and by listening to those most affected, I believe we can move closer to the truth.

Deconstructing Toxic Narratives is designed for a wide audience, including policymakers, public health professionals, medical practitioners, academic researchers, advocates, and journalists—anyone seeking to look beyond the headlines and understand the deeper systemic drivers of the opioid crisis. It is particularly relevant to professionals in pain and addiction medicine, public health, health policy, and medical sociology, as well as graduate and postgraduate students studying substance use, structural health disparities, and criminal justice. By integrating perspectives from public health, sociology, economics, and policy, the book offers a rigorous but accessible foundation for interdisciplinary coursework, policymaking, investigative reporting, and applied research.

Unlike works that narrowly attribute the opioid crisis to pharmaceutical misconduct or prescribing trends, this book challenges dominant narratives and exposes the toxic misconceptions that have misdirected policy and public understanding. It contains new data and methods, from econometric analyses to qualitative synthesis, revealing how structural inequality, social fragmentation, and economic dislocation drive substance use disorder (SUD). The data and illustrating visual elements are designed for critical discussion in academic, journalistic, and policy forums as the basis for lectures, policy simulation exercises, or interdisciplinary case studies on addiction, stigma, and health equity. The final chapter proposes forward-looking solutions—proposals not yet widely considered in public discourse—that push beyond harm reduction and toward systemic reform.

Deconstructing Toxic Narratives explores the structural and social-ecological contributors to drug use and SUD. Crucially, this focus is not meant to undervalue the strong role played by genetic vulnerability. This is an important point for families who have lost a child to SUD despite possessing strong support systems and none of the external risk factors highlighted here. Conversely, other families see no clear genetic link to their loved one's struggle. This book seeks to acknowledge these diverse experiences, recognizing that not every story of SUD fits neatly into a category of genetic vulnerability or social-structural disadvantage. Ultimately, the core message is that SUD is multifaceted, with no single cause. The core message is that we must consider multiple dimensions to effectively prevent harm and support those affected.

This book is my attempt to grapple with complexity and to offer a more accurate, compassionate, and evidence-informed narrative. I could not have done this alone. My co-author, Sarah Eichberg, brought deep research expertise and a sociological lens that served as the essential complement to my clinical and policy experience. Her analytical clarity and shared commitment to truth were vital in guiding this project toward a holistic understanding of the crisis and a vision for moving forward.

Salt Lake City, UT, USA Lynn R. Webster

AI Usage Statement for Lynn Webster

Lynn R. Webster: For some content, I wrote what I wanted to say and then submitted it to ChatGPT for editing and clarification. I created all of the content, but ChatGPT sometimes served as an editor before I sent it to a live editor for further clarification. Whenever I use AI assistance, I may go through a dozen iterations before I am satisfied with the product. I have learned not to trust ChatGPT. It may say the opposite of what I have written so I have to start over or tell it where it made a mistake. It requires careful reading.

AI Statement for Sarah Eichberg

During the preparation of this manuscript, I independently developed and drafted all scientific content, using ChatGPT (OpenAI) solely for language editing and clarification. All AI-assisted text was carefully reviewed, verified, and revised to ensure accuracy and alignment with my intended meaning. No AI tool was used to generate scientific ideas, analyze or interpret data, or influence the manuscript's conclusions. The final version of the manuscript was subsequently reviewed and edited by a human editor. I take full responsibility for the integrity of the content and conclusions presented here.

Acknowledgments

I am deeply grateful to those who supported the development and production of *Deconstructing Toxic Narratives: Data, Disparities, and a New Path Forward in the Opioid Crisis*.

I owe special thanks to my co-author, Sarah Eichberg. Her comprehensive understanding of the social, political, and structural forces shaping pain and addiction—and her unwavering commitment to intellectual rigor—provided the spine for many of this book's central themes. Her insight and clarity of thought were vital to transforming scattered ideas into a coherent and compelling narrative. Her collaborative spirit and tireless dedication were instrumental in bringing this complex volume to fruition.

My sincere thanks to Nishanthini Vetrivel, Production Editor at Springer Nature, for her invaluable guidance in preparing the manuscript and navigating the publishing process. I am also grateful to Gregory Sutorius, Executive Editor, whose support for a contrarian and evidence-based perspective on the opioid crisis made this book possible.

This book is directly informed by the foundational research of the broader scholarly community whose investigations of the socioeconomic, structural, and political drivers of substance use, overdose, and the opioid crisis paved the way for this work. Our analysis stands on their decades of empirical inquiry and critique and is intended as a direct continuation of their efforts to deconstruct toxic narratives through evidence-based scholarship.

I am especially indebted to my long-time friend and associate, Beth Dove, whose contributions to this book were both extensive and indispensable. She rigorously challenged the content and framing, identified inconsistencies in the narrative, and helped ensure that the data and arguments aligned with the evidence. She edited multiple versions of the manuscript and, ultimately, prepared the complete submission package for the publisher. Her insight, discipline, and persistence—including countless quiet interventions behind the scenes—were truly critical to making this book happen and elevated the work far beyond what I could have achieved alone.

I would also like to thank Samantha Elia, whose creation and refinement of several figures and graphics helped translate complex data and structural concepts into clear and accessible visuals.

My gratitude extends as well to Stacey Miller for her thoughtful editorial assistance. Her firm commitment to grammatical precision, clarity, and stylistic consistency was both needed and valued.

Above all, I owe a profound debt to the many people living with addiction and opioid use disorder whom I have cared for and learned from over the decades. They trusted me with their stories, their struggles, and their resilience. Much of what I understand about how addiction is created, sustained, and sometimes overcome has come from listening to them. Their courage and vulnerability are at the heart of this book.

Many others—colleagues, collaborators, reviewers, and advocates—contributed insights, encouragement, or lived experience that shaped this project. While I cannot name everyone individually, their influence is woven throughout these pages, and I remain sincerely thankful for their support.

Competing Interests The authors declare the following as potential competing interests:Lynn R. Webster reports having worked with industry in drug development, including professional activities that may include consulting and/or participation in industry-sponsored research. He has no affiliations with any religious or political entity that are relevant to the content of this book. He is an advocate for people with pain and addiction and writes about these subjects often. Sarah Eichberg has no competing interests to declare.

Contents

About the Authors

Sarah Eichberg PhD, is a sociologist, public health researcher, and policy consultant with over 30 years of experience advancing equity and addressing health disparities. Her insights on community health have appeared in the *New York Times*, *Bloomberg*, and *Newsday*, and been featured on NPR and CBS Radio. She believes research should engage communities and uplift voices, and that evidence can be a catalyst for healthier, more just societies. Her work connects universities and other institutions' resources with community priorities and translates research into practical strategies for underserved populations. A graduate of Smith College with a PhD in sociology from the University of Pennsylvania, she brings expertise in research design, data analysis, and policy development to initiatives that improve health and well-being across communities.

Lynn R. Webster MD, is a seasoned researcher, practitioner, and writer with expertise in addiction medicine, public health, and healthcare policy. He authored the award-winning book *The Painful Truth* (Oxford University Press) and co-produced the critically acclaimed television documentary of the same name, which was nationally distributed on public television. With decades of experience, he has published over 300 peer-reviewed articles, authored multiple books, and contributed to national dialogues on substance use and public health. Beyond his academic work, he has contributed to leading publications and broadcasts, including *The Wall Street Journal*, *The Washington Post*, *Bloomberg*, *NPR*, *ABC News*, *The New York Times*, and was a regular contributor to *The Hill*. Currently, he serves as a senior fellow at the Center for US Policy in Washington, DC. He is a past president of the American Academy of Pain Medicine and a senior editor for *Pain Medicine*. He is board-certified in anesthesiology, pain medicine, and addiction medicine.

1 Introduction

Not everything that is faced can be changed, but nothing can be changed until it is faced.

— James Baldwin (As Much Truth as One Can Bear, New York Times Book Review 1962; Also included in Baldwin J. As Much Truth as One Can Bear. In: The Price of the Ticket: Collected Nonfiction, 1948–1985. St. Martin's/Marek; 1962. p. 335–42.)

The dominant narrative concerning America's opioid epidemic[1] often centers on predatory pharmaceutical companies and unwitting physicians as primary culprits in the distribution of powerful opioid analgesics beginning in the 1990s. While the role of prescription opioids is undeniable, this narrative is incomplete and, in some ways, misleading. Conventional understanding of the crisis as an oversupply of prescription drugs does not account for its complex roots in long-term social and economic trends.

The long-term rise in overdose deaths sparked what is now a 30-year-long public health episode responsible for tremendous suffering and death, despite repeated regulatory and clinical interventions. Over the past 20 years (2003–2023), more than 750,000 Americans have died from opioid-related overdoses (both prescription and illicit), a 513% increase since 2003. Currently, most drug overdoses involve an opioid. In 2023 alone, 76% of the 105,007 drug overdose deaths in the United States (79,358 deaths) were opioid-related, primarily illegally manufactured fentanyl and fentanyl analogs, alone or in combination with another drug [1–3]. While these statistics underscore the devastating toll of the opioid crisis, they also raise questions about the effectiveness of current approaches to combat it (see Figs. 1.1 and 1.2).

[1] Use of the term "opioid epidemic" should not be read as acknowledgment that the epidemic is a discrete phenomenon untouched by social, political, and economic forces/interests.

L. R. Webster, S. Eichberg, *Deconstructing Toxic Narratives*,
https://doi.org/10.1007/978-3-032-23135-2_1

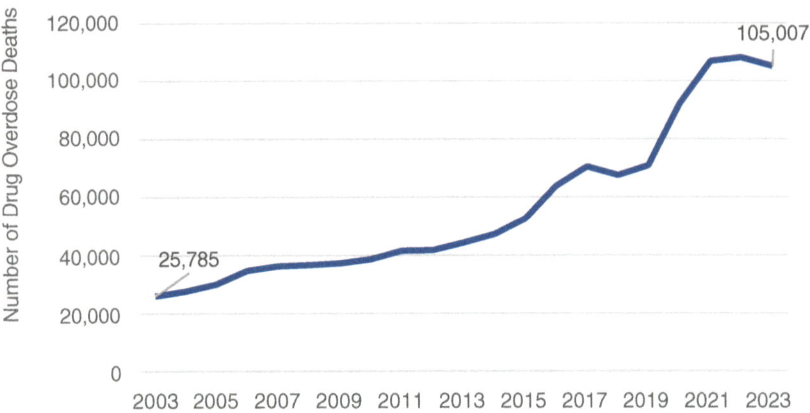

Fig. 1.1 Drug overdose deaths were identified using International Classification of Diseases, Tenth Revision underlying cause-of death codes X40–X44, X60–X64, X85, and Y10–Y14. Rates are age-adjusted per 100,000 Standard Population. (Source: National Center for Health Statistics, National Vital Statistics System, Multiple cause of death data on CDC Wonder)

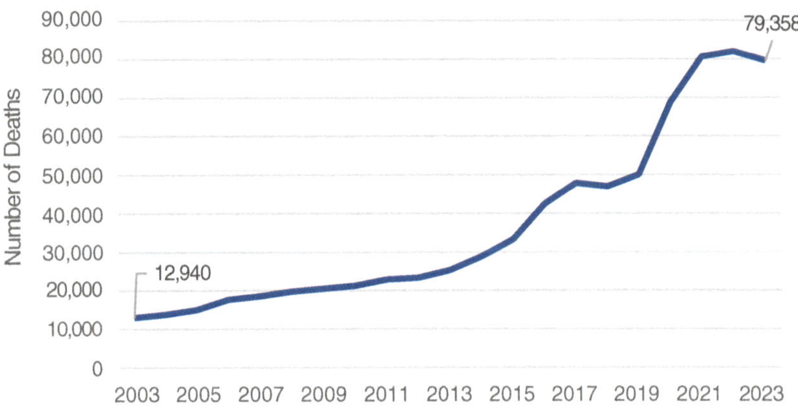

Fig. 1.2 Drug overdose deaths were identified using International Classification of Diseases, Tenth Revision (ICD–10) underlying cause-of-death codes X40–X44, X60–X64, X85, and Y10–Y14. Among these deaths, the following ICD–10 multiple cause-of-death codes indicate the drug type(s) involved: T40.0–T40.4, T40.6, any opioid; T40.1, heroin; T40.2, natural and semisynthetic opioids; T40.3, methadone; and T40.4, synthetic opioids other than methadone. Deaths involving more than one opioid category (e.g., a death involving both methadone and a natural and semisynthetic opioid) were counted in both categories. Natural and semisynthetic opioids include drugs such as morphine, oxycodone, and hydrocodone; and synthetic opioids other than methadone include drugs such as fentanyl, fentanyl analogs, and tramadol. Rates are age-adjusted per 100,000 Standard Population. (Source: National Center for Health Statistics, National Vital Statistics System, Multiple cause of death data on CDC Wonder)

The Centers for Disease Control and Prevention (CDC), the country's foremost public health agency, describes the opioid epidemic as a "three-wave" phenomenon in which mortality has been swept higher with each successive wave [4]. In the widely accepted but problematic CDC narrative, the epidemic's first wave occurred in the 1990s, marked by upsurges in opioid prescribing and prescription opioid overdose deaths. A second wave followed in 2010, propelled by heroin-involved overdose deaths after OxyContin reformulation and dose-curbing practice guidelines drove down prescribing rates and access to prescription opioids. The third wave, starting in 2013, has been driven by the surge in overdose deaths involving illegally manufactured fentanyl and other synthetic opioids introduced to the United States from China through Mexico (Fig. 1.3). Fentanyl and its analogs are used to spike other drugs, including different opioids, creating combinations that are stronger and deadlier. The CDC and other experts have also warned of a fourth wave, already underway, and characterized by increasing polysubstance use, particularly fentanyl mixed with stimulants, such as methamphetamine or cocaine (see Figs. 1.4 and 1.5).

This book challenges the dominant three-wave narrative. To be clear at the outset, it does not dispute that drug overdose deaths were in constant growth over the period described by the CDC. Rather, it posits that this long-term growth should be traced back well before the 1990s—to the 1970s—to capture various stages of an exponential rise in deaths caused by different types of drugs. The unremitting escalation reflects both the increasing lethality of the kinds and combinations of drugs being used *and* ever-shifting socioeconomic forces driving overdose fatalities.

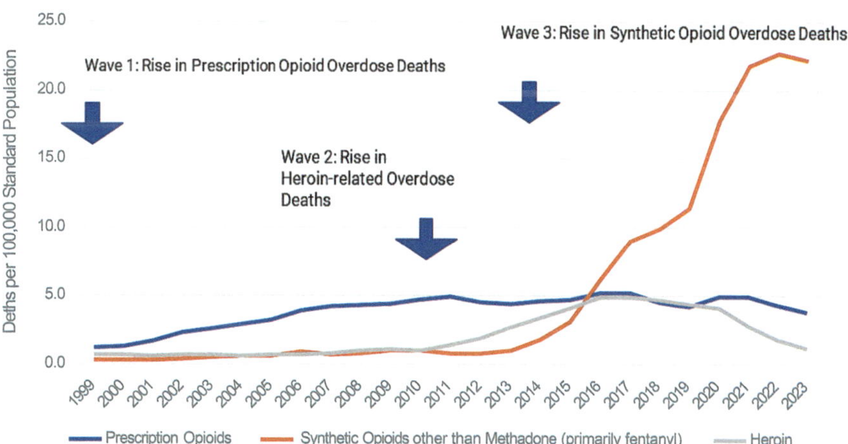

Fig. 1.3 Rates are age-adjusted per 100,000 standard population. Drug overdose deaths are identified using the International Classification of Diseases, 10th Revision (ICD–10) underlying cause-of-death codes X40–X44, X60–X64, X85, and Y10–Y14. Prescription Opioids: ICD-10 codes: T40.2-T40.3. Synthetic Opioids other than Methadone (primarily fentanyl): ICD-10 Code: T40.4; Heroin ICD-10 Code: T40.1. (Source: National Center on Health Statistics, National Vital Statistics System, Multiple cause of death data on CDC Wonder)

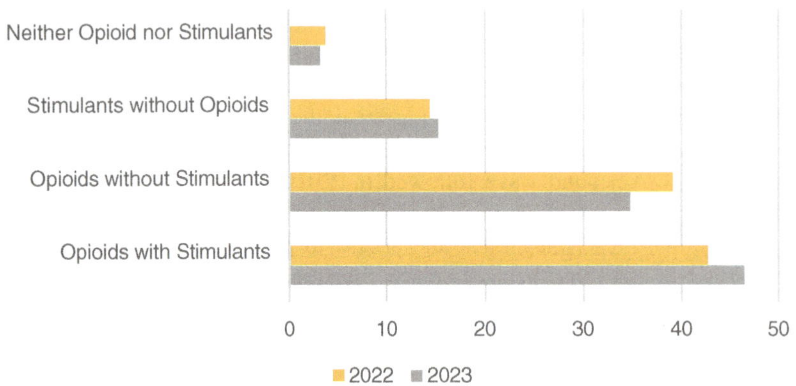

Fig. 1.4 CDC's Overdose Data to Action in States (OD2A-S) program supports 49 states and the District of Columbia to provide comprehensive data to the SUDOR. Each of these 50 funded jurisdictions collects and abstracts data on drug overdose deaths from death certificates, coroner/medical examiner reports, and postmortem toxicology reports for entry into a web-based CDC platform that is shared with the National Violent Death Reporting System (NVDRS). (Source: Centers for Disease Control (CDC), State Unintentional Drug Overdose Reporting System (SUDOR))

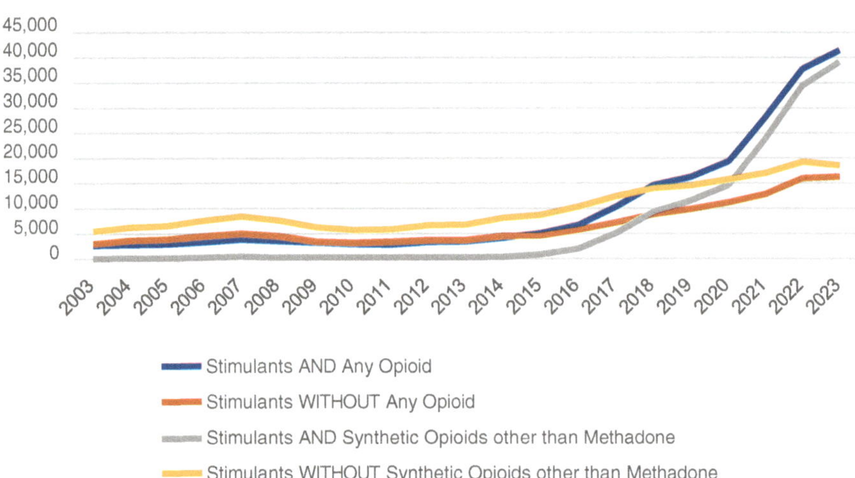

Fig. 1.5 ICD ICD-10 codes T40.5 and T43.6 Cocaine and psychostimulants, mainly methamphetamine. Mortality Rates are age-adjusted. (Source: Multiple Cause of Death Data at CDC Wonder)

Indeed, even as the CDC reports modest declines in overdose mortality, beginning in 2023, improving health outlooks, deaths remain at historically high levels. Meanwhile, the continued rise in deaths involving stimulants, cocaine, and other psychostimulants complicate any narrative of improvement and suggests that these declines may be temporary or influenced by situational factors—such as regional conditions or the easing of pandemic disruptions—that may not persist. The goal of this book is to offer sound empirical evidence to support these perspectives.

While the focus is primarily on the social, ecological, and policy dimensions of the crisis, it is essential to acknowledge that genetics also plays a significant role in opioid addiction risk. Twin, adoption, and family studies consistently estimate the heritability of opioid use disorder (OUD) to be between 40% and 60%, suggesting that inherited genetic differences contribute substantially to an individual's vulnerability to addiction [5]. Research has identified genetic variants across multiple neurobiological systems, including opioid receptor genes (e.g., OPRM1), stress regulation pathways (e.g., CRHR1), and reward circuitry components (e.g., COMT and HTR1B), which may shape individual responses to opioids and influence addiction trajectories [6].

Yet, genetic predisposition is not destiny. As neuroscientists and epidemiologists have emphasized, addiction emerges from the interaction of biological vulnerability and environmental exposure. Structural and social conditions, such as unstable housing, chronic stress, lack of access to health care, adverse childhood experiences, and economic dislocation, can act as catalysts, pushing those at genetic risk toward addiction. Conversely, supportive environments and equitable policy frameworks can serve as buffers that mitigate the expression of genetic vulnerability.

This book, therefore, takes a deliberate approach: it does not delve deeply into the complex genomics of addiction, not because these insights are unimportant, but because they are relatively less modifiable at a population level. We cannot change our genes, but we can change our environments. And it is precisely the structural environment—policies, institutions, and cultural discourses—that has enabled the opioid crisis to persist and evolve. Understanding and transforming these forces is the most effective path to preventing future suffering.

The concluding chapters will present potential demand-side solutions to the seemingly intractable opioid epidemic in the United States. For sustainable change to occur, certain elements must be in place. First, potential solutions must reflect the evolving nature of opioid misuse,[2] taking a multipronged approach to preventing or mitigating harm based on kind or combination of drugs. Policies and practices also must be rooted in social determinants of health frame and address the factors shaping opioid (mis)use across socioecological levels and social, cultural, and geographic contexts. Solutions must be equity-oriented and designed to promote racial and other forms of equality. As part of this approach, populations and communities with an excess burden of OUD or overdose, and who were excluded from earlier efforts, must be prioritized for prevention, treatment, and recovery and central to co-designing programs that address their needs.

Deconstructing toxic narratives means acknowledging that many prevailing interpretations of the opioid crisis are grounded more in ideology than in evidence. By unpacking the inconsistencies, oversights, and unintended consequences of dominant supply-side strategies, we can see how incomplete or misleading narratives can shape policy in damaging ways.

[2] There are many definitions for misuse in the addiction literature. Here, we define misuse as non-medical use or an unauthorized use of a prescription opioid.

References

1. Centers for Disease Control and Prevention. Drug overdose deaths in the United States, 2003–2023 [Internet]. [cited 2025 Sep 1]. Available from: https://stacks.cdc.gov/view/cdc/170565.
2. Garnett MF, Miniño AM. Drug overdose deaths in the United States, 2003–2023. NCHS Data Brief, no 522. Hyattsville: National Center for Health Statistics; 2024. doi:https://doi.org/10.15620/cdc/170565.
3. National Center on Health Statistics, National Vital Statistics System. Multiple cause of death data on CDC Wonder.
4. Centers for Disease Control and Prevention. Uncovering the Opioid Epidemic [Internet]. [cited 2025 Jul 29]. Available from: https://www.cdc.gov/museum/pdf/cdcm-pha-stem-uncovering-the-opioid-epidemic-lesson.pdf.
5. Ducci F, Goldman D. The genetic basis of addictive disorders. Psychiatr Clin North Am. 2012;35(2):495–519.
6. Mistry CJ, Bawor M, Desai D, Marsh DC, Samaan Z. Genetics of opioid dependence: a review of the genetic contribution to opioid dependence. Curr Psychiatr Rev. 2014;10(2):156–67.

Competing Narratives 2

The greatest obstacle to discovery is not ignorance—it is the illusion of knowledge.

—Daniel J. Boorstin (The 6 O'Clock Scholar: Librarian of Congress Daniel Boorstin And His Love Affair With Books, The Washington Post, 1984).

2.1 Introduction

In the complex landscape of public health crises, dominant narratives often shape policy responses, even when they present an incomplete picture. The prevalent understanding of America's opioid crisis, largely influenced by the Centers for Disease Control and Prevention's (CDC) "three-wave" narrative, has prioritized supply-side interventions like prescription limits and monitoring programs. However, what happens when policy based on such narratives yields mixed results or adverse unintended consequences?

This chapter examines the limitations of the prevailing supply-side approach to US drug policy. It explores the disconnect between falling prescription rates and persistently rising overdose deaths, revealing the inadequacies of current strategies. This chapter also scrutinizes the widely held belief that volume of prescription opioids is the primary driver of addiction, presenting evidence that challenges this conventional wisdom. By introducing multifactorial perspectives, including socioeconomic determinants, "deaths of despair," and racial disparities, this chapter encourages readers to evaluate how incomplete narratives can hinder effective policy, underscoring the need for a more comprehensive understanding of the opioid crisis.

L. R. Webster, S. Eichberg, *Deconstructing Toxic Narratives*,
https://doi.org/10.1007/978-3-032-23135-2_2

2.2 The Three-Wave Narrative: An Incomplete Picture

The widespread acceptance of the CDC's three-wave narrative among lawmakers has heavily influenced US drug policy, leading to a focus on the *supply* side of the drug market, which encompasses availability and pricing. Following guidance from public health organizations, particularly the CDC, most federal and state measures have prioritized law enforcement and public health surveillance. Predominant strategies include limits on how much and for how long opioids can be prescribed to patients and state prescription drug monitoring programs, which track patient data to flag for misuse of controlled substances [1]. Commitment to these strategies has been unwavering; yet, the results have been mixed at best.

Despite a 52% decrease in the per capita opioid prescribing rate from 2013 to 2023, opioid overdose deaths continued to rise for most of this period, exposing a flaw in expert causal thinking (Fig. 2.1) [2–5]. This disconnect between prescribing rates and overdose deaths suggests that the problem is more complex than simply the availability of prescription opioids. Meanwhile, chronic pain prevalence continued its long-term upward trajectory, further aggravated by new laws that led practitioners to abruptly reduce or discontinue long-term patients' dosages [6–8]. This change endangered the welfare of patients taking prescription opioids for pain and prompted some to replace prescription opioids with illicit drugs for pain relief, paradoxically exacerbating the very crisis supply-reduction measures were intended to prevent.

Yet, supply-side views continue to predominate. An editorial published in the *Washington Post* in 2019 by Keith Humphreys, a professor of psychiatry at Stanford University and former drug policy advisor in the Bush and Obama White Houses, rejects the need for alternative approaches (e.g., harm reduction and drug treatment)

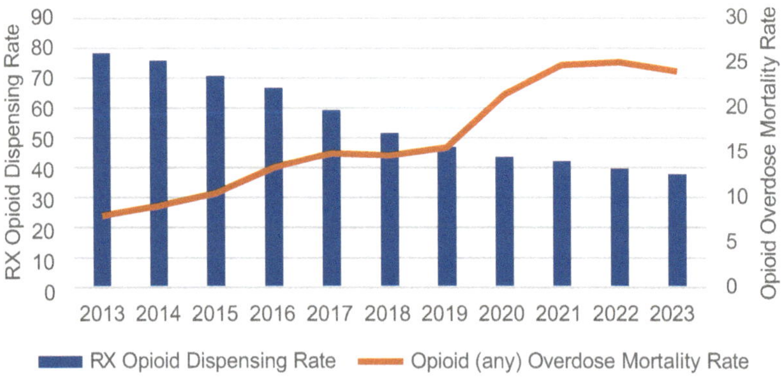

Fig. 2.1 IQVIA Xponent is drawn from a sample of approximately 50,400 retail (non-hospital) pharmacies, which dispense nearly 92% of all retail prescriptions in the United States. Opioid prescriptions include buprenorphine, codeine, fentanyl, hydrocodone, hydromorphone, methadone, morphine, oxycodone, oxymorphone, propoxyphene, tapentadol, and tramadol. (Source: Centers for Disease Control, Vital Statistics, Multiple Cause of Death Files, 1999–2020; 2018–2024; IQVIA Xponent (2013–2023))

and concludes: "We've repeatedly seen…that a rapidly rising supply of cheap, potent opioids leads to increased addiction and overdose rates. In short: Sometimes it's the drugs, stupid [9]."

However, a growing body of scholarship challenges this interpretation of clinical evidence and its application to the medical and legal requirements for opioid prescribing. These studies call into question the purported link between prescription opioid sales and overdose deaths proposed by Humphreys and others, highlighting the need for a more nuanced understanding of the issue.

2.3 Beyond Supply Side: Unpacking Multifactorial Causes

Watershed research by Aubrey and Carr is one example of moving beyond supply-side narratives. When the CDC's Guideline for Prescribing Opioids for Chronic Pain was released in 2016, the communication was highly impactful. Although not a directive, its recommendations for dispensing and managing opioids were quickly adopted as a standard of practice in laws across the United States [10]. To bolster its recommendations, the 2016 guideline cited a direct correlation between prescription opioid sales and opioid treatment admissions and prescription opioid overdose fatalities, using data from 1999 to 2010. Yet, when Aubrey and Carr re-evaluated these relationships, using data from the same sources for 2010–2019, they found that the positive relationships identified earlier had either reversed or disappeared [11]. Despite this, the CDC's revised guideline in 2022, which updated recommendations from 2016, retained the original discussion about the positive relationship between prescription opioid sales and overdose deaths [12]. What's more, the new version neglected to mention that the correlations were not present in the data 10 years later, a fact with resounding implications for pain management, addiction treatment, and public health policy.

Additional research has shown that for many people, nonmedical opioid use predates opioid use disorder (OUD). This stands as a competing narrative to a core myth of the mainstream opioid crisis narrative, namely that most individuals with OUD began with prescribed opioids for chronic and acute pain-related events [13, 14]. While there are undoubtedly patients who are susceptible to OUD under these conditions, it is actually a relatively rare pathway to addiction. As the first author of this book previously wrote, "If exposure alone were responsible for addiction, then the 50 million Americans who undergo an operation annually, or most Americans who undergo the nine [surgical] procedures in a lifetime, would develop an addiction [15]." In research on the experiences of "OxyContin addicts" entering rehab, Carise et al. found that close to 80% of respondents had never been prescribed opioids for any medical reason before undergoing treatment [14]. Studies following opioid-naïve adults prescribed opioid analgesics for post-surgical pain reveal that only a small percentage ever progress to chronic opioid use, varying by procedure and ranging from approximately 0.1% to 1.41% [16, 17].

Several sources have also raised questions about the accuracy and utility of dosage thresholds recommended in the CDC's guidelines.[1] In a study reviewing thousands of surgical claims, Brat et al. found no clear threshold of increased risk of negative outcomes, with daily dosages below 150 morphine milligram equivalents (MMEs) only weakly sensitive to misuse [18]. Dasgupta et al. made a similar discovery [19]. Examining the effect of high-dose opioid analgesics on overdose mortality, they detected a mortality rate of 0.022% over one year, but no distinct dosage risk threshold. On the other hand, they observed that mortality risk escalated for patients who were co-dispensed benzodiazepines (instead of opioids alone).

The studies above suggest that the narrative linking opioid misuse with pain prescriptions is nuanced, and that one-size-fits-all approaches to opioid management may be inadequate. The data imply (and future chapters will confirm) that addiction is a multifactorial process with various levels of risk varying across individuals/social groups and demographic features. The mixed results and conflicting evidence surrounding supply-side policies highlight the need for a broader perspective [20–22].

Additionally, opioid-related harm is not limited to OUD and misuse. Contributors to opioid-related overdose deaths include suicides, which are known to be undercounted in official reports, depression, and inadequately treated pain [23, 24].

2.4 System Dynamics Modeling: Revealing Unintended Consequences

In general, assessing policy impacts is difficult because long lags between implementation and behavioral outcomes, combined with unanticipated or intervening factors, can complicate analysis. System dynamics simulation modeling, which treats the opioid epidemic as a complex system with interacting factors, reveals that policies aimed at controlling supply of prescription opioids may yield unintended consequences. The models address complexity by depicting the opioid epidemic as a system, composed of stocks and flows and feedback loops, to evaluate adaptive response to internal and external influences, either *before* policy decisions are made or *after* results occur (Fig. 2.2). Parameter inputs include health and risk behaviors, environmental and social factors, and health-related resources and delivery systems [25].

In a recent study, Lim et al. tested a system dynamics model containing data on opioid initiation from 1999 to 2020 [26]. They observed that as a system, the opioid crisis' adaptation process did not necessarily produce behavioral outcomes aligned with drug policy aims. In fact, contrary to the conventional explanation, initiation of prescription opioid misuse dropped in the 2000s well before prescribing rates fell

[1] Both the 2016 and 2022 guidelines recommend that prescribers use caution when prescribing opioids. The 2016 guideline advises careful assessment of patients for treatment before prescribing ≥50 MME per day and warns against prescribing ≥90 MME per day. The 2022 guideline suggests that prescribers take care not to expose patients to greater harm than benefit.

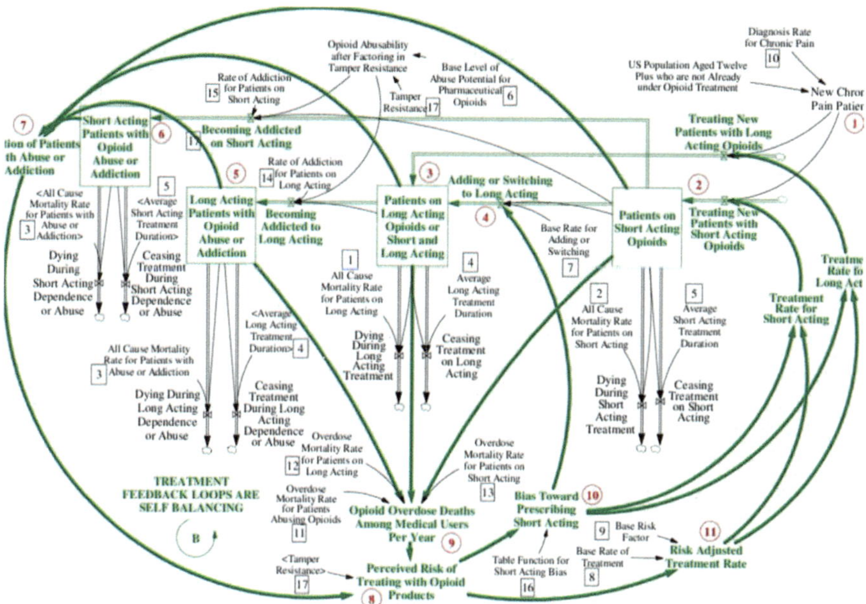

Fig. 2.2 Source: Wakeland, W., A. Nielsen, T. Schmidt, "System Dynamics Modeling of Medical Use, Nonmedical Use and Diversion of Prescription Opioid Analgesics," Proc. 30th Int'l Conf. System Dynamics Society, St. Gallen, Switzerland, July 2012

rather than after strict prescribing guidelines were in place. Failure by the CDC to recognize the actual transition order of phases of drug-related behavior left policy-makers ill-equipped to address the damage that followed.

Other system dynamics simulation models have exposed the potential for unintended outcomes from policies meant to control the dispensing of prescription opioids [27–29]. In a 2011 study, Wakeland et al.[2] modeled the effects of different interventions (e.g., physician education programs and tamper-resistant medications) on OUD and overdose deaths involving prescription opioids to treat patients with chronic pain [30]. They concluded that future decisions on policies to regulate pharmaceutical opioids must involve judicious "trade-offs" between outcome options. This is because any positive impacts, such as reduced mortality, are likely to be accompanied by negative effects on chronic pain patients' access to prescription opioid treatment. They reasoned that such supply disruption could produce dangerous results, including an increase in substitute drugs like heroin and fentanyl driving up overdose deaths.

Despite mounting evidence that the epidemic is multifaceted, the push for stronger supply-side laws and professional guidelines persists. As the outcome of the nation's drug policies continues to disappoint, it is more important than ever to question the relevance and utility of the interpretive framework that underlies such

[2] This research was partially funded by Purdue Pharmaceuticals.

regulations. Extant policies rarely consider the wider context in which the opioid crisis takes place. A truly comprehensive approach requires addressing demand-side factors, including the social and behavioral determinants that increase vulnerability to OUD and overdose and perpetuate disparities among different social groups. Without addressing both supply and demand, effective solutions will remain elusive.

2.5 A Demand-Side Perspective

Recognizing the limitations in mainstream accounts, a growing number of physicians and public health professionals are broadening their clinical and research scope to include social determinants of health (SDoH) (i.e., the societal conditions that shape and influence health outcomes) and other contextual factors when studying the opioid epidemic [31–36]. This broader perspective allows for a more integrated and multifactorial analysis over one that is unidimensional and ahistoric.

Considering SDoH leads to a more refined understanding of the epidemic's underpinnings and impacts, including barriers to treatment among diverse subpopulations and different places. These findings can be used to design evidence-based interventions that protect and promote the wellbeing of all people and communities.

One example of this approach is the socioecological model, already widely deployed in public health to capture the interplay of factors influencing quality of life across individual, interpersonal, community, and societal levels [35]. System dynamics simulation modeling also incorporates these multilevel influences. Figure 2.3 depicts a socioecological framework adapted to illustrate the factors producing and sustaining the opioid epidemic.

Multifactorial investigations have uncovered important insights that upend conventional understandings of the opioid crisis. Jalal et al.'s work challenges the notion that the opioid crisis is temporally bound [36]. Examining longitudinal data (N = 599,255 deaths from 1979 to 2016) on accidental drug poisonings, the authors exposed a 38-year exponential growth curve of drug mortalities resulting in more than one million estimated deaths. They conclude that the opioid crisis is part of a longer historical trajectory, encompassing multiple, yet discrete, sub-epidemics involving different drug classes across disparate populations and geographies. Linking the multiple sub-epidemics together into a smooth exponential curve may be essential to revealing deeper, underlying, causes of the opioid crisis.

Friedman et al. also take a long view of the crisis, examining how macroeconomic forces shape the community conditions that give rise to opioid overdose [33]. The authors posit various interactive upstream and downstream pathways to the epidemic, originating with what they call the "one-sided class war" or neoliberalism in the 1970s. At this time, free-market capitalism (re)emerged as the United States' dominant economic philosophy, leading to policies that shrank federal influence on the economy. (An extended definition of neoliberalism or free-market capitalism is provided in a later section.)

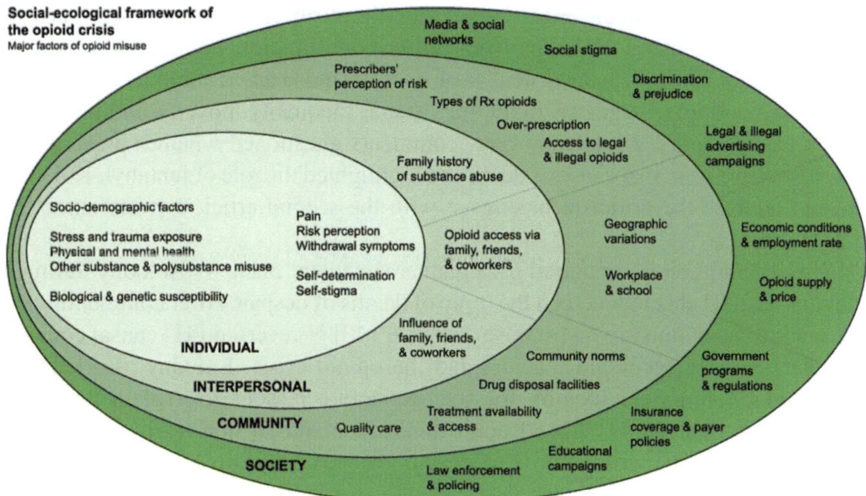

Fig. 2.3 Source: Jalali, M. S., Botticelli, M., Hwang, R. C., Koh, H. K., & McHugh, R. K. (2020). The opioid crisis: a contextual, social-ecological framework. *Health research policy and systems, 18* (1), 87

In Friedman et al.'s opinion, the implementation of free-market policies in the 1970s produced a socioeconomic environment downstream that set the epidemic on its current course. This move: (1) enabled pharmaceutical corporate misconduct with little accountability, (2) reinforced a culture of individualism, fueling despair and drug use, (3) undermined institutions that provided community support, and (4) eroded work place protections by reducing union power, undercutting remaining unions, and loosening enforcement of occupational safety and health regulations [33].

Perhaps the best-known work tracing the social origins of the US opioid crisis is Case's and Deaton's *Deaths of Despair and the Future of Capitalism* [37]. Their book documents the now widely reported link between economic decline and high death rates from suicide, alcoholism, and overdose of prescription opioids among less educated non-Hispanic white people. Case and Deaton argue that working-class white people develop OUD (or a disorder like alcoholism) to manage feelings of despair related to economic transformation, loss of work and community life, and social alienation. Despair in this case is derived not only from global capitalism's erosion of working-class wellbeing, but from structural forces that work through psychosocial factors—hopelessness, loss of purpose, and social isolation—to impact mortality.

Advocates for supply-side drug policies tend to ignore or dismiss the concept of deaths of despair. In 2018, Dr. Andrew Kolodny, Founder of Physicians for Responsible Opioid Prescribing, sparked debate on Twitter after posting an article describing a US drop in life expectancy due to the opioid crisis among young adults [38, 39]. Despite its heading, the article mentioned two studies that reached somewhat different conclusions. One explicitly attributed shortened lifespans to young people's misuse of/deaths from prescription opioids, heroin, and fentanyl, while the other acknowledged deaths of despair and blamed multifactorial influences for declining longevity, including "social inequality, poverty and declining health care quality." While followers' comments questioned whether prescription opioids were a principal cause of death and highlighted the role of fentanyl, Kolodny did not address the criticism or engage with the second article's focus on social determinants.

This assumption is supported by a plainer statement made by Kolodny during a webinar in 2021 that touched on the topic of deaths of despair. After commenting on the work of economists who propose a weaker [40] or reversed [41] causal connection between socioeconomic factors and the opioid crisis, Kolodny asserted that Case and Deaton were looking for socioeconomic reasons to explain the crisis because it is their field: "What I don't think Case and Deaton really understood, though, was that the vast majority of drug overdose deaths are occurring in people with the disease of opioid addiction, not necessarily people who are drinking or using drugs, driven by socioeconomic factors [42]." Kolodny further argued, "Social determinants of health are not a *cause* of the opioid crisis; certainly, though, social determinants of health impact morbidity and mortality in people with substance use disorders." However, such chicken-or-egg questions are not so easily settled, and despair, as deeper analysis will show, has components of trauma, isolation, and loss of social capital, not downward economic mobility alone.

> The increase in fentanyl use has disproportionately involved Black populations in urban areas; yet, research and policy remain fixed on prescription opioids and their threat to white rural and suburban Americans. This has happened partly because the drivers of the opioid crisis are not well known or understood. In this case, as in others, drivers matter because they change how the battle is fought, and whether it can ultimately be won.

Another notable criticism of *Deaths of Despair* is the book's singular focus on a white (sub)population, excluding other racial/ethnic groups from important policy conversations and outreach efforts. Indeed, race is central to how the opioid epidemic is framed, interpreted, and addressed. On the ground, structural racism shapes the lived experience of OUD for Black, Indigenous, and People of Color (BIPOC)[3] who are subject to systemic bias in the healthcare system as well as in other social,

[3] The term Black, Indigenous and People of Color (BIPOC) instead of People of Color (POC) is used in this book to acknowledge the distinct and disproportionate histories of structural racism, colonization, and state violence experienced by Black and Indigenous populations, which can be obscured under the broader term POC. Whenever data allow, we name racial and ethnic groups as specifically as possible (e.g., Black, Indigenous, or Chinese American), since aggregate terms like BIPOC and POC can mask important differences in experience, health outcomes, and access to care. It should be noted that both BIPOC and POC are contested terms; some critique POC for erasing specificity, while others view BIPOC as uneven or US-centric in its emphasis.

economic, and political domains. The increase in fentanyl use has disproportionately involved Black urban populations; yet, policymakers and the media remained fixed on prescription opioids, and their threat to white rural and suburban populations.

In a tendentious article, Keith Humphreys and co-authors argue that any short-term costs to patients with chronic pain from cutting the supply of prescription opioids, including increased heroin use or compromises in life quality, are outweighed by long-term positive health effects [43]. But who is benefiting and who is gaining when one means of death is exchanged for another, this time in BIPOC communities? A mismatch between real-world problems and popular policy prescriptions continues to take place because the drivers of the opioid crisis are not well known or understood. In this case, as in others, drivers matter because they change how the battle is fought, and whether it can ultimately be won.

The few studies examining the role of race in the opioid epidemic tend to uncover substantial knowledge gaps underscoring profound research needs. When unanticipated findings surface, they frequently call attention to limitations in established thinking about the epidemic. Reviewing mortality data from 1980 to 2015, Muennig et al. concluded that deaths of despair are not restricted to white Americans nor are they a recent phenomenon [44]. Instead, they are part of a protracted process of worsening health and life expectancy for all Americans due to widespread psychological distress, dissatisfaction, and hopelessness.

This position is supported in research by Friedman, Hansen, and Gone that revealed it is actually Native Americans who have the highest rate of midlife mortality from deaths of despair, signifying (again) that despair cuts across demographics [45]. Racial imbalances in deaths of despair are the result of myriad inequalities in socioeconomic conditions and public health. These include but are not limited to: differential access to mental health and substance misuse medications and treatment programs, increased rates of polysubstance use, and growing economic uncertainty and instability.

This insight is corroborated in the sociological literature, which measures an increase in despair in national surveys over the past 30–40 years. Like the opioid epidemic, the earlier crack cocaine and HIV/AIDS epidemics, while all but ignored in current narratives about despair, decreased life expectancy among Black Americans and widened disparities between white and Black people that is clearly reflected in the public health literature (Fig. 2.4) [46, 47].

With mental wellbeing deteriorating for white and BIPOC Americans alike, Muennig et al. close their article by arguing that exclusive focus on a white opioid crisis must be redirected. They assert: "We believe that the attention given to whites [in deaths of despair] is distracting researchers and policymakers from much more serious, longer term structural problems that affect all Americans [44]." In other words, sometimes it's not the drugs, it's the *structure*.

Most of the rest of this book will explore what is currently known about environmental, social, psychological, and economic factors driving the opioid epidemic, taking a transdisciplinary and multisource approach that incorporates qualitative research. Case and Deaton documented the explosion in deaths of despair through

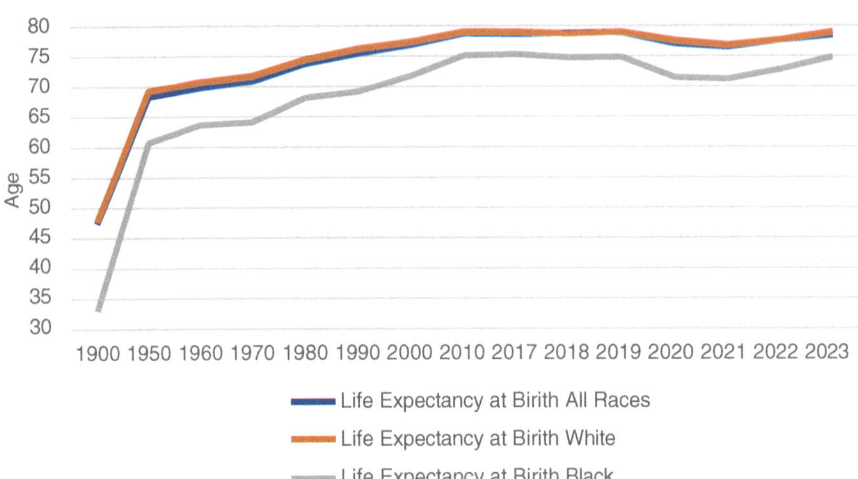

Fig. 2.4 Source: National Vital Statistics System, Multiple Cause of Death data on CDC Wonder; Sherry L. Murphy, B.S., Kenneth D. Kochanek, M.A., Jiaquan Xu, M.D., and Elizabeth Arias Ph.D. Mortality in the United States, 2023; Arias E, Xu JQ. United States life tables, 2020. National Vital Statistics Reports; vol 71 no 1. Hyattsville, MD: National Center for Health Statistics. 2022; Grove RD, Hetzel AM. Vital statistics rates in the United States, 1940–1960. 1968; National Center for Health Statistics. Vital Health Stat 2(152). 2010; United States life tables, 2001–2009 (using revised intercensal population estimates and a new methodology implemented with the final 2008 life tables) and United States life tables, 2010–2015 (based on a new methodology implemented with the final 2008 life tables and updated race and Hispanic-origin classification ratios)

analysis of CDC mortality data and other quantitative sources. While illuminating, their analysis did not investigate the underlying (and localized) mechanisms driving opioid overdoses in American communities. By including qualitative studies, we hope to provide insights into the social processes fueling the crisis as well as ways in which everyday people try to make sense of drug use in their lives and communities.

Understanding the structural and narrative roots of the opioid crisis requires not only interrogating the policies that emerged from dominant frameworks, but also examining the data used to formulate them. As Chap. 2 has shown, oversimplified causal claims have persisted despite conflicting evidence. In the next chapter, we turn our attention to the systems responsible for producing overdose data. We examine how flawed death reporting practices, inconsistent medical coding, and undercounting of suicides distort the reality of drug-related mortality, ultimately reinforcing harmful misconceptions and impeding effective, compassionate responses.

References

1. Soelberg CD, Brown RE Jr, Du Vivier D, Meyer JE, Ramachandran BK. The US opioid crisis: current federal and state legal issues. Anesth Analg. 2017;125(5):1675–81.
2. Bohnert ASB, Guy GP Jr, Losby JL. Opioid prescribing in the United States before and after the Centers for Disease Control and Prevention's 2016 Opioid Guideline. Ann Intern Med. 2018;169(6):367–75.
3. Centers for Disease Control and Prevention. United States dispensing rate maps [Internet]. Overdose Prevention 2024 Nov 7 [cited 2025 Jun 27]. Available from: https://www.cdc.gov/overdose-prevention/for-everyone/united-states-dispensing-rate-maps.html.
4. Centers for Disease Control and Prevention, National Center for Injury Prevention and Control. U.S. State Opioid Dispensing Rates, 2013 [Internet]. Atlanta: Centers for Disease Control and Prevention; 2020 Dec 7 [cited 2025 Sep 1]. Available from: https://archive.cdc.gov/www_cdc_gov/drugoverdose/rxrate-maps/state2013.html.
5. Guy GP Jr, Zhang K, Bohm MK, et al. Vital signs: changes in opioid prescribing in the United States, 2006–2015. MMWR Morb Mortal Wkly Rep. 2017;66(26):697–704. https://doi.org/10.15585/mmwr.mm6626a4.
6. Nahin RL, Sayer B, Stussman BJ, Feinberg TM. Eighteen-year trends in the prevalence of, and health care use for, noncancer pain in the United States: data from the medical expenditure panel survey. J Pain. 2019;20(7):796–809.
7. Zajacova A, Grol-Prokopczyk H, Zimmer Z. Pain trends among American adults, 2002-2018: patterns, disparities, and correlates. Demography. 2021;58(2):711–38.
8. Zimmer Z, Zajacova A. Persistent, consistent, and extensive: the trend of increasing pain prevalence in older Americans. J Gerontol B Psychol Sci Soc Sci. 2020;75(2):436–47.
9. Humphreys KN. We can't fight opioids by controlling demand alone. Washington Post. 2019 Jul 5 [cited 2025 Jun 30]. Available from: https://www.washingtonpost.com/outlook/we-cant-fight-opioids-by-controlling-demand-alone/2019/07/05/d025358e-7e2d-11e9-8ede-f4abf521ef17_story.html.
10. Dowell D, Haegerich TM, Chou R. CDC guideline for prescribing opioids for chronic pain - United States, 2016. MMWR Recomm Rep. 2016;65(1):1–49.
11. Aubry L, Carr BT. Overdose, opioid treatment admissions and prescription opioid pain reliever relationships: United States, 2010-2019. Front Pain Res (Lausanne). 2022;3:884674.
12. Dowell D, Ragan KR, Jones CM, Baldwin GT, Chou R. CDC clinical practice guideline for prescribing opioids for pain - United States, 2022. MMWR Recomm Rep. 2022;71(3):1–95.
13. Kertesz SG, Gordon AJ. A crisis of opioids and the limits of prescription control: United States. Addiction. 2019;114(1):169–80.
14. Carise D, Dugosh KL, McLellan AT, Camilleri A, Woody GE, Lynch KG. Prescription OxyContin abuse among patients entering addiction treatment. Am J Psychiatry. 2007;164(11):1750–6.
15. Webster L. The real reasons people become addicted. Pain News Network [Internet]. 2020 Jan 18 [cited 2025 Jun 30]. Available from: https://www.painnewsnetwork.org/stories/2020/1/18/the-real-reasons-people-become-addicted#google_vignette.
16. Sun EC, Darnall BD, Baker LC, Mackey S. Incidence of and risk factors for chronic opioid use among opioid-naive patients in the postoperative period. JAMA Intern Med. 2016;176(9):1286–93.
17. Rosenfeld S. Prolonged opioid use after surgery may burden public health. HCPLive. 2020. Available from: https://www.hcplive.com/view/prolonged-opioid-use-after-surgery-burden-public-health.
18. Brat GA, Agniel D, Beam A, Yorkgitis B, Bicket M, Homer M, et al. Postsurgical prescriptions for opioid naive patients and association with overdose and misuse: retrospective cohort study. BMJ. 2018;360:j5790.
19. Dasgupta N, Funk MJ, Proescholdbell S, Hirsch A, Ribisl KM, Marshall S. Cohort study of the impact of high-dose opioid analgesics on overdose mortality. Pain Med. 2016;17(1):85–98.

20. Dobkin C, Nicosia N. The war on drugs: methamphetamine, public health, and crime. Am Econ Rev. 2009;99(1):324–49.
21. Phillips JK, Ford MA, Bonnie RJ, National Academies of Sciences, Engineering, and Medicine. Evidence on strategies for addressing the opioid epidemic. In: Pain management and the opioid epidemic: Balancing societal and individual benefits and risks of prescription opioid use. National Academies Press (US); 2017.
22. Pollack HA, Reuter P. Does tougher enforcement make drugs more expensive? Addiction. 2014;109(12):1959–66.
23. Oquendo MA, Volkow ND. Suicide: a silent contributor to opioid-overdose deaths. N Engl J Med. 2018;378(17):1567–9.
24. Cheatle MD. Depression, chronic pain, and suicide by overdose: on the edge. Pain Med. 2011;12 Suppl 2(Suppl 2):S43–8.
25. Homer JB, Hirsch GB. System dynamics modeling for public health: background and opportunities. Am J Public Health. 2006;96(3):452–8.
26. Lim TY, Stringfellow EJ, Stafford CA, DiGennaro C, Homer JB, Wakeland W, et al. Modeling the evolution of the US opioid crisis for national policy development. Proc Natl Acad Sci USA. 2022;119(23):e2115714119.
27. Cerdá M, Jalali MS, Hamilton AD, DiGennaro C, Hyder A, Santaella-Tenorio J, et al. A systematic review of simulation models to track and address the opioid crisis. Epidemiol Rev. 2022;43(1):147–65.
28. Sharareh N, Sabounchi SS, McFarland M, Hess R. Evidence of Modeling impact in development of policies for controlling the opioid epidemic and improving public health: a scoping review. Subst Abuse. 2019;13:1178221819866211.
29. Frakt A. The opioid dilemma: Saving lives in the long run can take lives in the short run. The New York Times [Internet]. 2019 Mar 4 [cited 2025 Jun 30]. Available from: https://www.nytimes.com/2019/03/04/upshot/opioid-overdose-crisis-deaths.html.
30. Wakeland W, Schmidt T, Gilson AM, Haddox JD, Webster LR. System dynamics modeling as a potentially useful tool in analyzing mitigation strategies to reduce overdose deaths associated with pharmaceutical opioid treatment of chronic pain. Pain Med. 2011;12(Suppl 2):S49–58.
31. Dasgupta N, Beletsky L, Ciccarone D. Opioid crisis: no easy fix to its social and economic determinants. Am J Public Health. 2018;108(2):182–6.
32. El-Bassel N, Shoptaw S, Goodman-Meza D, Ono H. Addressing long overdue social and structural determinants of the opioid epidemic. Drug Alcohol Depend. 2021;222:108679.
33. Friedman SR, Krawczyk N, Perlman DC, Mateu-Gelabert P, Ompad DC, Hamilton L, et al. The opioid/overdose crisis as a dialectics of pain, despair, and one-sided struggle. Front Public Health. 2020;8:540423.
34. Singh GK, Kim IE, Girmay M, Perry C, Daus GP, Vedamuthu IP, et al. Opioid epidemic in the United States: empirical trends, and a literature review of social determinants and epidemiological, pain management, and treatment patterns. Int J MCH AIDS. 2019;8(2):89–100.
35. Jalali MS, Botticelli M, Hwang RC, Koh HK, McHugh RK. The opioid crisis: a contextual, social-ecological framework. Health Res Policy Syst. 2020;18(1):87.
36. Jalal H, Buchanich JM, Roberts MS, Balmert LC, Zhang K, Burke DS. Changing dynamics of the drug overdose epidemic in the United States from 1979 through 2016. Science. 2018;361(6408)
37. Case A, Deaton A. Deaths of despair and the future of capitalism. Princeton: Princeton University Press; 2020.
38. Kolodny A. X [Internet]. US sees drop in life expectancy, largely due to opioid crisis among young adults [Tweet]; 2018 Aug 23 [cited 2025 Aug 05]. Available from: https://x.com/andrewkolodny/status/1032415259443822592.
39. Pirani F. US sees drop in life expectancy due to opioid crisis among young adults. The Atlanta Journal-Constitution. 2018;
40. Ruhm CJ. Deaths of despair or drug problems? NBER Working Paper 24188 [Internet]. Cambridge, MA: National Bureau of Economic Research; 2018 [cited 2025 Jun 30]. Available from: http://www.nber.org/papers/w24188.

41. Krueger AB. Where have all the workers Gone? An inquiry into the decline of the U.S. Labor Force participation rate. Brook Paper Econ Act. 2017;2017(2):1–87.
42. Delivering whole person care: improving outcomes in opioid use disorder treatment [webinar]. 2021 May 25 [cited 2025 Jun 30]. Available from: https://ipro.webex.com/recordingservice/sites/ipro/recording/d1635cbe9f971039bfff0050568cc44f/playback.
43. Pitt AL, Humphreys K, Brandeau ML. Modeling health benefits and harms of public policy responses to the US opioid epidemic. Am J Public Health. 2018;108(10):1394–400.
44. Muennig PA, Reynolds M, Fink DS, Zafari Z, Geronimus AT. America's declining well-being, health, and life expectancy: not just a white problem. Am J Public Health. 2018;108(12):1626–31.
45. Friedman J, Hansen H, Gone JP. Deaths of despair and indigenous data genocide. Lancet. 2023;401(10379):874–6.
46. Harper S, Lynch J, Burris S, Davey Smith G. Trends in the black-white life expectancy gap in the United States, 1983-2003. JAMA. 2007;297(11):1224–32.
47. Levine RS, Foster JE, Fullilove RE, Fullilove MT, Briggs NC, Hull PC, et al. Black-white inequalities in mortality and life expectancy, 1933-1999: implications for healthy people 2010. Public Health Rep. 2001;116(5):474–83.

3 Reporting Data on Drug Overdose

It is easy to lie with statistics. It is hard to tell the truth without them.

—Andrejs Dunkels (Shore JE, Johnson RW. Axiomatic derivation of the principle of maximum entropy and the principle of minimum cross-entropy. IEEE Transactions on Information Theory. 1980;IT-26 (1):26–37.)

3.1 Introduction

Accurate, reliable data are critical inputs to solid research, public education, and policy design. But what happens when this information is incomplete, inaccurate, or misleading? To a certain extent, this is common. In large public health data systems, like those maintained by the Centers for Disease Control and Prevention (CDC), there are significant challenges to gathering complete information from multiple jurisdictional sources and organizing it in a conceptually meaningful manner. But whether data problems are intentional or unintentional, the ramifications of error can be enormous, both economically and in human terms.

This chapter examines persistent obstacles to accurate overdose mortality reporting, from errors to inconsistencies in classification systems to the role of death certificates. Later chapters will more directly confront how these issues distort reporting on fentanyl deaths, encouraging readers to evaluate the potential causes and institutional motives behind these distortions.

3.2 International Classification of Diseases Coding

A potential barrier to accurate opioid overdose death counts stems from disruptions to data in the World Health Organization's (WHO's) International Classification of Diseases (ICD), the medical coding system public health agencies use to report the

L. R. Webster, S. Eichberg, *Deconstructing Toxic Narratives*,
https://doi.org/10.1007/978-3-032-23135-2_3

underlying cause of death. Because the ICD is modified periodically to reflect changes in medicine, comparing codes over time can both confuse and mislead. Compressed mortality data at the CDC's WONDER database is presented in three separate files to manage this issue and prevent confusion. Data from 1968 to 1978 are classified using ICD 8 codes; data from 1979 to 1998 are classified using ICD 9 codes, which allows identification of accidental drug poisoning deaths; and data from 1999 to later are classified using ICD 10 codes, which enable identification of specific drugs as contributory causes of accidental overdose deaths. The CDC itself cautions against comparing data on cause of death across decades, noting that the differences "make direct comparisons of cause of death difficult and result in discontinuities in cause-of-death trends."

Keeping these constraints in mind, see Fig. 3.1, which illustrates trends in fatal drug and opioid overdose rates from 1968 to 2023. Interpreting these trends requires consideration of the changing coding systems.

Unfortunately, public access CDC data files do not allow for trend analysis of drug overdose deaths by drug class prior to 1999. However, national surveys like the National Household Survey on Drug Use and Health (NSDUH) and Monitoring the Future provide data extending back to the 1970s or 1980s allowing detection of changing patterns in substance use (although there is a data lag in their reporting) (Tables 3.1, 3.2, and 3.3) [1]. These surveys, while subject to their own limitations (including the reporting lags), can help contextualize mortality data. According to *Monitoring the Future*, after marijuana, cocaine had the highest reported use among substances in 1988, with 14.3% of individuals aged 19–30 reporting use that year before declining sharply to 4.9% by 1998. Sedative use was reported by 1.8% of people aged 19–30 in 1988 and decreased to 1.0% by 2024. Narcotic (opioid) use rose to 9.1% among people aged 19–30 and 4.7% among those aged 35–50 in 2008, followed by a gradual decline over the next 10–15 years. Hallucinogen use showed the opposite trend, increasing from 3.6% among 19–30-year-olds and 0.4% among 35–50-year-olds in 2008 to 9.7% and 5.0%, respectively, by 2024. Understanding these shifts in

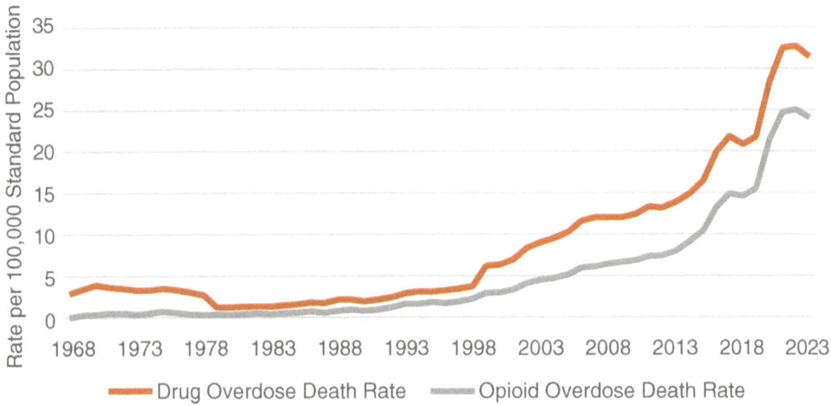

Fig. 3.1 Rates are age-adjusted per 100,000 standard population. (Source: National Center for Health Statistics, National Vital Statistics System, mortality data file)

Table 3.1 National household survey on drug abuse/drug use and health average usage rates per year among population aged 12+

	Average usage rate 1979–1988	Average usage rate 1990–1999	Average usage rate 2000–2009	Average usage rate 2010–2017	Single-year usage rate 2023
Pain relievers	2.97	2.38	6.89	5.59	3.0
Cocaine	6.25	2.14	2.77	2.14	1.8
Hallucinogens	2.36	1.75	3.28	2.77	3.1
Heroin	0.26	0.20	0.24	0.36	0.2
Inhalants	1.84	1.11	1.96	1.19	0.9
Sedatives	2.66	0.57	0.44	0.40	0.4
Stimulants	3.88	1.11	1.93	2.22	1.4
Tranquilizers	2.87	1.15	2.68	2.68	1.4

Usage rates are based on % of people age 12+ who have used a substance in the past year. (Source: SAMHSA, National Household Survey on Drug Abuse/Drug Use and Health)

Table 3.2 Monitoring the future survey, drug use over time, ages 19–30

Substance	1988	1998	2008	2018	2022	2023	2024
Marijuana	30.8	25.3	27.2	38.7	43.6	42.7	41.4
Cocaine	14.3	4.9	6.3	7.0	5.6	5.3	5.1
Heroin	0.2	0.4	0.5	0.4	0.2	0.0	0.1
Sedatives	1.8	2.2	4.6	2.8	1.4	1.0	1.2
Hallucinogens	3.6	4.4	3.6	5.3	7.8	8.9	9.7
Tranquilizers	4.2	3.6	6.8	4.4	2.3	2.1	2
Amphetamines	6.9	4.2	5.0	7.8	5.4	4.5	4.0
Narcotics (opioids other than heroin)	2.5	3.1	9.1	3.9	1.8	1.3	0.5

Based on % of people who have used a substance in the past year. (Source: Patrick et al. [1])

Table 3.3 Monitoring the future, drug use over time, ages 35–50

Substance	2008	2018	2022	2023	2024
Marijuana	12.2	19.0	27.9	29.2	26.6
Cocaine	2.8	2.7	2.9	2.9	3.2
Heroin	0.2	0.2	0.3	0.2	0.2
Sedatives	3.3	2.5	2.2	2.0	1.7
Tranquilizers	4.1	4.0	3.6	3.5	2.7
Hallucinogens	0.4	1.4	4.1	4.2	5.3
Amphetamines	0.9	2.1	3.2	2.6	2.9
Narcotics (opioids other than heroin)	4.7	4.7	3.1	2.7	1.9

Based on % of people who have used a substance in the past year. (Source: Patrick et al. [1])

substance use over time can provide valuable insights into potential changes in overdose patterns, even when detailed mortality data are unavailable. Such longitudinal survey data offer a broader perspective on evolving drug use behaviors and help to identify potential factors contributing to fluctuations in overdose rates.

The challenges inherent in collecting and interpreting overdose mortality data are linked to the limitations in relying solely on death certificates and the complexities introduced by the evolving ICD coding systems. These limitations highlight the importance of considering data from other sources, such as national surveys on drug use, to gain a more complete understanding of substance use trends. In addition, these limitations and complexities are crucial to keep in mind when considering the data presented in later chapters, particularly those concerning the reporting of fentanyl-related deaths.

3.3 Death Certificates

Obstacles to reporting accurate counts of drug overdose mortality begin with the data source: the death certificate. This document is compiled in a manner that presents numerous opportunities for error. Typically, physicians, coroners, and medical examiners in local areas are responsible for certifying cause and manner of death and sending this information to the state, which then forwards relevant information to the National Center for Health Statistics (NCHS) at the CDC. However, differences in personnel's experience and training as well as state laws governing the reporting of accidental and suspicious deaths lead to delays, omissions, and inaccuracies; in hospital death certificates, the frequency of error broadly ranges from 17.7% to 96% [2]. This wide range underscores the unreliability of death certificates as sole data sources and illustrates the urgent need for standardized training and reporting practices.

One proposed standardization approach to improved data is a new death certificate proposed by Webster and Dasgupta [3]. Understanding the limitations and distortions in overdose data reporting is essential not only for accurate historical analysis but also for interpreting the impact of real-time crises and for the development of interventions based on true causes of the problem.

As noted above, the reliability of opioid-related mortality data is an inconsistent and inadequate system for gathering and documenting information on death certificates. Webster and Dasgupta argue that these documents frequently fail to differentiate between opioids that caused a death, contributed to it, or were simply present at the time [3]. Moreover, toxicology reports lack consistency, and postmortem drug levels are often misinterpreted due to redistribution after death. The ICD-10 coding system, while more detailed than its predecessors, still fails to distinguish among opioid types, formulations, and routes of administration. These limitations hinder the ability to trace overdose deaths to their root causes.

To address these issues, Webster and Dasgupta recommend redesigning death certificates to include critical contextual information: type and route of drug administration, co-ingested substances, legitimacy of prescription, and relevant patient characteristics like mental health status, pain history, and substance use disorder [3]. They also call for expanding toxicology coding to better capture patterns of drug use. Without such enhancements, regulatory efforts may be based on misleading data, potentially harming patients who use opioids appropriately for pain management. Accurate postmortem data are thus a cornerstone of informed opioid policy and overdose prevention. Today's technology and data collection platforms should make it easier than ever to collect this type of data.

These structural data problems are compounded by how overdose deaths are categorized by intent—an issue that raises further concerns about accuracy, particularly with respect to suicide misclassification.

3.4 Misclassification and the Silent Toll of Drug Overdose Suicides

Accurate classification of overdose deaths is essential for public health surveillance; yet, mounting evidence reveals that a substantial proportion of these deaths are misclassified—particularly when they involve drug self-intoxication with potential suicidal intent. The line between "unintentional" overdose and suicide is often blurred, especially in populations with chronic pain, substance use disorders, and psychiatric comorbidities. This misclassification not only distorts epidemiological data but also hinders the deployment of appropriate prevention strategies tailored to the psychological and behavioral drivers of these deaths.

The CDC reporting on opioid overdose deaths and the media reporting of the deaths from prescription opioids have relied on data that may not be as accurate as widely believed. A foundational concern is the inadequacy of current death investigation systems in discerning intent in drug-related fatalities. In their landmark article, Rockett et al. argue that traditional death certification protocols fail to capture the behavioral reality behind many overdose deaths [4]. The authors propose a new classification—Death from Drug Self-Intoxication (DDSI)—to describe fatalities that result from recurrent, high-risk drug use behaviors regardless of explicit intent to die. They show that in 2011, a staggering 91% of drug intoxication deaths were labeled "accidental," despite often involving behaviors incompatible with accident, such as polydrug use or known psychiatric risk factors. It is worth noting that this coincides with the peak of prescription opioid prescribing raising questions about the accuracy of reporting on overdose causality. The absence of affirmative evidence—like suicide notes—often leads medical examiners and coroners to default to "accidental" classifications, masking the true nature of many overdose deaths [4].

Building on this concern, Rockett et al. conducted an empirical analysis of how suicides are classified based on the presence or absence of psychological evidence [5]. Their findings show that suicide classification for drug-related deaths is disproportionately dependent on explicit indicators such as notes or psychiatric history. A suicide note increased the odds of a drug-related death being classified as suicide by a factor of 45, compared to a much lower threshold for deaths involving firearms or hanging. This evidentiary asymmetry reflects systemic bias and resource constraints in the death investigation process, contributing to a chronic undercounting of drug-related suicides and consequently an overcounting of prescription opioid overdose deaths that are assumed to result from overprescribing or opioid use disorder (OUD). An additional consequence is that overdose deaths with likely suicidal origins are systematically stripped of their psychological context, further decoupling data from reality [5].

Volkow and Oquendo reinforce these concerns from a clinical and policy-oriented lens, describing suicide as a "silent contributor" to the opioid overdose crisis [3]. They cite evidence that only 54% of emergency department visits for opioid overdose were classified as unintentional, with the remainder deemed intentional or undetermined. Epidemiologic studies show that people with OUD have dramatically elevated suicide risk—up to six times the general population rate among veterans—even when controlling for other psychiatric conditions. The authors argue that diminished motivation to live, common in addiction, may drive high-risk use that sits on a spectrum between passive self-neglect and overt suicidal intent. As Webster (the first author) wrote in 2017, "Recognizing that death from drug self-intoxication may be passively awaited is important for prevention, as factors associated with suicide and other adverse outcomes with opioids are also risk factors for passively awaited deaths" [6]. Without accurate classification, this spectrum remains invisible in national surveillance data, undermining both suicide prevention and addiction treatment efforts [3].

Together, these studies point to a structural flaw in how overdose deaths are documented and interpreted. The rigid binary classification between suicide and accident fails to capture the complex, often ambiguous realities of drug-related mortality. The result is a surveillance system that systematically underestimates the psychosocial dimensions of the overdose epidemic.

Rectifying these structural inadequacies in data acquisition demands not only improved death investigation protocols, including expanded access to psychological autopsies and standardized classification guidelines but also a broader conceptual shift in how risk and intent are understood in the context of substance use.

These persistent inaccuracies in classifying overdose deaths underscore systemic weaknesses in our public health surveillance system. As the next chapter reveals, this issue was further exacerbated during the COVID-19 pandemic, which intensified overdose mortality and further strained our ability to accurately track and respond to drug-related deaths. Understanding how the pandemic magnified existing disparities and distorted data systems is essential to interpreting recent trends and identifying the structural forces shaping today's opioid crisis.

References

1. Patrick ME, Miech RA, Johnston LD, O'Malley PM. Monitoring the future panel study annual report: National Data on substance use among adults ages 19 to 65, 1976–2024, Monitoring the future monograph series. Ann Arbor: Institute for Social Research, University of Michigan; 2025.
2. Schuppener LM, Olson K, Brooks EG. Death certification: errors and interventions. Clin Med Res. 2020;18(1):21–6.
3. Oquendo MA, Volkow ND. Suicide: a silent contributor to opioid-overdose deaths. N Engl J Med. 2018;378(17):1567–9.
4. Rockett IRH, Smith GS, Caine ED, Kapusta ND, Hanzlick RL, Larkin GL, et al. Confronting death from drug self-intoxication (DDSI): prevention through a better definition. Am J Public Health. 2014;104(12):e49–55.
5. Rockett IRH, Caine ED, Connery HS, D'Onofrio G, Gunnell DJ, Miller TR, et al. Discerning suicide in drug intoxication deaths: paucity and primacy of suicide notes and psychiatric history. PLoS One. 2018;13(1):e0190200.
6. Webster LR. Risk factors for opioid-use disorder and overdose. Anesth Analg. 2017;125(5):1741–8.

4 COVID-19 and the Opioid Epidemic

COVID-19 has been likened to an X-ray, revealing fractures in the fragile skeleton of the societies we have built.

—António Guterres (Nelson Mandela Annual Lecture. 2020 July 18; New York New York)

4.1 Introduction

The COVID-19 pandemic significantly worsened the opioid crisis in the United States, though its impact varied across different groups. While overdose deaths increased overall, certain groups experienced disproportionately high rates and increases. Examining how the pandemic affected people who misuse opioids (PWMO) underscores the powerful role of social and economic forces in shaping drug-related behavior and outcomes, especially for populations most at risk. It also helps to situate and interpret long-term socioeconomic trends within the fast-changing dynamics of today's opioid crisis.

It is important to emphasize that this book's data, including the statistics cited here, come from observational studies that cannot establish cause-and-effect between variables, only associations. However, taken together, the statistics point to an opportunity to understand how the COVID-19 pandemic exposed pre-existing divides and disparities that are central to addressing the opioid crisis.

4.2 Impact on Overdose Trends and Intervention Access

The World Health Organization (WHO) declared the virus a pandemic in March 2020, warning that it posed a significant threat to global health. A period of social and economic volatility followed, but key developments, including access to a vaccine, eventually allowed a return to social and economic stability. While COVID-19 remains a public health concern, in March 2023, WHO announced that the disease

L. R. Webster, S. Eichberg, *Deconstructing Toxic Narratives*,
https://doi.org/10.1007/978-3-032-23135-2_4

was no longer a public health emergency. The federal government followed in May of the same year with a similar announcement.

The COVID-19 pandemic aggravated drug overdose mortality worldwide. In the United States, overdose deaths rose substantially during the pandemic's peak, with fatalities soaring across all 50 states [1–3]. Deaths involving any drug climbed 30% between 2019 and 2020 and another 16% between 2020 and 2021. Growth in overdose deaths slowed between 2021 and 2022, with rates plateauing. Between 2022 and 2023, deaths fell by 2.7% (107,941 to 105,007), and the rate fell by 4% (32.6 to 31.3), but both measures remained above pre-pandemic levels [4]. Provisional CDC data indicate a continued downward trend into 2024, though the figures are incomplete and likely underestimate final counts (Fig. 4.1) [4].

Illicit fentanyl and fentanyl analogs accounted for a large share of these overdose deaths. Between 2019 and 2023, overdose deaths involving synthetic opioids rose by 105%, and the rate increased by 94.7% (Fig. 4.2). From 2022 to 2023, both measures declined slightly: deaths by 1.4% and the rate by 2.3% [5]. Provisional CDC data indicate the downward trend continued into 2024, but the estimates remain preliminary and may be adjusted prior to finalization (Fig. 4.3) [4].

Methamphetamine and cocaine, alone or in combination with other substances, also contributed to worsening mortality during the pandemic (Figs. 4.4 and 4.5) [6]. In addition, overdoses involving prescription opioids and heroin were increasingly likely to be contaminated with illicit fentanyl and other adulterants (e.g., benzodiazepines, tranquilizers) [7].

Experts point to several reasons for the dramatic uptick in overdose deaths during the pandemic. These include diminished access to interventions and mental health supports and greater social isolation and heightened feelings of hopelessness.

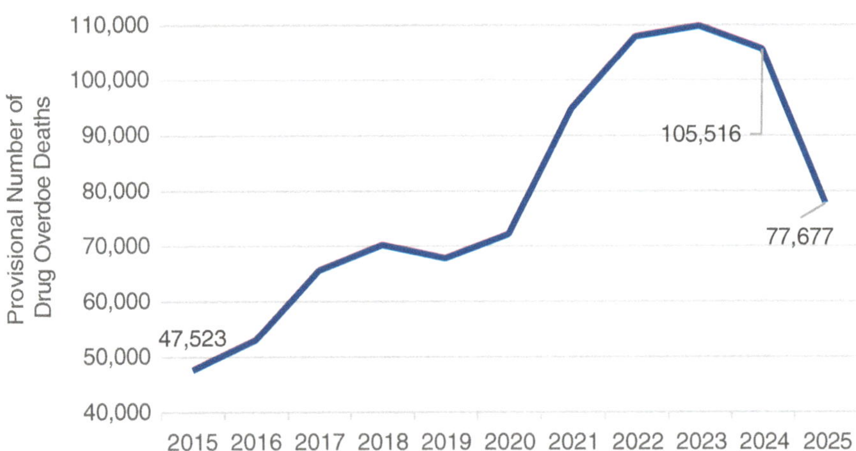

Fig. 4.1 The counts represent the numbers of deaths due to drug overdose occurring in the 12-month period ending in the month indicated. Estimates for 2024 and 2025 are based on incomplete reporting. The predicted value of deaths for January 2024 is 110,909; the predicted value for January 2025 is 82,138. (Source: Ahmad et al. [4])

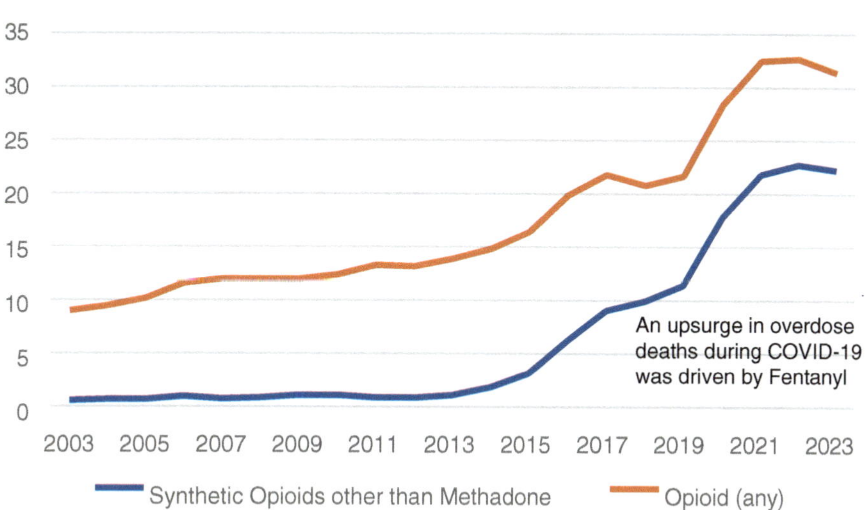

Fig. 4.2 Rates are age-adjusted per 100,000 population. (Source: CDC, NCHS, National Vital Statistics System, Provisional Drug Overdose Counts; Multiple Cause of Death data on CDC Wonder)

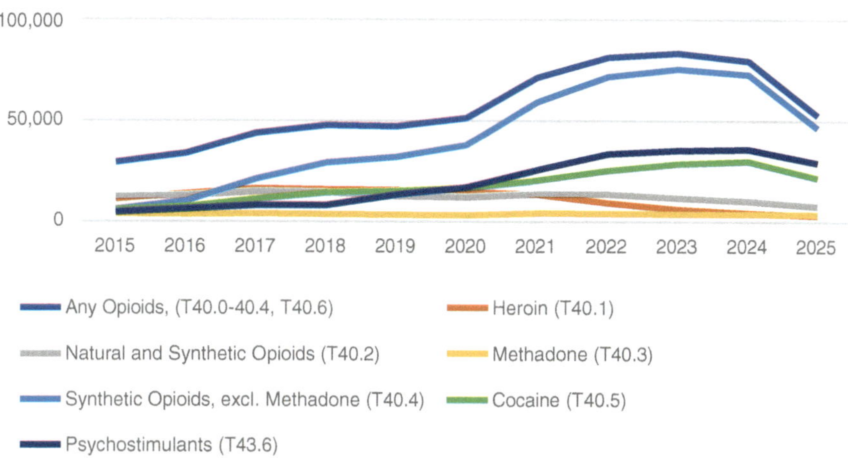

Fig. 4.3 Provisional data include deaths occurring within the 50 states and the District of Columbia as of the date specified. (Source: Ahmad et al. [4])

At the outset, the pandemic disrupted conventional in-person modes of screening, treatment, and recovery, as primary care visits, individual counseling, and group recovery meetings were halted to prevent contagion. Without direct access to healthcare providers, many patients struggled to obtain medications for opioid use disorder (OUD). While health systems established telehealth programs to uphold essential services, these interactions were dependent on technology (e.g., smartphones, broadband internet, computers) not always available or affordable in

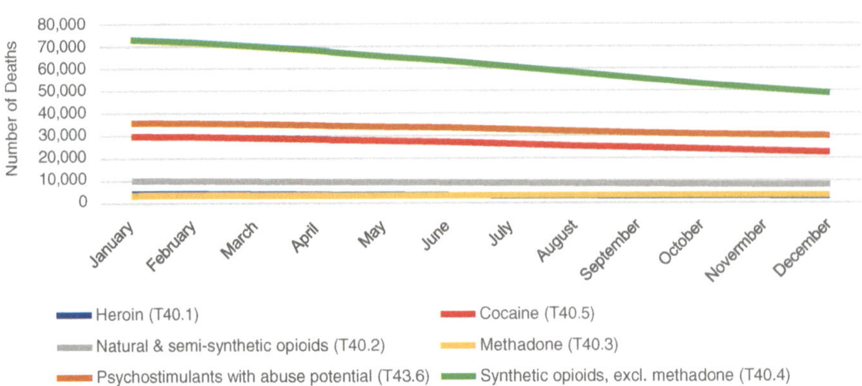

Fig. 4.4 Provisional data include deaths occurring within the 50 states and the District of Columbia as of the date specified. (Source: Ahmad et al. [4])

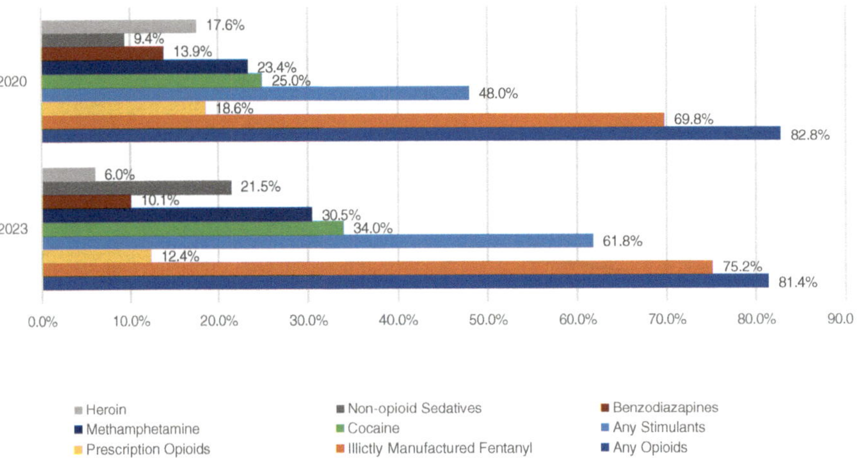

Fig. 4.5 SUDORS covers deaths from 49 states and the District of Columbia. However, reporting is incomplete, due to missing data. Some states report data from only a subset of counties. (Source: Centers for Disease Control and Prevention. State Unintentional Drug Overdose Reporting System (SUDORS). Final Data. Atlanta, GA: US Department of Health and Human Services, CDC; [2025, August 28] Access at: https://www.cdc.gov/overdose-prevention/data-research/facts-stats/sudors-dashboard-fatal-overdose-data.html)

underserved communities. This service gap deprived many at-risk individuals of vital care and support systems, deepening prevailing health disparities. Dramatic cuts to Medicaid in the 2025 congressional One Big Beautiful Bill Act are likely to further exacerbate the problem [8].

Emotional distress is a known stressor for substance use disorders (SUDs), making it likely that the damaging psychosocial effects of the pandemic exacerbated OUD relapse and overdose among at-risk populations [2, 9]. Indeed, multiple studies report rising rates of poor mental health among people who misuse drugs during the COVID-19 emergency [10–12]. Although necessary to contain spread of the virus, social distancing measures were one reason for poor mental health outcomes among PWMO, contributing to worsening substance dependency and solitary drug use [13, 14]. Economic uncertainty, due to un- and under-employment after business closures in 2020, may also have triggered heightened drug misuse. Overall, the pandemic eroded recent advances in combatting the drug epidemic, particularly as public health workers redirected their attention to managing the virus.

Persons with OUD are highly susceptible to COVID-19; their weakened lung function and respiratory depression, common side effects of opioid use, increase their chances of contracting the virus, which involves respiratory distress [15]. They are also prone to contracting the illness given higher prevalence of chronic disease. A review of the electronic health records of over 73 million patients (12,030 had been diagnosed with COVID-19 in the past year) found that individuals with a recent SUD were over eight times more likely to contract COVID-19 than those without an SUD; people with OUD were the most vulnerable of all substance users [16]. Other studies show that PWMO exhibit high rates of hospitalization and mortality compared to other people who misuse drugs [17–19].

4.3 Exacerbating Disparities in the Pandemic Era

Racial and ethnic minorities were especially hard hit as fatal drug overdoses and increases were disproportionately high during the pandemic in vulnerable and/or structurally marginalized populations. The country's highest drug overdose death rates were recorded for Non-Hispanic American Indian or Alaska Native (AIAN) and Black Americans from 2020 to 2023 (See Fig. 4.6) [20, 21].

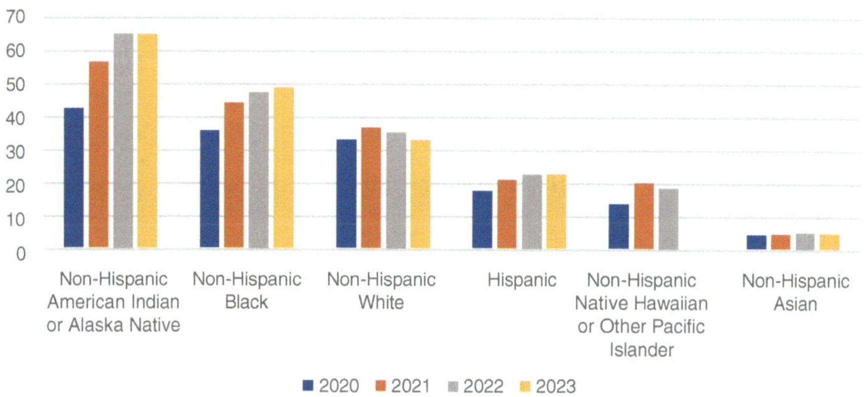

Fig. 4.6 Drug overdose deaths were identified using International Classification of Diseases, Tenth Revision underlying cause-of-death codes X40–X44, X60–X64, X85, and Y10–Y14. Rates are age-adjusted per 100,000 Standard population. (Source: CDC. National Center for Health Statistics, National Vital Statistics System, Multiple Cause of Death Data at CDC Wonder)

COVID-19 amplified stressors concentrated in BIPOC communities, including economic distress and social isolation, compounding already rising rates of opioid overdose deaths.

From 2019 to 2020, opioid overdose death (OOD) rates rose twice as much for Black people as for white people, 44% versus 22%, respectively [22, 23]. This disparity continued from 2020 to 2021, with rates increasing 26% for Black people compared to 11% for white people [24]. By 2021 to 2022, as impact of COVID lessened, inequities persisted: OOD rates fell 3.3% among white Americans but rose 7.5% among Black Americans. Although overall national rates declined from 2022 to 2023, the racial gap persisted, with rates falling 7.6% among white individuals but rising 2.7% among Black individuals [21].

Disparities in infection, hospitalization, and death among AIAN and Black persons were aggravated by long-standing social and economic inequalities (Table 4.1) [25, 26]. The greater prevalence of pre-existing health conditions, such as hypertension, diabetes, and heart disease, also predisposed members of these groups to sickness and death from COVID-19 [27–29].

COVID-19 amplified stressors concentrated in BIPOC communities, including economic distress and social isolation, compounding already rising rates of OOD [30, 31]. Lack of treatment services during COVID-19 also exacerbated long-term racial disparities in access to medication and substance misuse treatment and are at least partially responsible for the prevalence of COVID-19 among BIPOC people with OUD. At the height of COVID-19, Black, Hispanic, and biracial individuals were 8–10 times more likely than non-Hispanic white people to report reduced access to harm reduction services, specifically naloxone and sterile syringes [32].

The pandemic also affected age groups in distinct ways. Although drug overdose deaths increased for all age groups, young people, ages 15–24, experienced the

Table 4.1 Rate ratios in infection, hospitalization, and death by race/ethnicity, March 1, 2020–May 13, 2023

Rate ratios compared to white, non-Hispanic persons	American Indian or Alaska Native, non-Hispanic persons	Asian, non-Hispanic persons	Black, non-Hispanic persons	Hispanic persons
Cases[1]	1.6×	0.8×	1.1×	1.5×
Hospitalization[2]	2.4×	0.7×	2.0×	1.8×
Death[3]	2.0×	0.7×	1.6×	1.7×

Source: CDC, Risk for COVID-19 Infection, Hospitalization, and Death By Race/Ethnicity; CDC Archive. [1]Case level surveillance data from state, local and territorial public health jurisdictions (data through April 19, 2023). Numbers are ratios of age-adjusted rates standardized to the 2019 US intercensal population estimate. Calculations use only 65% of case reports that have race and ethnicity; this can result in inaccurate estimates of the relative risk among groups. [2]Data source: COVID-NET (March 1, 2020 through May 13, 2023). Numbers are ratios of age-adjusted rates standardized to the 2020 US standard COVID-NET catchment population. [3]Data Source: CDC, NCHS Provisional Death Counts (data through April 15, 2023). Numbers are ratios of age-adjusted rates standardized to the 2019 US intercensal population estimate

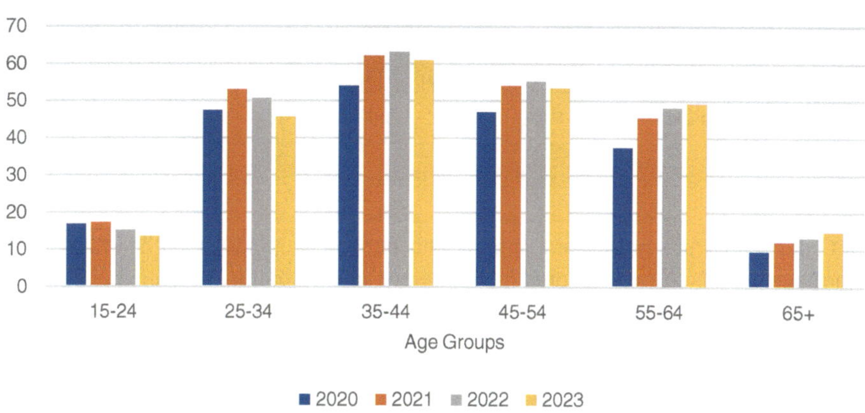

Fig. 4.7 Drug overdose deaths were identified using International Classification of Diseases, Tenth Revision underlying cause-of-death codes X40–X44, X60–X64, X85, and Y10–Y14. Rates are age-adjusted per 100,000 population. (Source: CDC, National Center for Health Statistics, National Vital Statistics System, Multiple Cause of Death data at CDC Wonder)

sharpest increase from 2019 to 2020, with fatalities and overdose rates both climbing 49% [5]. However, this group saw a 12.2% *decrease* in the drug overdose death rate in 2021–2022 followed by a 10.9% decline in 2022–2023. In contrast, older adults (65+) experienced the steepest growth, with rates rising in 2020–2021 and 2021–2022, including a 10% increase from 12.0 to 13.2 in the latter period; this upward trend persisted into 2022–2023 (see Fig. 4.7) [5].

COVID-19 was detrimental to young people's emotional wellbeing in several ways. School closures to contain the virus were one source of impacts, although public health advances (e.g., vaccines) and relaxation of social distancing policies eventually permitted normal school hours and activities to resume. When online learning replaced in-person classes, this new mode of instruction presented learning difficulties and limited peer interaction and social support opportunities. These conditions may have induced feelings of isolation, anxiety, and depression or magnified existing health disorders in youth, increasing risk for OUD. Indeed, studies show a relationship between heightened emotional strain caused by the pandemic and increases in mental health-related emergency department visits and suicide ideation and attempts among adolescents [33, 34]. As noted in the U.S. Surgeon General's advisory on protecting youth mental health, US emergency department visits for suspected suicide attempts were 51% higher for adolescent girls and 4% higher for adolescent boys in early 2021 compared to the same time period in early 2019 [34].

Like young people, older people (65+) experienced emotional distress during the pandemic. Social distancing policies intensified social isolation, already a strong risk factor for unhealthy substance use among older adults [35]. In addition, disruptions to healthcare access impeded some older adults from taking advantage of telemedicine to address psychiatric symptoms [36].

Drug overdose deaths increased for all age groups during the height of the pandemic, but people aged 15–24 experienced the largest percentage increase from 2019 to 2020, while those aged 65+ had the fastest rate of growth from 2020 to 2021.

Older adults are prescribed opioids and benzodiazepines at higher rates than other age groups to treat chronic pain, anxiety, and insomnia, heightening risk for dependence. Interruptions to routine medical visits during the pandemic may have increased obstacles to effective pain management and addiction treatment; for older persons already engaged in treatment, care disruptions may have blocked access to methadone, buprenorphine, or naloxone. These barriers (in combination with social isolation) were likely a stressor for addiction, relapse, and overdose among older persons [37].

In summary, the existing vulnerabilities are clear. Studies have confirmed higher rates of hospitalization and death from COVID-19 among PWMO. BIPOC people, already facing systemic inequalities, were disproportionately affected. The pandemic highlighted the unique vulnerabilities of both young people and older adults, demonstrating the importance of tailored interventions. Although these statistics reflect *associations*, not necessarily direct cause-and-effect, the data strongly suggest that the pandemic aggravated existing vulnerabilities related to socioeconomic status, race, and age, showing that the opioid crisis is not simply a matter of opioid availability, but a complex issue deeply intertwined with social and economic determinants.

The COVID-19 pandemic did not cause the opioid crisis, but it illuminated and accelerated many of its underlying drivers. Overdose mortality surged during the pandemic not only because of increased drug potency or supply-side factors, but also because long-standing social and economic vulnerabilities—such as unstable housing, inadequate healthcare access, systemic racism, and social isolation—were magnified under pandemic conditions. These same vulnerabilities are not new. They are structural forces that have shaped the contours of the opioid crisis for decades. In this sense, COVID-19 acted as a stress test for a society already fractured along lines of inequality. Understanding how these fractures contributed to pandemic-era overdose patterns helps to clarify that the opioid crisis is less about drugs themselves and more about the conditions in which people live and suffer.

Chapter 5 builds on this insight by examining the root causes of the opioid crisis through the lens of social determinants of health. Drawing on data and research across multiple dimensions—including race, gender, socioeconomic status, veteran status, housing, and geography—the chapter unpacks how social position and environmental context influence who is most at risk for opioid misuse, addiction, and death. The reader will learn how deeply entrenched disparities, often invisible in conventional policy responses, are central to the persistence and escalation of the crisis. This shift from individual behavior to structural conditions sets the stage for a more comprehensive and just framework for prevention and intervention.

References

1. Ochalek TA, Cumpston KL, Wills BK, Gal TS, Moeller FG. Nonfatal opioid overdoses at an urban emergency department during the COVID-19 pandemic. JAMA. 2020;324(16):1673–4.
2. Slavova S, Rock P, Bush HM, Quesinberry D, Walsh SL. Signal of increased opioid overdose during COVID-19 from emergency medical services data. Drug Alcohol Depend. 2020;214:108176.
3. Soares WE 3rd, Melnick ER, Nath B, D'Onofrio G, Paek H, Skains RM, et al. Emergency department visits for nonfatal opioid overdose during the COVID-19 pandemic across six US health care systems. Ann Emerg Med. 2022;79(2):158–67.
4. Ahmad FB, Cisewski JA, Rossen LM, Sutton P. Provisional drug overdose death counts. National Center for Health Statistics; 2025. https://doi.org/10.15620/cdc/20250305008.
5. Centers for Disease Control and Prevention (CDC), National Center for Health Statistics. Multiple cause of death data on CDC WONDER [Internet]. Atlanta: Centers for Disease Control and Prevention (CDC); [cited 2025 Oct 07]. Available from: https://wonder.cdc.gov/mcd.html.
6. Schneider KE, Martin EM, Allen ST, Morris M, Haney K, Saloner B, et al. Volatile drug use and overdose during the first year of the COVID-19 pandemic in the United States. Int J Drug Policy. 2024;126:104371.
7. American Medical Association. Issue brief: Nation's drug-related overdose and death epidemic continues to worsen [Internet]. 2021 Nov 12 [cited 2025 Jul 2]. Available from: https://www.ama-assn.org/system/files/issue-brief-increases-in-opioid-related-overdose.pdf.
8. Congress HR. 1: one big beautiful bill act, 119th Congress. [Internet]. Washington DC: U.S. Government Publishing Office; 2025 Jul 4 [cited 2025 Sep 4]. Available from: https://www.congress.gov/bill/119th-congress/house-bill/1.
9. National Institute on Drug Abuse. Co-occurring disorders and health conditions. Bethesda: National Institute on Drug Abuse; 2024. Available from: https://nida.nih.gov/research-topics/co-occurring-disorders-health-conditions. Accessed 29 Jul 2025.
10. Czeisler M, Howard ME, Rajaratnam SMW. Mental health during the COVID-19 pandemic: challenges, populations at risk, implications, and opportunities. Am J Health Promot. 2021;35(2):301–11.
11. Bennett AS, Townsend T, Elliott L. The COVID-19 pandemic and the health of people who use illicit opioids in new York City, the first 12 months. Int J Drug Policy. 2022;101:103554.
12. Stack E, Leichtling G, Larsen JE, Gray M, Pope J, Leahy JM, et al. The impacts of COVID-19 on mental health, substance use, and overdose concerns of people who use drugs in rural communities. J Addict Med. 2021;15(5):383–9.
13. Linas BP, Savinkina A, Barbosa C, Mueller PP, Cerdá M, Keyes K, et al. A clash of epidemics: impact of the COVID-19 pandemic response on opioid overdose. J Subst Abus Treat. 2021;120:108158.
14. Heimer R, McNeil R, Vlahov D. A community responds to the COVID-19 pandemic: a case study in protecting the health and human rights of people who use drugs. J Urban Health. 2020;97(4):448–56.
15. National Institute on Drug Abuse. People with SUDs have increased risk for COVID-19 and worse outcomes [Internet]. 2021 Jan 13 [cited 2025 Jul 2]. Available from: https://tinyurl.com/mr35aa26.
16. Wang QQ, Kaelber DC, Xu R, Volkow ND. COVID-19 risk and outcomes in patients with substance use disorders: analyses from electronic health records in the United States. Mol Psychiatry. 2021;26(1):30–9.
17. Baillargeon J, Polychronopoulou E, Kuo YF, Raji MA. The impact of substance use disorder on COVID-19 outcomes. Psychiatr Serv. 2021;72(5):578–81.
18. Board AR, Kim S, Park J, Schieber L, Miller GF, Pike J, et al. Risk factors for COVID-19 among persons with substance use disorder (PWSUD) with hospital visits - United States, April 2020-December 2020. Drug Alcohol Depend. 2022;232:109297.

19. Venkatesh AK, Janke AT, Kinsman J, Rothenberg C, Goyal P, Malicki C, et al. Emergency department utilization for substance use disorders and mental health conditions during COVID-19. PLoS One. 2022;17(1):e0262136.
20. Centers for Disease Control and Prevention (US), National Center for Health Statistics. CDC WONDER: multiple cause of death 2018-2023 [Internet]. Atlanta: Centers for Disease Control and Prevention; [cited 2025 Jul 8]. Available from: https://wonder.cdc.gov/.
21. Garnett MF, Miniño AM. Drug overdose deaths in the United States, 2003–2023. NCHS Data Brief, no 522. Hyattsville: National Center for Health Statistics; 2024. https://doi.org/10.15620/cdc/170565.
22. Kariisa M, Davis NL, Kumar S, et al. Vital signs: drug overdose deaths, by selected sociodemographic and social determinants of health characteristics — 25 states and the District of Columbia, 2019–2020. MMWR Morb Mortal Wkly Rep. 2022;71:940–7. Available from: https://doi.org/10.15585/mmwr.mm7129e2.
23. Centers for Disease Control and Prevention (US), National Center for Health Statistics. CDC WONDER: National vital statistics system, provisional drug overdose counts; multiple cause of death data [Internet]. Atlanta: Centers for Disease Control and Prevention; [cited 2025 Jul 2]. Available from: https://wonder.cdc.gov/.
24. Spencer MR, Garnett MF, Miniño AM. Drug overdose deaths in the United States, 2002–2022. NCHS Data Brief, no 491. Hyattsville: National Center for Health Statistics; 2024. Available from: https://doi.org/10.15620/cdc:135849.
25. Chowkwanyun M, Reed AL Jr. Racial health disparities and Covid-19 - caution and context. N Engl J Med. 2020;383(3):201–3.
26. Centers for Disease Control and Prevention (US). Risk for COVID-19 infection, hospitalization, and death by race/ethnicity [Internet]. Atlanta: Centers for Disease Control and Prevention (US); 2023 May 25 [cited 2025 Oct 7]. Available from: https://archive.cdc.gov/#/details?url=https://www.cdc.gov/coronavirus/2019-ncov/covid-data/investigations-discovery/hospitalization-death-by-race-ethnicity.html.
27. Arena PJ, Malta M, Rimoin AW, Strathdee SA. Race, COVID-19 and deaths of despair. EClinicalMedicine. 2020;25:100485.
28. Pan D, Sze S, Minhas JS, Bangash MN, Pareek N, Divall P, et al. The impact of ethnicity on clinical outcomes in COVID-19: a systematic review. EClinicalMedicine. 2020;23:100404.
29. Price-Haywood EG, Burton J, Fort D, Seoane L. Hospitalization and mortality among black patients and white patients with Covid-19. N Engl J Med. 2020;382(26):2534–43.
30. James K, Jordan A. The opioid crisis in black communities. J Law Med Ethics. 2018;46(2):404–21.
31. Khatri UG, Pizzicato LN, Viner K, Bobyock E, Sun M, Meisel ZF, et al. Racial/ethnic disparities in unintentional fatal and nonfatal emergency medical services-attended opioid overdoses during the COVID-19 pandemic in Philadelphia. JAMA Netw Open. 2021;4(1):e2034878.
32. Rosales R, Janssen T, Yermash J, Yap KR, Ball EL, Hartzler B, et al. Persons from racial and ethnic minority groups receiving medication for opioid use disorder experienced increased difficulty accessing harm reduction services during COVID-19. J Subst Abus Treat. 2022;132:108648.
33. Meade J. Mental health effects of the COVID-19 pandemic on children and adolescents: a review of the current research. Pediatr Clin N Am. 2021;68(5):945–59.
34. Office of the U.S. Surgeon General. Protecting youth mental health: the U.S. Surgeon General's advisory. Washington: U.S. Department of Health and Human Services; 2021. Available from: https://www.hhs.gov/sites/default/files/surgeon-general-youth-mental-health-advisory.pdf.
35. Satre DD, Hirschtritt ME, Silverberg MJ, Sterling SA. Addressing problems with alcohol and other substances among older adults during the COVID-19 pandemic. Am J Geriatr Psychiatry. 2020;28(7):780–3.
36. Tsamakis K, Tsiptsios D, Ouranidis A, Mueller C, Schizas D, Terniotis C, et al. COVID-19 and its consequences on mental health (review). Exp Ther Med. 2021;21(3):244.
37. Konakanchi JS, Sethi R. The growing epidemic of opioid use disorder in the elderly and its treatment: a review of the literature. Prim Care Companion CNS Disord. 2023;25(1)

Opioids and Social Determinants of Health

5

If access to health care is considered a human right, who is considered human enough to have that right?

—Paul Farmer (Pathologies of Power: Health, Human Rights, and the New War on the Poor. University of California Press, 2004)

5.1 Introduction

In some parts of America, opioid overdoses now claim more lives than cancer or car accidents. But the crisis isn't just chemical—it's structural. This chapter argues that overdose deaths are not random tragedies, but predictable outcomes of poverty, racism, social isolation, and policy neglect. We need to stop asking what's wrong with people who misuse opioids and start asking what's wrong with the systems around them.

Everything discussed thus far points to the importance of socioeconomic determinants in understanding and addressing the opioid crisis. Particular attention should be paid to social determinants of health (SDoH), broadly defined as "the conditions in the environments where people are born, live, learn, work, play, worship, and age that affect a wide range of health, functioning, and quality-of-life outcomes and risks" [1]. Current policy largely addresses symptoms "downstream," neglecting root causes. This chapter argues that SDoH are critical public health priorities that significantly shape opioid misuse and overdose risks as well as health outcomes.

Drawing from insights on proactive problem-solving, this chapter advocates for an "upstream" approach to the opioid epidemic, moving beyond short-sighted interventions. It explores how SDoH operate across multiple levels, encompassing micro-level factors such as race, gender, age, and socioeconomic status, alongside macro-level structural factors including poverty, unemployment, and systemic racism. By centering these fundamental drivers, the chapter highlights how deeply

L. R. Webster, S. Eichberg, *Deconstructing Toxic Narratives*,
https://doi.org/10.1007/978-3-032-23135-2_5

entrenched disparities, often overlooked in conventional policy responses, are key to the crisis's persistence, setting the stage for comprehensive prevention and intervention frameworks.

5.2 Upstream Thinking and Social Determinants of Health

Author Dan Heath observes that we typically respond to pressing social problems (like health crises) reactively rather than deliberately thinking issues through to their source. As a result, critical resources are directed downstream to manage harms instead of upstream to the problem's roots as a pre-emptive deterrent. Heath suggests two strategies to move beyond the stale cycle of reflexive problem solving. First, he proposes making long-term commitments to problem resolution and, second, he advises incorporating systemic thinking into the problem-solving process from the start [2].

Heath's insights are applicable to disentangling the thorny elements perpetuating the opioid epidemic. As discussed previously, most policy fixes to date have been short-sighted and partial rather than far-reaching and systemic.

Because SDOH operate across multiple levels of influence to shape health and health disparities, they account for up to 90% of health outcomes [3, 4]. SDoH are often the root cause of many health issues: for example, poverty can lead to food insecurity, poor housing, and limited access to health care, all of which contribute to poor health outcomes. SDoH affect entire populations and have a wide and lasting impact on community health. Given the primacy of their role, resolving SDoH is a public health priority. One example of incorporating SDoH with innovative thinking is the proposal to create community-based solutions that address the crisis' fundamental drivers by operating outside of health care and addiction treatment systems [5].

The relationship between SDoH and health is not always direct but may involve interactions among multiple/moderating variables. Examples of micro-level or personal SDoH correlates include race/ethnicity, gender, age, and socioeconomic status. Macro-level structural factors include poverty rates, unemployment rates, racial/ethnic composition, structural racism, housing affordability, and income inequality [5–8]. Bivariate relationships (between a single correlate and an opioid--related outcome) are useful for identifying associations but cannot establish causality and may be influenced by unmeasured confounding factors. They offer insight into possible mechanisms, including social processes, but must be interpreted with caution.

5.3 Bivariate Correlates of Opioid Outcomes

To humanize the often-dry discussion of data, clinical vignettes have been developed. While some are hypothetical in their specific details, all are rooted in the lived experiences of real patients, kept anonymous to protect individual identities.

5.3.1 Differential Pain and Risk (Sex)

Maria, a 42-year-old mother of three, sustained a back injury at work. Her doctor prescribed opioids for a few months, but when the prescription ended, the pain remained. Without access to alternative treatments, she began taking leftover pills from a friend, just to get through her day.

Women and men exhibit different drug (mis)use and overdose patterns. Women experience chronic pain more often than men and are more likely to be administered prescription opioids for longer periods of time [9]. They also tend to consume prescription opioids without a prescription to manage pain, even when their pain levels are similar to those of men. Women are more likely to misuse prescription opioids by self-medicating for anxiety or tension [10]. In 2023, 4.3 million females (aged 12+) reported misusing opioids, excluding illicitly manufactured fentanyl, in the past year, with 93.5% reporting misuse of pain relievers alone without other substances [11].

Men are more likely to self-report any opioid misuse, including prescription opioids, to "feel good or get high" [12]. They also experience a higher opioid-involved overdose death(s) (OOD) rate than women (34.5 per 100,000 vs. 14.4, respectively), accounting for more than 70% of fatalities in 2023. From 2022 to 2023, OOD rates dropped 2.4% for men and 4.4% for women, following a period of mostly rising rates for both groups from 2003 to 2023 (Figs. 5.1 and 5.2) [13].

Overall, men are more likely than women to die from OOD. Women are more likely to misuse prescription opioids with a motive to manage pain or a mental health condition, while men's misuse is more often driven by efforts to feel good or "high." Pain is sexed—and so too is disbelief.

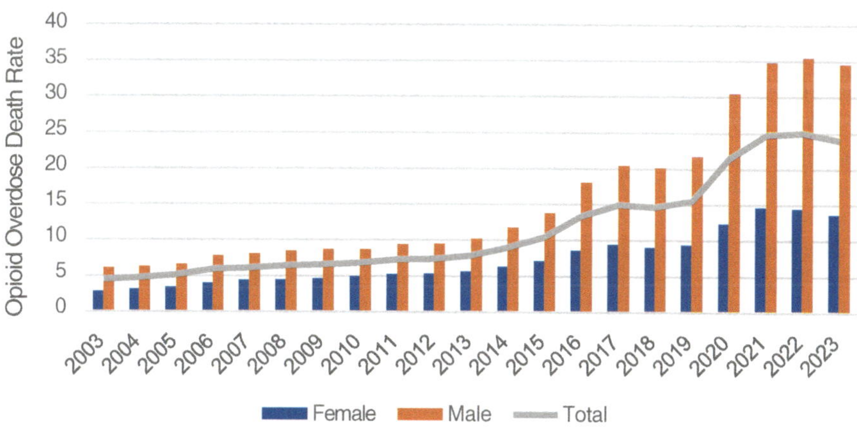

Fig. 5.1 Rates are age-adjusted per 100,000 population. Source: CDC, National Center for Health Statistics, National Vital Statistics System, Multiple Cause of Death data at CDC Wonder

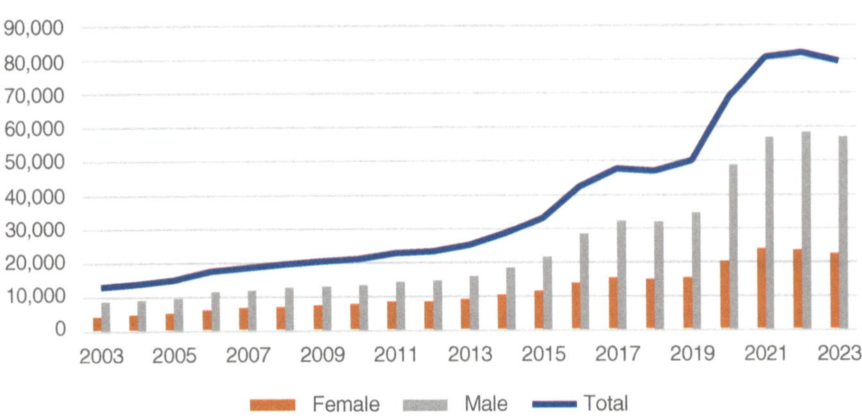

Fig. 5.2 Source: CDC, National Center for Health Statistics, National Vital Statistics System, Multiple Cause of Death data at CDC Wonder

Research on pain differences between men and women has traditionally focused on biological sex. However, many studies use sex and gender interchangeably, despite their distinct yet overlapping meanings: sex refers to biological and physiological characteristics, while gender encompasses social and cultural identities, roles, behaviors, and expectations linked to masculinity and femininity [14, 15].

5.3.2 Identity, Stress, and the Weight of Stigma (LGBTQIA+)

Consider Kai, a 17-year-old transgender teen in Tennessee. Every day, he skipped lunch to avoid harassment in the school cafeteria. At night, the anxiety followed him home. When Kai first misused a leftover pain pill, it wasn't to get high—it was to feel numb. Like so many others navigating fear, rejection, and systemic discrimination, his story is far from uncommon.

Lesbian, gay, bisexual, transgender, queer, and other LGBTQIA+ populations have higher rates of opioid misuse than their heterosexual and cisgender peers. In 2023, among persons aged 12+, 1.2 million LGB people reported misusing opioids in the past year; 98.5% reported misuse of prescription pain relievers. Past-month opioid misuse was reported by 0.3% of lesbians, 0.7% of gay men, 1.7% of bisexuals, 1.8% of LGB people using another identity term, and 1.7% of bisexual women (Fig. 5.3). Disparities among lesbian, gay, and bisexual populations stem from minority stress, which includes stigma, harassment, violence, and discrimination in healthcare settings [16–18].

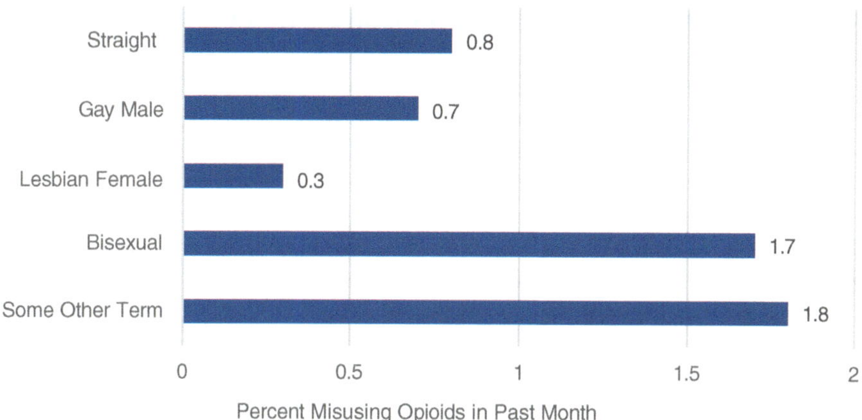

Fig. 5.3 The percentage of misuse of opioids by sexual identity in the 2023 National Survey on Drug Use and Health (NSDUH) cannot be compared to prior years. The 2023 survey was revised to be more inclusive and to include all respondents, regardless of age. (Source: SAMHSA NSDUH, 2023)

Less is known about the mechanics of opioid use among transgender and other gender-diverse individuals, although the few existing studies show high prevalence of illicit drug use among this social group. In a survey focused on transgender students exclusively, 35% reported using substances to cope with verbal and physical harassment at school [19].

In the current political and social climate, hostility toward transgender and non-binary people is intensifying, heightening risks for mental health disorders and substance use. In 2024, more than 20% of victims of single-bias hate crimes were LGBTQ+, with 4% targeted specifically for gender identity [20]. State laws and policies prohibiting or restricting transgender youths' rights have proliferated in recent years. In 2023, more than 250 pieces of legislation were introduced nationwide to ban or constrain minors' access to bathrooms, sports participation, or gender-affirming care (GAC) [21–23]. By 2025, 27 states had enacted restrictions on GAC for minors, leaving 40% of transgender youth (aged 13–17) living in a state with limited or no access. A study published in 2023 found that exposure to news stories about anti-trans laws or policies was associated with poorer mental and physical health among trans/nonbinary youth and adults [24]. And a 2023 national survey conducted by the Trevor Project reported that nearly one in three LGBTQIA+ youth described their mental health as poor "most of the time or always" due to anti-LGBTQIA+ policies and legislation [25].

Minority stress fuels higher rates of opioid misuse and mental health struggles in LGBTQIA+ populations. Reducing stigma and discrimination is crucial to improving the wellbeing of these communities. When society makes identity itself a risk factor, it creates conditions for despair.

5.3.3 Older, Overlooked, and Overexposed (Age)

Walter, 72, underwent a hip replacement and was prescribed opioids for post-surgical pain. Living alone and increasingly isolated, he continued refilling his prescription well after the pain subsided. He didn't realize how dependent he had become until he ran out—and withdrawal set in.

Opioid use disorder (OUD) and OOD can affect people of all ages. As previously described, the COVID-19 pandemic exposed evolving risks and vulnerabilities within different populations even as increases in opioid overdose fatalities were seen in all age groups. Initially, younger adults saw a sharp rise in opioid misuse and overdose fatalities, especially during the pandemic's peak, whereas older adults were affected to a lesser extent [26]. However, recent data reveal a concerning trend: while overdose deaths among younger individuals have slightly decreased, older adults, particularly those aged 65 and older, are undergoing a significant rise in opioid-related fatalities, with synthetic opioids playing a major role.

In 2023, adults aged 35–44 continued to have the highest drug overdose rates among individuals 15 and older, though their rate fell modestly from the prior year. Within this group, the OOD rate was 60.8 per 100,000—a 3.7% decline from 2022. Adults aged 15–24 and 25–34 also saw small reductions. By contrast, rates increased among those aged 55–64 and especially among adults 65 and older. For individuals 65+, the OOD rate reached 14.7 per 100,000 in 2023, representing an 11.4% increase from 2022 and a 56.4% increase since 2020 (Fig. 5.4).

Older people face several challenges that interact and contribute to opioid-related risk. Aging can lead to social and physical changes that heighten the risk for substance misuse. One reason older adults are at risk for OUD is that with age, medications take longer to leave people's systems resulting in more severe side effects. Other risk factors that can increase the toxicity of opioids include comorbid

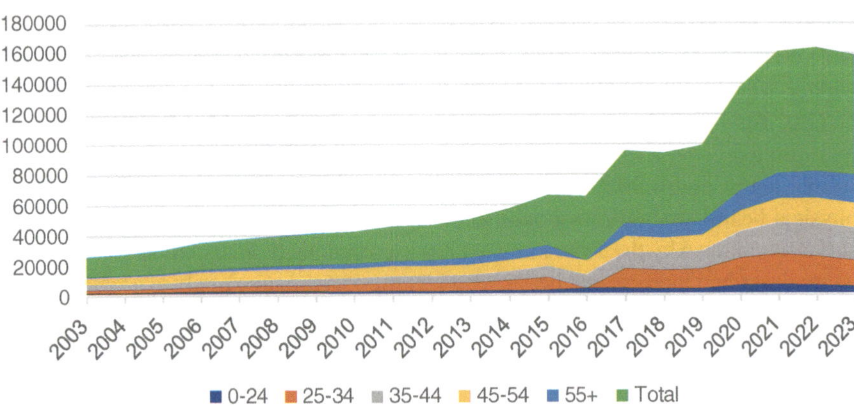

Fig. 5.4 Drug overdose deaths were classified using the International Classification of Disease, Tenth Revision (ICD-10). Opioids = T40.0, T40.1, T40.2, T40.3, T40.4, or T40.6. Missing data for some age groups in certain years result in inconsistent trend lines. (Source: CDC, National Center for Health Statistics. Data are from the Multiple Cause of Death Files, 1999–2020 and 2018–2023)

conditions, such as obesity, heart disease, mental health disorders, and concurrent use of other medications. Growing old shouldn't mean growing invisible, but for many older adults in pain, it does.

Several additional factors may account for the rise in overdose deaths among older adults. First, barriers to in-person medical care during COVID-19 may have motivated older adults to substitute illicit drugs for pharmaceutical analgesics to manage pain. Drug surveillance and access controls may also play a role, through items such as tamper-resistant medications, prescription drug monitoring programs (PDMPs), and artificial intelligence clinical decision support (CDS) tools.

For example, CDS tools, like Bamboo Health's Narxcare, employ algorithms to assign overdose risk scores to patients by analyzing PDMP data. Narxcare is widely implemented across the United States but has come under attack for lacking both evidence of clinical benefit and FDA approval. Critics charge that overreliance on risk scores can result in pain management decisions that are harmful to patients and increase disparities for marginalized or stigmatized populations, including older people with chronic complex health conditions [27–29]. Reliance on algorithmic CDS tools, like Narxcare, for overdose risk assessment raises concerns about potential biases and detrimental impacts on patient care [30].

The foregoing analysis makes clear that older adults are facing escalating risks due to unique age-related factors. Substance use in older adults is often underrecognized and underdiagnosed. Disruptions in healthcare access for patients with chronic pain can alter opioid use patterns, particularly among older people. In addition, technological solutions such as CDS tools require careful analysis to avoid unintended consequences and ensure equitable patient care across all age groups.

5.3.4 Not Just a White Crisis (Race/Ethnicity)

Jamal, a 29-year-old Black warehouse worker in Baltimore, sustained an injury on the job and was prescribed painkillers. When the prescription stopped, he turned to the street. Jamal died from fentanyl-laced heroin. His death never made the news—but it mirrored thousands of others.

Media attention to the problem of opioid addiction disproportionately centers on prescription opioids, creating the impression that the (prescription) opioid epidemic exists only in white communities [31, 32]. In reality, OOD rates have risen more rapidly among nearly all other racial and ethnic groups than among white Americans—with the exception of Asian Americans—though some stabilization and modest declines have occurred since the end of the COVID-19 pandemic.

In 2023, the age-adjusted opioid overdose mortality rate was highest among American Indian or Alaska Native (AIAN) persons (49.4 per 100,000) and lowest among Asian persons (3.2) [33]. Between 2022 and 2023, rates declined 7.6% for white Americans and remained unchanged for Asians, while increasing slightly for Black (2.7%) and Hispanic persons (1.7%). The steepest increase was among Native Hawaiian and other Pacific Islanders (NHPI), whose OOD rates rose by 88% (Fig. 5.5) [33, 34].

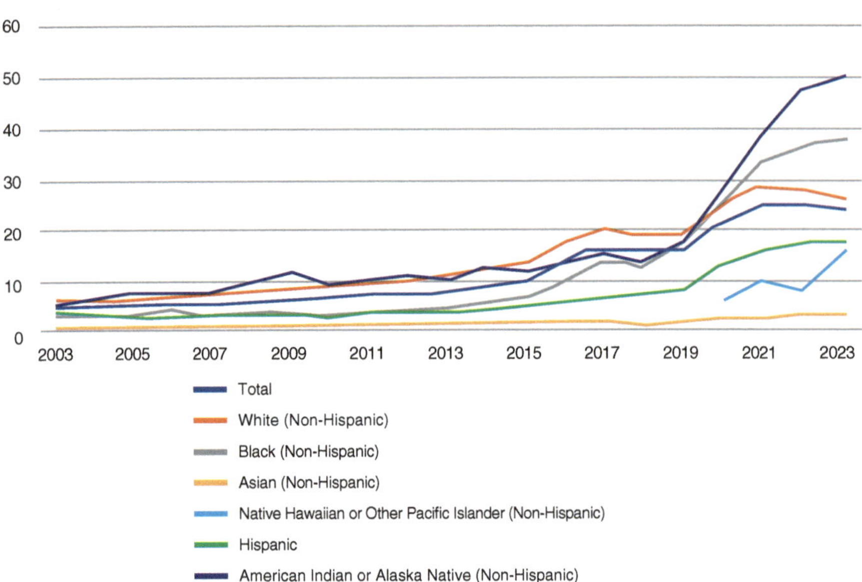

Fig. 5.5 Any Opioid ICD-10 codes: T40.0–T40.4, T40.6 Rates are age-adjusted per 100,000 population. (Source: CDC, National Center for Health Statistics. Data are from the Multiple Cause of Death Files, 1999–2020 and 2018–2023)

Distinguishing between synthetic and prescription opioids is critical when interpreting these numbers. Elevated OOD rates reflect a surge in synthetic OODs among all race/ethnic groups except for Asian Americans. In 2023, AIAN people had the highest rate (46.5) of fatal overdoses involving synthetic opioids followed by Black (36.1) and white individuals (23.2) (Figs. 5.6 and 5.7) [33].

The *type* of opioid involved matters, as synthetic opioids are a major contributor to the high rates observed among AIAN and Black individuals. While many Black, Indigenous, and People of Color (BIPOC) have higher rates of OOD, misuse of substances such as heroin and prescription pain relievers does not differ significantly across racial or ethnic groups; percentages for prescription pain medication range from 2.3% (Asians) to 6.6% (multiracial) [11]. Racial disparities in OOD rates stem from the greater lethality of synthetic opioids, differences in cultural knowledge, and local histories, sociostructural inequalities in health care, and other domains disproportionately affecting racial/ethnic minorities.

In the current political moment, lawmakers around the country are proposing bills to limit diversity, equity, and inclusion (DEI) programs, which are designed to promote racial equity and fairness in schools and workplaces. These measures target DEI offices, mandatory diversity training, diversity statements in hiring, and the consideration of identity factors in admissions or hiring decisions. Since 2023, 131 bills undermining DEI initiatives were introduced in 31 states and at the federal level; 29 have been signed into law, affecting public colleges, community colleges,

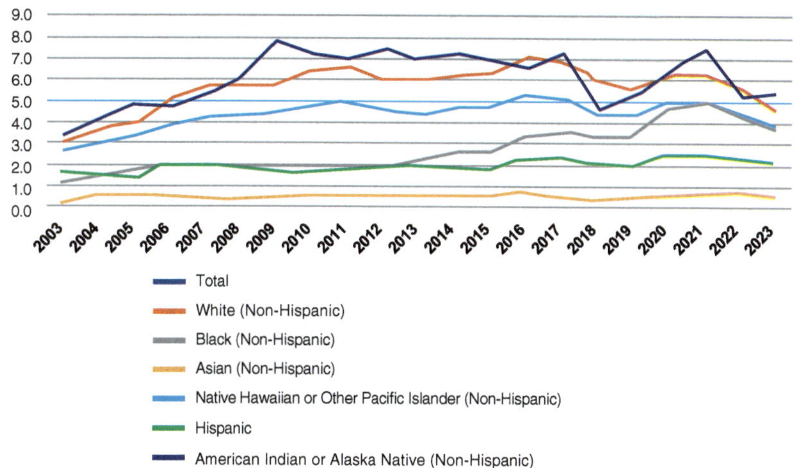

Fig. 5.6 Rates are age-adjusted per 100,000 population. (Source: CDC, National Center for Health Statistics. Data are from the Multiple Cause of Death Files, 1999–2020 and 2018–2023)

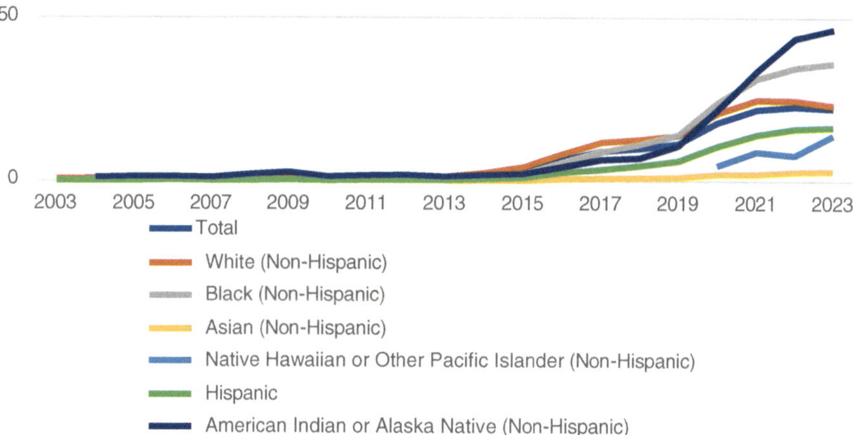

Fig. 5.7 Synthetic Opioids other than Methadone (Primarily Fentanyl) ICD-10 Code: T40.4. Rates are age-adjusted per 100,00 standard population. (Source: CDC, National Center for Health Statistics. Data are from the Multiple Cause of Death Files, 1999–2020 and 2018–2023)

and state agencies [35]. As with anti-trans laws, research suggests that proposing or passing bills to eliminate DEI programs can worsen the physical and mental health of those targeted—specifically BIPOC children and adults [36]. Such political attacks on equity parallel the dynamics of the opioid crisis: while the crisis may appear white on the front page, its burden falls disproportionately on BIPOC populations.

5.3.5 Poverty Isn't Just a Risk Factor—It's a Death Sentence (Socioeconomic Status)

Diane worked two jobs but still struggled to keep the lights on. She rationed her insulin and skipped meals so her kids could eat. When a neighbor gave her an opioid to dull the pain of the untreated tooth abscess, she took it—and found temporary relief. That moment marked the start of her descent into addiction.

The opioid crisis is often described as an "equal opportunity" problem for people from all socioeconomic backgrounds, but this framing masks the disproportionate risk for OUD and its consequences among people with lower socioeconomic status (SES) [37]. Across studies, opioid-related overdose is associated with a range of SES metrics, both individual determinants (e.g., income) and composite measures, combining several indicators of social and economic wellbeing [38]. Policies such as Medicaid expansion, income support, or improved educational access may help to mitigate these risks. Later chapters will expand upon these concepts as potential solutions to the opioid crisis.

People with lower educational attainment face a higher risk of fatal opioid overdose. In one study, 35.4% of OODs took place among people whose highest educational attainment was a high school diploma or GED, and 23.7% involved those who did not complete high school [39]. In an assessment of the probability of a fatal overdose, the study found that people with a high school degree or GED had statistically significant elevated hazard ratios compared to people with graduate degrees.

Lower income is also associated with opioid-related harm. The National Survey on Drug Use and Health (NSDUH) (2015–2018) found that individuals with a household income under $20,000 per year were more likely to report OUD (31.4%) than those in higher income brackets (16.5%) [26]. Another study found that people living in poverty were faced with a higher likelihood of dying from opioid overdoses than people with incomes at least five times above the poverty line [39].

Income level is also associated with the specific type of drug involved in overdose. A study of drug overdose in San Francisco found that people who died in high-poverty areas were more likely to die from methadone and cocaine, while those in higher income areas were more likely to die from oxycodone and benzodiazepines [40].

At an aggregate or community level, there is often a relationship between income/SES measures and OUD [41]. In a cross-sectional study of ZIP codes in 17 states, from 2002–2014, elevated rates of prescription opioid overdose were observed in disadvantaged ZIP codes, regardless of urbanicity [42]. For heroin overdose deaths, urbanicity altered the relationship, with economic disadvantage having a greater effect on urban than rural areas. In an overdose crisis, despair is not a symptom, it's a precondition.

Insurance status acts as a proxy for poverty or low income. Individuals eligible for Medicaid, which is means tested, are more likely to be prescribed opioid analgesics than are other populations; in addition, the pills are prescribed at higher doses and for longer periods of time [43, 44]. Medicaid covers nearly 40% of nonelderly adults with OUD. Overdose deaths are also disproportionately higher among populations eligible for Medicaid [45]. Poverty doesn't just increase vulnerability, it manufactures it.

5.3.6 Is a Paycheck the Strongest Opioid Antagonist? (Unemployment)

Carlos lost his factory job during the pandemic. Without income or purpose, depression set in. He started using opioids recreationally, then habitually. It wasn't until he found a job through a local reentry program that he began to recover—proving that employment isn't just economic but therapeutic. His experience reflects the vulnerability faced by those in post-industrial regions where job loss and disconnection from the formal labor market often precede problematic opioid use.

A substantial literature demonstrates an association between unemployment and OUD/OOD. However, the relationship's strength is diluted by two factors: (1) effect sizes tend to be small, and (2) unemployment appears to act through mediating variables to affect outcomes. The quality and implications of econometric research are explored in more detail in a future chapter. Basic bivariate relationships are described below.

In a county-level study, researchers found that a 1% increase in the unemployment rate was associated with a 3.6% increase in the opioid-related death rate, and a 7% increase in the opioid-related emergency department utilization rate [46]. Employment has a protective effect on drug treatment outcomes and is predictive of greater treatment completion. One investigation showed that an increase in months of employment was the best predictor of post-treatment recovery at 6 months [47]. Another longitudinal study on people with heroin use disorder reported a strong association between employment and abstinence: 56% were employed in the group with five or more years of abstinence compared to 15% in the group with less than 5 years. Employment may be the strongest opioid antagonist we haven't fully deployed.

A paycheck doesn't just pay the bills—it affirms purpose. Without it, despair can fill the void. In communities where the factories shut down, opioid use moved in, not as a moral failure, but as a coping mechanism.

Across these populations, from women and LGBTQIA+ youth to the working poor, a pattern emerges—systemic exclusion begets vulnerability. The SDoH are not merely correlates of risk, but preconditions for exposure, trauma, and neglect.

5.3.7 The Silent Epidemic (Disability)

Lena, who lives with multiple sclerosis, faces daily pain and fatigue. Her doctor prescribed opioids, but as prescribing restrictions tightened, she was abruptly cut off. Still in pain and desperate, Lena turned to illicit pills—unpredictable and dangerous.

People with disabilities are particularly susceptible to harmful opioid prescribing practices and experience OUD more often than those without a disability [48, 49]. From 1993 to 2014, adults with disabilities, particularly those who were middle-aged and low-income, comprised the majority of hospitalizations for prescription opioid and heroin overdoses [50].

Opioid misuse commonly begins shortly after individuals file worker compensation claims and continues throughout the duration of the claims [49]. Disability often co-occurs with depression and anxiety, which are themselves risk factors for OUD and overdose [51–53]. Disability also creates barriers to substance use disorder (SUD)/OUD treatment, and people with disabilities are less likely to receive medications for OUD [54]. On top of this, disability limits or bars engagement in work activities, aggravating a series of risk factors for OUD, including SES, social connectedness, and emotional wellbeing [55–57].

While disability doesn't cause addiction, abandonment related to disability can increase vulnerability and risk. As prescribing tightened, many disabled people were left not with safer care but with fewer options and more suffering.

5.3.8 Wounded Warriors and Prescription Scars (Veteran Status)

Marcus, a decorated Iraq veteran, returned home with a Purple Heart—and post-traumatic stress disorder. His chronic back pain earned him a steady supply of prescribed opioids but little mental health support. When his dose was tapered too quickly, he turned to heroin to manage the pain that never left.

Most studies examining OODs among US veterans focus on patients in treatment at the Veterans Health Administration (VHA) [58, 59]. This group has greater prevalence of chronic pain than the overall US adult population and veterans not treated at the VHA, exposing them to higher risk for substance misuse and overdose deaths [60]. In addition, many veterans receiving care at the VHA have complex diagnoses related to their service, including post-traumatic stress disorder, traumatic brain injury, and other mental health disorders that may induce them to self-medicate [61].

In 2023, 14% of veterans aged 18 and older, or 2.8 million veterans, reported an SUD in the past year on the NSDUH, a federal household interview survey that is not VHA-based [62]. Among these, 1.8% reported a prescription pain reliever disorder and 0.3% reported a heroin use disorder, totaling 407,000 veterans. The survey found no significant differences in prevalence of SUD between veterans and non-veterans [63].

Shifts in opioid overdose rates among the veteran population mirror broader trends. As with other subpopulations, the OOD rate among veterans rose (53.4%) from 19.8 to 30.3 from 2010 to 2019 (with a slight decrease from 2017 to 2019). Rates of overdose deaths involving synthetic opioids other than methadone and involving psychostimulants grew continuously throughout 2010–2019. Mortality rates for other types of opioids declined during this time, including fatalities from methadone (61%) and natural/semisynthetic opioids (17%) (Fig. 5.8) [64].

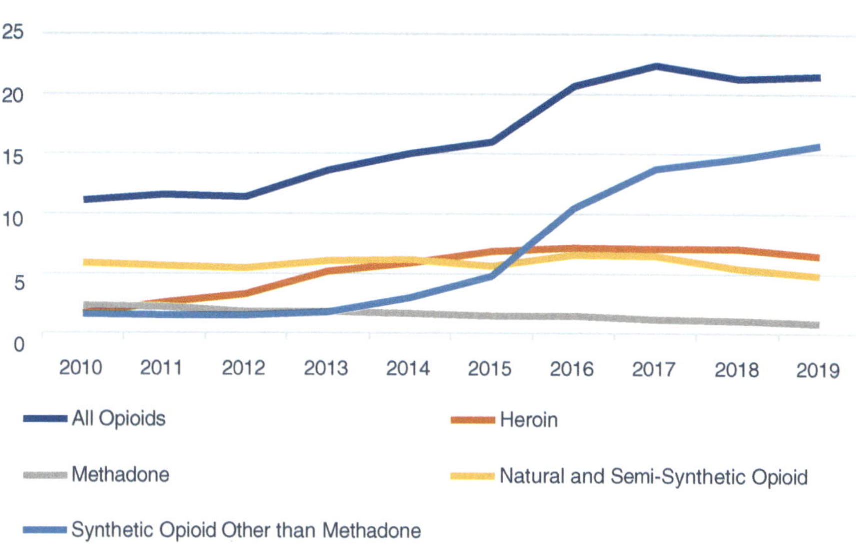

Fig. 5.8 Sources: Veterans Affairs (VA) medical records, the VA/Department of Defense Mortality Data Repository, Multiple Cause of Death data at CDC WONDER and Begley et al. [64]

Change in the type of opioid involved in overdose deaths has been observed across studies. In a recent investigation of VHA veterans, half of those who overdosed in 2010 had filled an opioid pain prescription within 3 months before death. By 2016, only a quarter of veterans had done the same. As with other populations, the increase in OODs was driven by substantial increases in overdose deaths involving synthetic opioids and heroin [58].

The research paints a complex picture of OODs among US veterans. While VHA-based studies show higher risk due to chronic pain and service-related mental health conditions, broader national survey data found no significant difference in SUDs between veterans and non-veterans. What is clear is that OOD rates among veterans have risen, mirroring national trends, with a shift from prescription opioids to synthetic opioids and psychostimulants fueling the increase. Policymakers would do well to recognize the evolving nature of the opioid crisis within the veteran population and to address both prescription and illicit drug use with a focus on the underlying mental health and pain conditions driving substance misuse.

5.3.9 No Home, No Safety Net (Housing)

Tasha has been living in her car for six months. Evicted after losing her job, she now uses opioids to get through cold nights and crowed shelters. With no address, no access to treatment, and no stable environment, recovery feels out of reach.

Housing insecurity is associated with a range of negative health outcomes, including OUD and overdose death. A recent study found that people who own a home with a mortgage face a lower risk of OUD than people in other housing situations [39].

Research in Massachusetts found a correlation between homelessness and OOD. People who have experienced homelessness are 30 times more likely than those who have not to die from an overdose [65]. A key ingredient in recovery is something far more basic than medication: a place to sleep.

5.3.10 Uncovered and Overdosing (Insurance)

Paul lost his health insurance after being laid off. When his chronic pain worsened, he couldn't afford a doctor. He turned to pills from a friend, then a dealer. Insurance might not have prevented his addiction, but the lack of it made it likelier.

In the United States, persons without insurance tend to have less access to health care, receive lower quality medical care, and experience poorer health outcomes, such as a greater likelihood of OUD and opioid-involved overdose death when compared to those with insurance. About 18% of nonelderly adults with OUD are uninsured [66].

Analysis of data from the National Inpatient Sample for 2012–2014 and 2016–2017 showed that patients with no payment method (classified as no charge) were admitted to the hospital more often than patients with other methods of payment. Only the Medicaid hospitalization rate increased over time compared to rates for other payer groups (Fig. 5.9) [67]. In the United States, treatment often depends not on need, but on network.

5.3.11 Geography as Destiny (Place of Residency)

Ella, a mother in rural West Virginia, lives 90 miles from the nearest addiction specialist. When her son overdosed, the local emergency room stabilized him—but

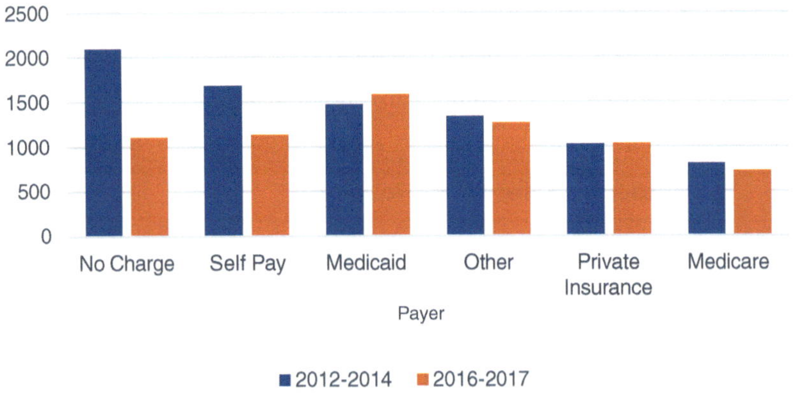

Fig. 5.9 Source: Sulley and Ndanga [67]

there was no follow-up care, no medications, no counseling. Rural often means abandoned. Her isolation is emblematic of the geographic healthcare deserts that limit access to care, harm reduction, and life-saving treatment options.

Opioid-involved overdose death rates differ by US urban and rural counties and have shifted over time. CDC data from 1999 to 2020 show that overdose deaths involving prescription opioids were, at first, higher in rural than in urban counties; however, by 2018, as rural rates decreased, the rates became more comparable. Rates for overdose deaths involving synthetic opioids were similar or marginally higher in rural than in urban counties through 2014. However, from 2015 to 2019, this trend reversed and, by 2020, the rate of deaths involving synthetic opioids was noticeably higher in urban counties (18.3) than in rural counties (14.3) (Figs. 5.10 and 5.11) [68].

In 2023, the NSDUH reported that past-year illicit drug use among people aged 12 and older was highest in large metro areas (25.3%), compared to 22.4% in non-metro areas and 17.5% in completely rural non-metro areas [62]. Fatal opioid

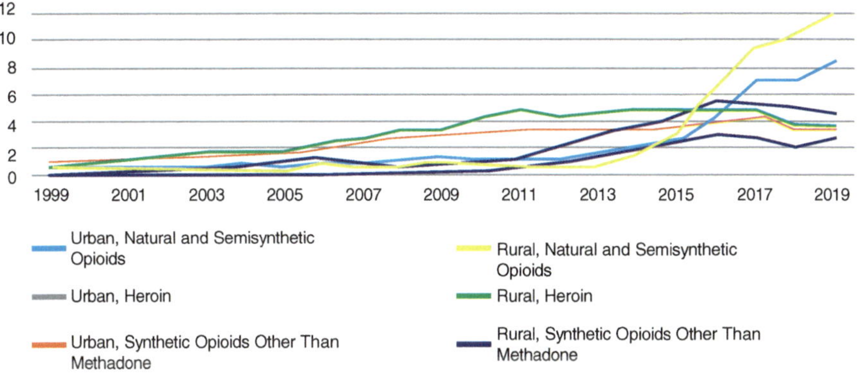

Fig. 5.10 Source: National Center for Health Statistics, National Vital Statistics System, Mortality

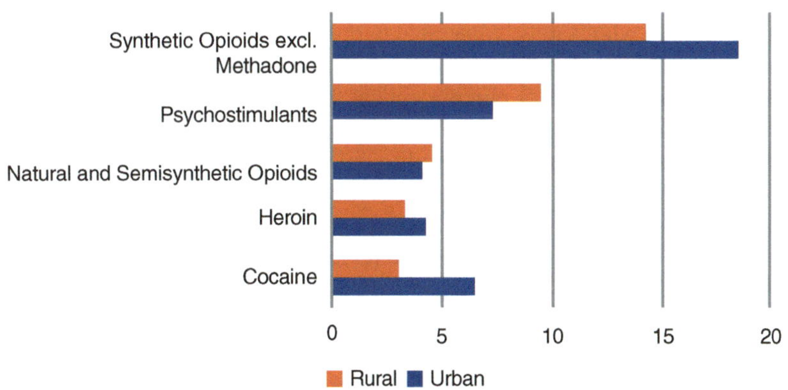

Fig. 5.11 Source: National Center for Health Statistics, National Vital Statistics System, Mortality

Table 5.1 Opioid overdose mortality by urbanization category, 2022 and 2023

Region	Deaths 2022	Percentage of total deaths 2022	Deaths 2023	Percentage of total deaths 2023
Large central metro	28,309	34	28,389	35.8
Large fringe metro	18,711	22.9	17,323	21.8
Medium metro	18,885	23.1	17,924	22.6
Small metro	6799	8.3	6557	8.3
Micropolitan (nonmetro)	6184	7.6	5885	7.4
Noncore (nonmetro)	3418	4.2	3280	4.1
Total	81,806	1000	79,358	100

Decedent's county of residence classified as urban or rural based on the 2013 NCHS Classification Scheme for Urban–Rural Counties. Deaths may involve other drugs in addition to opioids. Source: CDC, National Center for Health Statistics. Data are from the Multiple Cause of Death Data, 2018–2023

overdose rates showed a similar pattern: in 2022, rates were 27.8 per 100,000 in large metro areas versus 18.3 in non-metro (non-core) areas (Table 5.1) [13].

It is important to note that strictly dichotomous urban/rural comparisons can obscure important regional differences related to the degree of rurality, population characteristics, healthcare infrastructure, and local economic conditions. For example, even as opioid-related hospitalizations, emergency department visits, and overdose deaths are considerably higher in certain rural states. (e.g., Maine, Kentucky, and West Virginia), they are lower in others (e.g., Iowa, Nebraska, Idaho, and the Dakotas). This issue and a call for more granular analysis of geographic settings will be explored in detail in a later chapter. ZIP code has become a stronger predictor of overdose deaths than genetic code.

5.4 Understanding Disparities

Taken together, the statistics in this chapter illustrate that the opioid crisis is not an "equal opportunity" problem. SDoH, including sex, sexual orientation, gender identity, age, race, socioeconomic status, housing, insurance, and location, all play a significant role in who is most vulnerable to opioid misuse and overdose.

Understanding SDoH reveals that opioid misuse and overdose are not simply the result of individual choices or pharmaceutical supply. They are the predictable outcomes of structural inequality and social neglect. Yet, the prevailing narrative has long focused on controlling drug supply while ignoring the broader context that fuels demand. *This chapter* dismantles this reductive lens.

Each overdose death is more than a data point; it's a mirror reflecting the inequities embedded in our systems. The patterns revealed through social determinants are not coincidental, they are consequences of structural neglect, disinvestment, and discrimination. To focus solely on the substance, while ignoring the scaffolding of poverty, racism, housing instability, and social isolation, is to treat the fever and ignore the infection. An intersectional lens is also critical, as individuals facing multiple forms of marginalization—such as LGBTQIA+ persons of color or low-income veterans—may be particularly vulnerable to opioid harms. If we want to stem the tide of opioid harm, we must look not only at who is dying, but where, how, and why. The answers don't lie in individual pathology but in the policies and the environments that shape lives long before the first pill is taken.

The next chapter traces the historical and ideological roots of dominant addiction models, particularly the moral and disease frameworks, showing how they have shaped and often distorted public understanding. By exposing these frameworks as incomplete or misleading, we move closer to a more accurate and humane account of addiction, one that centers social context over scapegoats.

References

1. Office of Disease Prevention and Health Promotion (US). Healthy people: social determinants of health [Internet]. Washington, DC: U.S. Department of Health and Human Services; [cited 2025 Jul 2]. Available from: https://tinyurl.com/5reahpr4.
2. Heath D. Upstream: the quest to solve problems before they happen. New York: Avid Reader Press/Simon & Schuster; 2020.
3. Alegría M, NeMoyer A, Falgàs Bagué I, Wang Y, Alvarez K. Social determinants of mental health: where we are and where we need to go. Curr Psychiatry Rep. 2018;20(11):95.
4. Magnan S. Social determinants of health 101 for health care: five plus five. NAM Perspectives. Discussion Paper. Washington (DC): National Academy of Medicine; 2017. https://doi.org/10.31478/201710c.
5. Dasgupta N, Beletsky L, Ciccarone D. Opioid crisis: no easy fix to its social and economic determinants. Am J Public Health. 2018;108(2):182–6.
6. King NB, Fraser V, Boikos C, Richardson R, Harper S. Determinants of increased opioid-related mortality in the United States and Canada, 1990-2013: a systematic review. Am J Public Health. 2014;104(8):e32–42.
7. Singh GK, Kim IE, Girmay M, Perry C, Daus GP, Vedamuthu IP, et al. Opioid epidemic in the United States: empirical trends, and a literature review of social determinants and epidemiological, pain management, and treatment patterns. Int J MCH AIDS. 2019;8(2):89–100.
8. Park JN, Rouhani S, Beletsky L, Vincent L, Saloner B, Sherman SG. Situating the continuum of overdose risk in the social determinants of health: a new conceptual framework. Milbank Q. 2020;98(3):700–46.
9. Campbell CI, Weisner C, Leresche L, Ray GT, Saunders K, Sullivan MD, et al. Age and gender trends in long-term opioid analgesic use for noncancer pain. Am J Public Health. 2010;100(12):2541–7.
10. McHugh RK, Devito EE, Dodd D, Carroll KM, Potter JS, Greenfield SF, et al. Gender differences in a clinical trial for prescription opioid dependence. J Subst Abus Treat. 2013;45(1):38–43.
11. Substance Abuse and Mental Health Services Administration (US). NSDUH 2022 highlighted population slides [Internet]. 2023 [cited 2025 Jul 8]. Available from: https://www.samhsa.gov/data/report/nsduh-2022-highlighted-population-slides.
12. Silver ER, Hur C. Gender differences in prescription opioid use and misuse: implications for men's health and the opioid epidemic. Prev Med. 2020;131:105946.
13. Centers for Disease Control and Prevention (US), National Center for Health Statistics. CDC WONDER: Multiple Cause of Death 2018-2023 [Internet]. Atlanta (GA): Centers for Disease Control and Prevention; [cited 2025 Jul 8]. Available from: https://wonder.cdc.gov/.
14. Boerner KE, Chambers CT, Gahagan J, Keogh E, Fillingim RB, Mogil JS. Conceptual complexity of gender and its relevance to pain. Pain. 2018;159(11):2137–41.

15. Strath LJ, Sorge RE, Owens MA, Gonzalez CE, Okunbor JI, White DM, et al. Sex and gender are not the same: why identity is important for people living with HIV and chronic pain. J Pain Res. 2020;13:829–35.
16. Hatzenbuehler ML, Pachankis JE. Stigma and minority stress as social determinants of health among lesbian, gay, bisexual, and transgender youth: research evidence and clinical implications. Pediatr Clin N Am. 2016;63(6):985–97.
17. Paschen-Wolff MM, Kidd JD, Paine EA. The state of the research on opioid outcomes among lesbian, gay, bisexual, transgender, queer, and other sexuality- and gender-diverse populations: a scoping review. LGBT Health. 2023;10(1):1–17.
18. Slater ME, Godette D, Huang B, Ruan WJ, Kerridge BT. Sexual orientation-based discrimination, excessive alcohol use, and substance use disorders among sexual minority adults. LGBT Health. 2017;4(5):337–44.
19. Grant JM, Mottet LA, Tanis J, Harrison J, Herman JL, Keisling M. Injustice at every turn: a report of the national transgender discrimination survey. National Center for Transgender Equality and National Gay and Lesbian Task Force: Washington; 2011.
20. Federal Bureau of Investigation (US). UCR summary of reported crimes in the nation: 2024 [Internet]. Washington (DC): Federal Bureau of Investigation (US); 2025 [cited 2025 Oct 7]. Available from: https://cde.ucr.cjis.gov/LATEST/webapp/#/pages/explorer/crime/special-reports.
21. Barbee H, Deal C, Gonzales G. Anti-transgender legislation-a public health concern for transgender youth. JAMA Pediatr. 2022;176(2):125–6.
22. Mallory C, Redfield E. The impact of 2023 legislation on transgender youth [Internet]. Los Angeles (CA): Williams Institute, UCLA School of Law; 2023 Oct [cited 2025 Jul 8]. Available from: https://williamsinstitute.law.ucla.edu/publications/2023-trans-legislative-summary/.
23. Federal Bureau of Investigation (US). Crime Data Explorer [Internet]. Washington (DC): Federal Bureau of Investigation; 2023 [cited 2025 Jul 8]. Available from: https://cde.ucr.cjis.gov/LATEST/webapp/#/pages/home.
24. Dhanani LY, Totton RR. Have you heard the news? The effects of exposure to news about recent transgender legislation on transgender youth and young adults. Sex Res Soc Policy. 2023:1–15.
25. Trevor Project. U.S. National Survey on the Mental Health of LGBTQ Young People [Internet]. 2023 [cited 2025 Jul 8]. Available from: https://www.thetrevorproject.org/survey-2023/.
26. Haider MR, Brown MJ, Gupta RD, Karim S, Olatosi B, Li X. Psycho-social correlates of opioid use disorder among the US adult population: evidence from the National Survey on Drug Use and Health, 2015-2018. Subst Use Misuse. 2020;55(12):2002–10.
27. Center for U.S. Policy. CUSP FDA Citizen Petition to Protect Patients [Internet]. 2023 Apr 28 [updated 2023 May 11; cited 2025 Jul 9]. Available from: https://centerforuspolicy.org/fdacp2023-2/.
28. Buonora MJ, Axson SA, Cohen SM, Becker WC. Paths forward for clinicians amidst the rise of unregulated clinical decision support software: our perspective on NarxCare. J Gen Intern Med. 2024;39(5):858–62.
29. Oliva J. Prescribing algorithmic discrimination [video]. In: Conferences and symposia; no. 1011. Case Western Reserve University School of Law, Scholarly Commons; 2023 Apr 5. Available from: https://scholarlycommons.law.case.edu/law_videos_general/1011/.
30. Kabella D, Apollonio D, Young H, Knight KR. The rise of clinical decision support algorithms in pain management 2009–2024. J Gen Intern Med. 2025;40(10):2423–32.
31. U.S. Department of Health and Human Services Substance Abuse and Mental Health Services Administration. The Opioid Crisis and the Black/African American Population: An Urgent Issue [Internet]. 2020. [cited 2025 Jul 9]. Available from: https://store.samhsa.gov/sites/default/files/pep20-05-02-001.pdf.
32. PBS News Hour. How racial inequity is playing out in the opioid crisis [Internet]. 2019 Jul 18. [cited 2025 Jul 9]. Available from: https://www.pbs.org/newshour/health/how-racial-inequity-is-playing-out-in-the-opioid-crisis.

33. Centers for Disease Control and Prevention, National Center for Health Statistics. Multiple Cause of Death Files, 1999–2020 and 2018–2023.
34. Garnett MF, Miniño AM. Drug overdose deaths in the United States, 2003–2023. NCHS Data Brief, no 522. Hyattsville (MD): National Center for Health Statistics; 2024. https://doi.org/10.15620/cdc/170565.
35. The Chronicle of Higher Education. DEI Legislation Tracker [Internet]. Washington (DC): The Chronicle of Higher Education; 2025 Aug 22 [cited 2025 Oct 7]. Available from: https://www.chronicle.com/article/here-are-the-states-where-lawmakers-are-seeking-to-ban-colleges-dei-efforts?sra=true.
36. Fairbank R. Psychologists persevere in EDI work despite growing backlash against racial equity efforts. Monitor on Psychology [Internet]. 2024 Jan 1 [cited 2025 Jul 9];55(1). Available from: https://www.apa.org/monitor/2024/01/trends-anti-equity-diversity-inclusion-laws.
37. Volkow N, Benveniste H, McLellan AT. Use and misuse of opioids in chronic pain. Annu Rev Med. 2018;69:451–65.
38. van Draanen J, Tsang C, Mitra S, Karamouzian M, Richardson L. Socioeconomic marginalization and opioid-related overdose: a systematic review. Drug Alcohol Depend. 2020;214:108127.
39. Altekruse SF, Cosgrove CM, Altekruse WC, Jenkins RA, Blanco C. Socioeconomic risk factors for fatal opioid overdoses in the United States: findings from the mortality disparities in American Communities Study (MDAC). PLoS One. 2020;15(1):e0227966.
40. Visconti AJ, Santos GM, Lemos NP, Burke C, Coffin PO. Opioid overdose deaths in the City and County of San Francisco: prevalence, distribution, and disparities. J Urban Health. 2015;92(4):758–72.
41. Rudolph KE, Kinnard EN, Aguirre AR, Goin DE, Feelemyer J, Fink D, et al. The relative economy and drug overdose deaths. Epidemiology. 2020;31(4):551–8.
42. Pear VA, Ponicki WR, Gaidus A, Keyes KM, Martins SS, Fink DS, et al. Urban-rural variation in the socioeconomic determinants of opioid overdose. Drug Alcohol Depend. 2019;195:66–73.
43. Edlund MJ, Martin BC, Fan MY, Braden JB, Devries A, Sullivan MD. An analysis of heavy utilizers of opioids for chronic noncancer pain in the TROUP study. J Pain Symptom Manag. 2010;40(2):279–89.
44. Platts-Mills TF, Hunold KM, Bortsov AV, Soward AC, Peak DA, Jones JS, et al. More educated emergency department patients are less likely to receive opioids for acute pain. Pain. 2012;153(5):967–73.
45. Whitmire JT, Adams GW. Unintentional overdose deaths in the North Carolina Medicaid Population: prevalence, prescription drug use, and medical care services. Raleigh (NC): State Center for Health Statistics, North Carolina Department of Health and Human Services; 2010 Aug. SCHS Study No. 162.
46. Hollingsworth A, Ruhm CJ, Simon K. Macroeconomic conditions and opioid abuse. J Health Econ. 2017;56:222–33.
47. Sahker E, Ali SR, Arndt S. Employment recovery capital in the treatment of substance use disorders: six-month follow-up observations. Drug Alcohol Depend. 2019;205:107624.
48. Pitcher MH, Von Korff M, Bushnell MC, Porter L. Prevalence and profile of high-impact chronic pain in the United States. J Pain. 2019;20(2):146–60.
49. Webster BS, Verma SK, Gatchel RJ. Relationship between early opioid prescribing for acute occupational low back pain and disability duration, medical costs, subsequent surgery and late opioid use. Spine (Phila Pa 1976). 2007;32(19):2127–32.
50. Song Z. Mortality quadrupled among opioid-driven hospitalizations, notably within lower-income and disabled white populations. Health Aff (Millwood). 2017;36(12):2054–61.
51. Whitney DG, Hurvitz EA, Peterson MD. Cardiometabolic disease, depressive symptoms, and sleep disorders in middle-aged adults with functional disabilities: NHANES 2007-2014. Disabil Rehabil. 2020;42(15):2186–91.
52. Cho J, Spence MM, Niu F, Hui RL, Gray P, Steinberg S. Risk of overdose with exposure to prescription opioids, benzodiazepines, and non-benzodiazepine sedative-hypnotics in adults: a retrospective cohort study. J Gen Intern Med. 2020;35(3):696–703.

53. Ford JA, Hinojosa MS, Nicholson HL. Disability status and prescription drug misuse among U.S. adults. Addict Behav. 2018;85:64–9.
54. Lauer EA, Henly M, Brucker DL. Prescription opioid behaviors among adults with and without disabilities - United States, 2015-2016. Disabil Health J. 2019;12(3):519–22.
55. De Souza L, Frank AO. Patients' experiences of the impact of chronic back pain on family life and work. Disabil Rehabil. 2011;33(4):310–8.
56. Hughes C, Avoke SK. The elephant in the room: poverty, disability, and employment. Res Pract Persons Severe Disabil. 2010;35(1–2):5–14.
57. Wilson HD, Mayer TG, Gatchel RJ. The lack of association between changes in functional outcomes and work retention in a chronic disabling occupational spinal disorder population: implications for the minimum clinical important difference. Spine (Phila Pa 1976). 2011;36(6):474–80.
58. Lin LA, Peltzman T, McCarthy JF, Oliva EM, Trafton JA, Bohnert ASB. Changing trends in opioid overdose deaths and prescription opioid receipt among veterans. Am J Prev Med. 2019;57(1):106–10.
59. Warfield SC. Characteristics and patterns of opioid-related overdoses among veterans [Doctoral dissertation]. Morgantown (WV): West Virginia University; 2019.
60. Meffert BN, Morabito DM, Sawicki DA, Hausman C, Southwick SM, Pietrzak RH, et al. US veterans who do and do not utilize Veterans Affairs Health Care Services: demographic, military, medical, and psychosocial characteristics. Prim Care Companion CNS Disord. 2019;21(1).
61. Sandbrink F. What is special about veterans in pain specialty care? Pain Med. 2017;18(4):623–5.
62. Substance Abuse and Mental Health Services Administration (US). Key substance use and mental health indicators in the United States: results from the 2023 National Survey on drug use and health [Internet]. Rockville (MD): Substance Abuse and Mental Health Services Administration; 2024 Jul [cited 2025 Jul 8]. Available from: https://www.samhsa.gov/data/report/2023-nsduh-annual-national-report.
63. Substance Abuse and Mental Health Services Administration. 2023 National Survey on drug use and health (NSDUH) releases [Internet]. Rockville, MD: Substance Abuse and Mental Health Services Administration; 2023. [cited 2025 Oct 10]. Available from: https://www.samhsa.gov/data/data-we-collect/nsduh-national-survey-drug-use-and-health/national-releases/2023#highlighted-population-slides.
64. Begley MR, Ravindran C, Peltzman T, Morley SW, Stephens BM, Ashrafioun L, et al. Veteran drug overdose mortality, 2010-2019. Drug Alcohol Depend. 2022;233:109296.
65. Massachusetts Department of Public Health. An Assessment of Fatal and Nonfatal Opioid Overdoses in Massachusetts (2011–2015). Boston (MA): Massachusetts Department of Public Health; 2017. Available from: https://www.mass.gov/files/documents/2017/08/31/legislative--report-chapter-55-aug-2017.pdf.
66. Orgera K, Tolbert J. Key facts about uninsured adults with opioid use disorder. San Francisco (CA): KFF; 2019. Available from: https://www.kff.org/uninsured/issue-brief/key-facts-about--uninsured-adults-with-opioid-use-disorder/ [Accessed 2025 Jul 29].
67. Sulley S, Ndanga M. Inpatient opioid use disorder and social determinants of health: a Nationwide analysis of the National Inpatient Sample (2012-2014 and 2016-2017). Cureus. 2020;12(11):e11311.
68. Hedegaard H, Spencer MR. Urban–rural differences in drug overdose death rates, 1999–2019. NCHS Data Brief, no 403. Hyattsville (MD): National Center for Health Statistics; 2021.

Models of Addiction

6

It is tempting, if the only tool you have is a hammer, to treat everything as if it were a nail.

—Abraham Maslow (The Psychology of Science: A Reconnaissance. New York: Harper & Row, 1966)

6.1 Introduction

The understanding and treatment of addiction have historically been shaped by societal biases as much as scientific advancements. Throughout the twentieth century, addiction was viewed as either moral failing or individual disease, largely neglecting the critical role of social context and root causes. While the "brain disease model of addiction" (BDMA) has gained prominence, defining addiction as a chronic brain disorder, it faces criticism for potentially oversimplifying complex behaviors by focusing solely on neuroscience. Critics argue that the BDMA may inadvertently reinforce stigma, deny individual agency, and divert attention from crucial social, psychological, and environmental determinants of substance use. Conversely, social science perspectives increasingly highlight that drug demand frequently stems from trauma, isolation, economic precarity, and lack of opportunity. Examining historical context reveals how scientific and medical conceptions of addiction are intimately linked with the social world, shaping research and its application. By deconstructing individualizing narratives and focusing on systemic drivers of vulnerability, this chapter advocates for a more comprehensive and equitable approach to understanding and addressing addiction, setting the stage for an examination of capitalism's role in the crisis. How we define addiction determines how we treat it, whom we blame, and who receives funding or compassion. Models of addiction are not neutral; they serve political, economic, and social agendas. By analyzing these frameworks critically, we can begin to understand not just what they say about addiction, but what they obscure.

L. R. Webster, S. Eichberg, *Deconstructing Toxic Narratives*,
https://doi.org/10.1007/978-3-032-23135-2_6

6.2 Historical Context and Addiction Models

Placing public health models in social and historical context matters for understanding evolving conceptions of health and illness and their impact on people's everyday life. By applying this kind of analysis to competing etiological paradigms in drug addiction, it is possible to uncover unknown or underappreciated influences on the opioid epidemic, opening up discussion. With this knowledge, policy and decision makers can come to the table with more information to design policies that improve outcomes for all people who misuse opioids (PWMO).

A rich historiography captures the complex sociocultural dynamics behind shifting scientific/medical conceptions of addiction as well as their implications for drug treatment and control. These studies draw on multiple forms of data, including archival sources, such as medical and scientific articles, and oral histories from scientists, physicians, and drug users, to present a nuanced account that combines two interrelated domains: the scientific and the social. Historian Nancy Acker explains why making this connection is crucial analytically [1]:

> …the laboratory, far from being an isolated and impermeable space, is intimately linked with the social world around it. Influence flows in both directions. Patronage, public expectation and more help shape research directions and methods. As findings emerge from the laboratory, they are selectively adopted and adapted; their application depends on alterations to physical and social structures and processes that enable scientific findings to work in the world (p. 71).

The two hegemonic—and polarized—frameworks on substance misuse common to the twentieth century illustrate this narrative. The first model depicted addiction as a form of deviance and a sign of moral failure, subject to social condemnation and castigation. The second model portrayed addiction as a disease over which addicts had little-to-no control. Both models emphasize personal choice and ignore contextual factors affecting behavior, positioning drug use as an individual pathology [2, 3].

Within the past 30 or so years, the disease model of addiction ascended among mainstream scientists and physicians but has been disparaged by social scientists, patient advocates, and unorthodox physicians. Detractors charge that the disease model, linked with drug recovery programs emphasizing abstinence, blocks discovery of more appropriate scientific and political solutions to addiction [3–5].

In past battles over addiction policy, institutional actors have attempted to consolidate power and gain legitimacy by distinguishing between the legal (i.e., medicinal and therapeutic) and the illegal [1]. The binary constructs have been closely intertwined with dominant discourses on race, class, and gender, giving rise to harsh moral judgment about drug users and drug policies that strengthen prevailing social hierarchies [4, 6, 7]. Regardless of time period, perceptions about opiate users have been colored by the users' socioeconomic status as well as by broader sociopolitical currents [4]. To determine changes in medical discourse over time, Cooper performed a content analysis of 297 medical articles on opiate addiction during two time periods: 1880–1920 and 1955–1975 [6]. In both eras, she examined perspectives on the etiology of addiction and beliefs about drug users' race/ethnicity, social class, and gender. Historian Nancy Campbell writes [4]: "What American publics and institutions define as worthy cures for drug addiction depends on who is perceived to be addicted, on what drugs addicts depend, on the meanings attributed to addiction, and on patterns of social status (p. 12)."

6.3 Medical Discourse and Drug Control Over Time

A medical misunderstanding with lasting consequences emerged in the aftermath of the Civil War. Tens of thousands of Union and Confederate soldiers were treated with opium, laudanum, and later morphine for pain, injury, and dysentery. In the years following the war, physicians observed that many of these veterans experienced intense withdrawal symptoms when the drugs were abruptly stopped. Without a modern understanding of physical dependence, clinicians interpreted these symptoms as signs of moral failing and "addiction"—a term not yet clearly defined. As a result, veterans who were physically dependent, were often lumped together with those who used opioids for emotional or psychological relief, a behavior more consistent with today's clinical criteria for addiction. Physicians lacked both the conceptual framework and tapering protocols to manage withdrawal, and so they often blamed the patient rather than the treatment. This era cemented the association between opioid use and character weakness, and it illustrates how inadequate definitions, and poor clinical guidance can fuel stigma—especially when war, trauma, and medicine collide. Even today, historians and journalists mischaracterize the post-Civil War problem of opiate use as exclusively a problem of addiction [8–10]. Addiction was not born on the battlefield, but confusion about it was.

By the late-nineteenth century, opium use was widespread in American society. Physicians relied on it heavily during the Civil War as a pain management tool, but its use grew beyond the battlefield. Roughly 1 in 200 Americans was addicted to opium by century's end [11]. As addiction, or what was perceived to be addiction, became more visible, doctors began to debate publicly what constituted legitimate medical use versus moral failing. Opiates remained acceptable for certain groups, usually patients who were white and middle or upper class, especially women, who by then made up more than 60% of people identified as addicted. Physicians often attributed their chronic opiate use to stress of modern life and medical conditions of womanhood, distinguishing them from others whose use was considered deviant or criminal [4, 6, 11]. This racialized and gendered view of addiction foreshadowed the discriminatory patterns that would shape drug policy for generations to come.

Opiate users who were poor, foreign, and/or non-white (e.g., Chinese Americans, Black Americans) and acquired drugs in illicit settings (e.g., opium dens) were cast as members of a new urban "underclass," who were presumed to use drugs for sinister non-medical purposes. In medical journals of the day, the desire to use illicit drugs was ascribed to individual pathology, such as "mental deficiencies" and a predilection for vice [6].

Under this new medical framework, moral entrepreneurs joined policymakers and doctors in the late-nineteenth century to advocate for tighter controls on opium use through prohibition and policing [4, 6, 7, 12]. These efforts intensified in the early-twentieth century and, in response, consumption of opiates decreased [12]. Passage of the Harrison Act in 1914, which criminalized possession of drugs for recreational use, officially marked the start of America's "classic era of narcotics control," which spanned roughly half a century [7, 13]. The time period was notable for ever growing uncertainty and punishment for nonmedical drug users, even as doctors retained the ability to distribute morphine and heroin, albeit more conservatively and judiciously than before [14]. When medicine lacked understanding, it substituted morality.

Highly racialized characterizations of illicit drug users continued into the classic era. Medical journals from the 1950s described addicts as "regressive" and prone to "psychiatric disturbances," such as "passivity," "dependency," and "emotional immaturity" [6] (p. 440). Some articles argued that "slum conditions" contributed to drug use by providing easy access to drugs but maintained that only the pathologized individuals living in these environments were susceptible to drug use [6].

In stark contrast to the illicit "black market," a "white market" for drugs began to flourish due to lax government and law enforcement oversight. Physicians legally dispensed prescription drugs to middle- and upper-class white patients, first barbiturates and opioids, and by mid-twentieth century, sedatives and stimulants [7]. Prescription pill rates soared and overdoses from legal pharmaceuticals exceeded heroin overdoses, sustaining the white market system throughout the decades after WW II [7, 15]. It was within this white market that pharmaceutical companies first asserted themselves as major players in the political conflict over drugs.

By the mid-1960–1970s, attitudes toward drugs had begun to change, as US society responded to insistent social protest and moved, at least marginally, toward more equitable social relations [16, 17]. This occurred alongside growing recognition by scientists and policymakers that illicit drug use was routine among some white, middle-class young people (e.g., soldiers in Vietnam).

The mid-twentieth century also saw the emergence of contemporary addiction science. Abandoning moralizing, experts medicalized the language of addiction through the paradigm of metabolic disease. The metabolic disease model proposed that heroin caused permanent biochemical changes in the brain, requiring ongoing drug use to maintain homeostasis; thus, addiction became a serious medical concern, and methadone was the course of treatment [6, 18]. The other major theory of the era, the communicable disease model, embraced notions of individual psychopathology and susceptibility to heroin use. Authors disagreed on the relative influence of different elements in the public health triad—the agent (heroin), the host (person), and the environment (social milieu)—in spreading the disease, which was typically associated with poor Black, Indigenous, and People of Color groups [6].

6.4 The Disease Model

In 1974, the National Institute on Drug Abuse (NIDA) was established, eventually becoming the lead federal agency supporting scientific research on drug use and addiction. Throughout the 1990s, NIDA promoted the BDMA, which soon took hold in the field. Anchored in neuroscience, the BDMA proposed addiction as a chronic relapsing brain disorder, characterized by altered brain structure and function and expressed through compulsive behavior, like substance use [19]. Leveraging this framework, the paradigm achieved dominance and raised the profile of addiction research. Once considered more of a "soft" science, the BDMA unified addiction scientists around a single, potent framework and drew on the cachet of neuroscience to secure research funding [4] (p. 200) [20, 21].

BDMA supporters argue that the model offers benefits to people who misuse drugs (PWMD) by destigmatizing addiction, diminishing personal and social judgment, and broadening access to clinical treatments and supportive services [22, 23]. They liken addiction to conventional neurological disorders, such as Alzheimer's or schizophrenia, portraying PWMD as targets of errant brain activity, lacking agency, control, and responsibility for their actions [20, 24]. Neuroscientist and former drug user Marc Lewis explains: "[it] makes sense of the helplessness addicts feel and encourages them to expiate their guilt and shame by validating their belief that they are unable to get better by themselves [25] (p. 163)."

Although the BDMA appears to offer a more compassionate approach to addiction, the model has its critics who cite unintended consequences produced through discursive tactics that marginalize PWMD and reinforce feelings of shame and stigma [26–30]. By positing addiction as a biological and immutable characteristic, the disease model denies PWMD's agency, trapping them in an uncontrollable behavior cycle that makes them seem untrustworthy, menacing, or burdensome to others [31–33]. This perception can then be used to legitimize the exclusion of PWMD from social life [34].

In addition, while medication helps some people manage substance-related behavior cycles, it is not a cure-all and may amplify depression and helplessness for those who do not respond to pharmaceuticals [20]. Ultimately, critics are uneasy with the BDMA because it directs researchers and policymakers solely toward neuroscientific solutions, obscuring social, psychological, or environmental forces and obstructing the discovery of interventions to address the broad span of incentives for drug use.

This biomedicalization of addiction is a key reason why federal and state policy efforts to control prescription opioids have been short-sighted. For example, stringent restrictions intended to curb opioid misuse have left many physicians ill-equipped to address opioid use disorder, particularly the social conditions that enable and encourage addiction. Most physicians are trained solely in pharmacology, unable to offer alternative modalities to treat addiction, including harm reduction and holistic interventions to meet diverse psychosocial needs [35]. As a result, some patients were driven to the illicit market, exacerbating the problem.

As a letter in *The Lancet* pointed out, long-term deficits in medical education, particularly in pain, addiction, and disability, permitted pharmaceutical companies to exploit physicians' professional lack of knowledge, contributing to the opioid crisis [36]. We contend that the nation's insufficient regulatory framework worsened matters, allowing pharmaceutical companies to perform like all capitalistic enterprises do when government oversight is lacking. Later, these same conditions exacerbated the adverse health and social consequences that developed when prescribing was abruptly curtailed. For example, a study of buprenorphine prescribers in private practice in New York revealed that regulations to control access to prescription opioids, including stricter prescriber surveillance rules, discouraged doctors from continuing opioid addiction management in their practices [35]. Feeling unsupported and betrayed in the doctor–patient relationship, many patients turned to illicit markets to self-medicate, worsening morbidity and mortality rather than mitigating them.

6.5 The Social Science of Addiction

While the disease model and its variations have dominated addiction discourse for decades, social scientists have increasingly emphasized the importance of environmental context. With the emergence of the disease model in the 1960s, epidemiologists began integrating social science into their analyses of addiction, responding to the era's unrest and social movements. There was growing criticism of science's disregard for pressing social issues, such as economic inequality and environmental harm, and its practice of separating empirical facts from human principles [37]. By the 1990s, epidemiology was meaningfully challenging the individual-level biological and behavioral "risk factor" theories of addiction, mainly through the Social determinants of health framework. As epidemiologists turned their attention to environmental factors in etiological models, *place* began to play an important role in addiction research [38]. Linear thinking about risk factors and outcomes was replaced with a new appreciation for the dynamic interactions taking place between humans and their environments.

While much public discourse and policy have focused on control of the supply of drugs, the evidence suggests that demand, rooted in trauma, isolation, economic precarity, and lack of opportunity, is the more powerful driver of substance use. People rarely seek out drugs in a vacuum; they are often responding to emotional pain, social exclusion, or structural abandonment. This insight exposes the limitations of biomedical models that reduce addiction to a brain disorder and dismantles moral models that frame it as a failure of character. These frameworks, while influential, obscure structural and economic forces that shape vulnerability to addiction. The next chapter builds on this critique by exploring the broader political economy that sustains such narratives, specifically, the role of free-market capitalism in creating the social and economic conditions that fuel despair and substance use.

References

1. Acker CJ. How crack found a niche in the American Ghetto: the historical epidemiology of drug-related harm. BioSocieties. 2010;5(1):70–88. https://doi.org/10.1057/biosoc.2009.1.
2. Pickard H, Ahmed SH, Foddy B. Alternative models of addiction. Front Psychiatry. 2015;6:20.
3. Frank LE, Nagel SK. Addiction and moralization: the role of the underlying model of addiction. Neuroethics. 2017;10(1):129–39.
4. Campbell ND. Discovering addiction: the science and politics of substance abuse research [Internet]. Ann Arbor (MI): University of Michigan Press; 2007 [cited 2025 Jul 10]. Available from: https://doi.org/10.3998/mpub.269246.
5. Fisher CE. The urge: our history of addiction [Internet]. New York: Penguin Random House; 2022 [cited 2025 Jul 10]. Available from: https://www.penguinrandomhouse.com/books/598209/the-urge-by-carl-erik-fisher/.
6. Cooper HL. Medical theories of opiate addiction's aetiology and their relationship to addicts' perceived social position in the United States: an historical analysis. Int J Drug Policy [Internet]. 2004 Dec [cited 2025 Jul 10];15(5):435–45. Available from: https://doi.org/10.1016/j.drugpo.2004.05.006.
7. Herzberg D. White market drugs: big pharma and the hidden history of addiction in America. First Edition. Chicago: University of Chicago Press; 2020. 400 p.
8. Brown A. The Civil War's opioid crisis. The Washington Post. 2021 Dec 1. Available from: https://www.washingtonpost.com/history/2021/12/01/opioid-crisis-civil-war-addiction/.
9. Medical Historical Library, Yale University. At great risk for opium-eating: how Civil War-era doctors reacted to prescription opioid addiction [Internet]. 2021 [cited 2025 Jul 30]. Available from: https://library.medicine.yale.edu/blog/great-risk-opium-eating-how-civil-war-era-doctors-reacted-prescription-opioid-addiction.
10. Virginia Museum of History & Culture. Opiate addiction in the Civil War's aftermath [Internet]. [cited 2025 Jul 30]. Available from: https://virginiahistory.org/learn/opiate-addiction-civil-wars-aftermath.
11. Trickey E. Inside the story of America's 19th-century opiate addiction. Smithsonian Magazine [Internet]. 2018 Jan 4 [cited 2025 Jul 10]. Available from: https://www.smithsonianmag.com/history/inside-story-americas-19th-century-opiate-addiction-180967673/.
12. Courtwright DT. A short history of drug policy or why we make war on some drugs but not on others [Internet]. 2012 [cited 2025 Jul 10]. (History Faculty Research and Scholarship; 23). Available from: https://digitalcommons.unf.edu/ahis_facpub/23.
13. Acker CJ. Creating the American junkie: addiction research in the classic era of narcotic control. Baltimore: Johns Hopkins University Press; 2002. 276 p.
14. Musto DF. The American disease: origins of narcotic control. 3rd ed. New York: Oxford University Press; 1999. 432 p.
15. Herzberg D. Happy pills in America: from Miltown to Prozac. Baltimore: Johns Hopkins University Press; 2009.
16. Garrow DJ. Bearing the Cross: Martin Luther King Jr., and the Southern Christian Leadership Conference. New York: Vintage Books; 1988.
17. Zinn H. A people's history of the United States: 1492-present. New York: Harper Perennial; 1995.
18. Courtwright DT. The prepared mind: Marie Nyswander, methadone maintenance, and the metabolic theory of addiction. Addiction. 1997;92(3):257–65.
19. Volkow N. Fiscal Year 2010 Budget Request before the Senate Subcommittee on Labor-HHS-education Appropriations. Testimony to U.S. Congress, May 21, 2009.
20. Satel S, Lilienfeld SO. Addiction and the brain-disease fallacy. Front Psych. 2013;4:141.
21. Vrecko S. Birth of a brain disease: science, the state and addiction neuropolitics. Hist Human Sci. 2010;23(4):52–67.
22. Volkow ND, Koob GF, McLellan AT. Neurobiologic advances from the brain disease model of addiction. N Engl J Med. 2016;374(4):363–71.

23. Leshner AI. Addiction is a brain disease, and it matters. Science. 1997;278(5335):45–7.
24. Schüll ND. Addiction by design: machine gambling in Las Vegas. Princeton: Princeton University Press; 2014. 456 p.
25. Lewis M. The biology of desire: why addiction is not a disease. Reprint ed. New York: PublicAffairs; 2016. 256 p.
26. Heather N. Q: Is addiction a brain disease or a moral failing? A: Neither. Neuroethics. 2017;10(1):115–24.
27. Meurk C, Carter A, Partridge B, Lucke J, Hall W. How is acceptance of the brain disease model of addiction related to Australians' attitudes towards addicted individuals and treatments for addiction? BMC Psychiatry. 2014;14:373.
28. Trujols J. The brain disease model of addiction: challenging or reinforcing stigma? Lancet Psychiatry. 2015;2(4):292.
29. Hall W, Carter A, Forlini C. The brain disease model of addiction: is it supported by the evidence and has it delivered on its promises? Lancet Psychiatry. 2015;2(1):105–10.
30. Walker LJ. The chronic disease concept of addiction: helpful or harmful? Addict Res Theory. 2015; https://doi.org/10.3109/16066359.2014.987760.
31. Clark TW. Determinism and destigmatization: mitigating blame for addiction. Neuroethics. 2021;14(2):219–30.
32. Merrill JO, Rhodes LA, Deyo RA, Marlatt GA, Bradley KA. Mutual mistrust in the medical care of drug users: the keys to the "narc" cabinet. J Gen Intern Med. 2002;17(5):327–33.
33. Pescosolido BA, Martin JK, Long JS, Medina TR, Phelan JC, Link BG. "A disease like any other"? A decade of change in public reactions to schizophrenia, depression, and alcohol dependence. Am J Psychiatry. 2010;167(11):1321–30.
34. Lie AK, Hansen H, Herzberg D, Mold A, Jauffret-Roustide M, Dussauge I, et al. The harms of constructing addiction as a chronic, relapsing brain disease. Am J Public Health. 2022;112(S2):S104–s8.
35. Mendoza S, Rivera-Cabrero AS, Hansen H. Shifting blame: buprenorphine prescribers, addiction treatment, and prescription monitoring in middle-class America. Transcult Psychiatry. 2016;53(4):465–87.
36. Kertesz SG, Varley AL, Fuqua LA, Gordon AJ. The North American opioid crisis: educational failures and incautious stoppage. Lancet. 2022;400(10361):1402.
37. Krieger N. Epidemiology and social sciences: towards a critical reengagement in the 21st century. Epidemiol Rev. 2000;22(1):155–63.
38. Cooper HL, Tempalski B. Integrating place into research on drug use, drug users' health, and drug policy. Int J Drug Policy. 2014;25(3):503–7.

7 Free-Market Capitalism and the Opioid Crisis

Markets on their own often lead to excessive inequality.

—Joseph Stiglitz (People, Power, and Profits. W.W. Norton & Company, 2019)

7.1 Introduction

The opioid crisis is not only about drugs but reflects deeper societal problems rooted in free-market capitalism. While promoting individual choice, free-market policies prioritize profit and deregulation, producing harmful consequences like declining wages, job losses from globalization, weakening unions, and a growing sense of powerlessness among ordinary people. These factors foster despair, which can manifest in various ways, including substance misuse.

During the mid-twentieth century, economic stability was fostered through a collaboration between government and organized labor, an arrangement that began to erode from the 1970s onward with the rise of neoliberalism. This shift accelerated deindustrialization, especially in regions hard hit by the opioid crisis, and contributed to stagnant wages and widening income inequality, particularly impacting lower and middle-income workers and certain racial groups. Additionally, declining union power, a perceived "democratic deficit" where corporate interests overshadow public voice, and increased political polarization have all weakened social cohesion. This chapter argues that free-market capitalism, through its pursuit of profit and deregulation, created conditions ripe for pharmaceutical exploitation and systemic neglect, ultimately fueling despair and the opioid crisis.

L. R. Webster, S. Eichberg, *Deconstructing Toxic Narratives*,
https://doi.org/10.1007/978-3-032-23135-2_7

7.2 Neoliberalism and the Sociohistorical Approach

Early on, this book introduced Friedman et al.'s sociohistorical approach to the opioid epidemic, linking upstream and downstream factors to explain the myriad pathways to overdose deaths. Friedman et al.'s article offers a helpful diagram to illustrate these processes, which originated with what they call the "one-sided class war" or neoliberalism [1]. The term neoliberalism is most often used in academic contexts and takes on somewhat different meanings or implications depending on an author's standpoint or a text's intended audience. However, in its most general sense, it is categorized as a free-market philosophy coupled with limited government. Free-market policies limit (but do not entirely eliminate) government influence on the economy through efforts to lower trade barriers, deregulate capital markets, privatize government functions, and reduce fiscal support for public programs. While free-market philosophy promotes smaller government, it also endorses another core idea: maximum individual choice. Emphasizing human agency, this ethos creates challenges for people who fail to meet capitalism's normative expectations of success; they are held personally responsible for their circumstances without recognition of the system in which they are embedded [2].

Friedman et al.'s sociohistorical account aligns with other explanations that (1) trace the origin of the opioid crisis and (2) expose the links between free-market capitalism and economic inequality and social exclusion in the United States today [3, 4].

Figure 7.1 depicts Friedman et al.'s sociohistorical framework [1].

We now delve deeper into Friedman et al.'s sociohistorical model, which links neoliberalism to the opioid epidemic, by tracing how specific upstream factors related to free-market capitalism diminished workers' quality of life and moderated public reaction, allowing the crisis to proliferate. Shortly, this chapter will attempt to tie these upstream factors to downstream factors to trace the epidemic's socioeconomic origins more thoroughly. It's useful to note at the start that the data informing this story cannot show definitive cause and effect between upstream and downstream determinants. In other words, more work is needed to show conclusively how and when (through what mechanisms) economic stagnation, declining incomes, and unemployment sabotaged social and civic life and enabled damage to emotional wellbeing, provoking despair-related behaviors. Nevertheless, a trove of information across disciplines—sociology, psychology, economics, and public health—allows the piecing together of a plausible account of what took place. Altogether, these data help to uncover critical forces behind the epidemic that are rarely considered in public health policy but are urgently in need of attention.

7.3 The Rise of Free-Market Capitalism

From the post-World War II era to the mid-1970s, economic stability was sustained through compromise between labor, management, and government in most of the world's industrialized societies. This broad consensus is referred to as the Keynesian

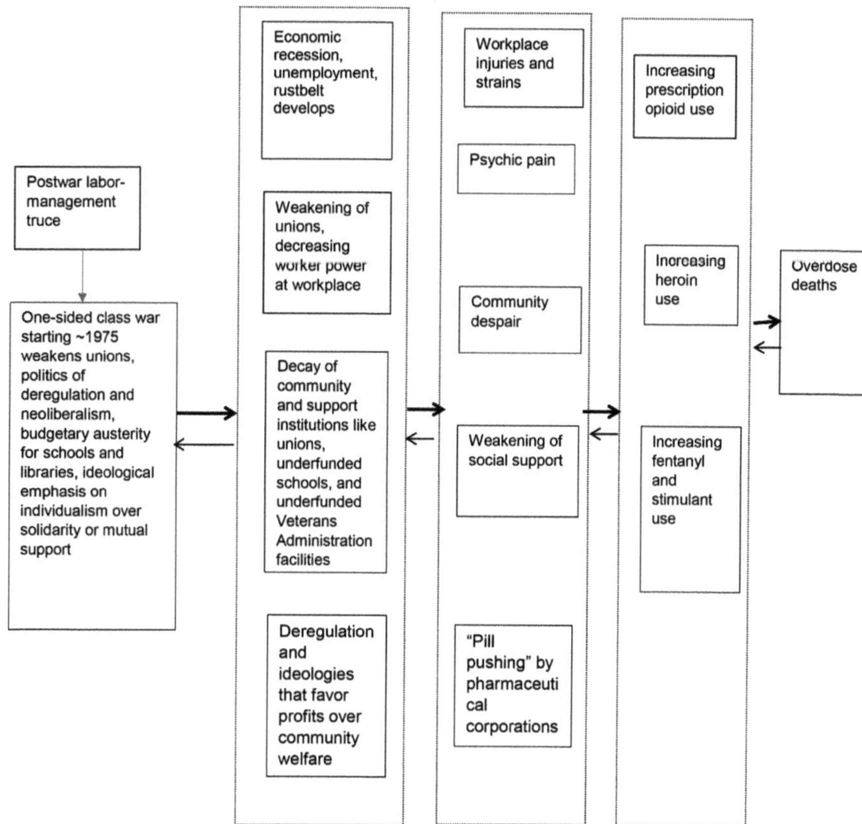

Fig. 7.1 Friedman et al.'s Socio-Historical Framework. Systemic progression from the postwar labor-management truce to overdose deaths, mapping the cascading effects of neoliberal policy and economic recession on community support systems and opioid use. (Source: Friedman et al. [1])

welfare state, a system of regulated capitalism and state service provision that increased the government's role in managing the political economy [5–8]. In America, the New Deal ushered in the first elements of the welfare state, which paused during World War II and expanded after the war ended, through policies such as Truman's Fair Deal and Johnson's Great Society. The era granted Americans unprecedented prosperity, with full or near full employment and shared improvement in living standards, despite a substantial tax rate for the wealthy [9].

However, this system weakened amid global economic shifts and the rise of neoliberal ideology. Abandonment of the welfare state for free-market capitalism first gained traction in the 1970s. There are several reasons for this ideological sea change. A standard structural explanation is that a series of global crises, including the oil crisis and stagflation, destabilized the postwar Keynesian consensus, clearing the way for a new ethos of fiscal discipline and corporate governance [10, 11]. This turn was spearheaded by a coalition of institutional actors, including big business, the super-rich, and the right political machine (e.g., conservative think tanks), who took advantage of developments to promote unchecked market capitalism [12–14]. These parties had been gathering on the sidelines since the New Deal and were thus poised to capitalize on any discontent with the Keynesian economic order. Given an entry point in the 1970s, capitalists and their right-wing allies actively engaged in efforts to eradicate existing policies and practices (unions) that they felt threatened corporate earnings and market control. Much of the public, in a conservative mindset after the cultural unrest of the 1960s, tended to be receptive to these events [9]. The radical individualism ("freedom of choice") endorsed by neoliberalism also coincided with the nation's Cold War mindset, which disparaged collective economic action and repudiated limitations on market capitalism [11].

After gaining a foothold, free-market capitalism's influence grew in the 1980s and 1990s. By the start of the millennium, it was firmly in place and found support among Republican and Democratic administrations alike. Throughout this time, a series of policies, agreements, and bills chipped away at workers' rights and standard of living, leading to stark income inequality and economic uncertainty for countless Americans. This shift had profound impacts on the American worker.

7.4 Globalization and Industrialization

Globalism describes a belief in free trade across borders. Globalism began in the 1970s as previously isolated, often less developed countries with manufacturing capabilities opened up trade with industrialized nations. This form of free-market capitalism accelerated deindustrialization throughout much of the United States. American companies soon took advantage of cheap and exploitable labor abroad, undermining union influence and gutting living wages at home [15]. Globalism gained momentum in the 1990s with the passage of the North American Free Trade Agreement (NAFTA) and the emergence of China as a global trading partner. An unintended consequence of NAFTA, which was expected to stimulate economic growth and job production, was that manufacturing companies opted to "offshore" production of their products overseas to reduce costs and achieve higher profit margins [16]. With companies offshoring labor to increase profits, many US factories closed down and the communities dependent on these businesses were devastated as work opportunities disappeared [17]. Often, it was the small towns and rural communities where the opioid crisis first emerged in the Midwest, Appalachia, New England, and other regions that fell victim to free-market policies and deindustrialization. This loss of economic stability created a sense of hopelessness and contributed to the rise of despair-related behaviors, including opioid misuse.

The following is an example of the consequences of unemployment or deindustrialization [18]:

Jonathan Guffey, 32, from Muncie, Indiana, worked several factory jobs—but each ended once opioid dependence took hold. Once vibrant and employed, he recounted how he "lived and breathed drugs," prioritizing addiction over work and slipping entirely out of the labor force. His history reflects a broader regional crisis: community labor pools hollowed out by despair as much as by economic transformation.

7.5 Stagnant Wages

Under free-market capitalism, wage growth has been slow and uneven for many American workers. Between 1979 and 2019, real wages rose for high-wage workers (90th percentile) but fell for those at the middle and bottom of the wage distribution (50th and 10th percentile, respectively), amplifying income inequality (Figs. 7.2 and 7.3) [19, 20]. Over the same period, the wage gap shrank between men and women but grew between Black and white, and between Hispanic and non-Hispanic workers. Wages for workers with a high school diploma or less also declined at the top, middle, and bottom of the wage distribution) [21].

In 2020, COVID-19 temporarily disrupted the US economy, but its effects were short-lived. After a period of wage instability, average hourly earnings began rising in 2021. Surging inflation, however, led to negative real wage growth and reduced purchasing power for most workers in 2022 and 2023 [22]. Despite this, between 2019 and 2023, workers in the bottom tenth percentile of the wage distribution experienced historically high wage growth, reversing a four-decade trend favoring higher earners (Fig. 7.3) [19]. Even amid inflation, these low-wage workers saw a 13.2% increase in earnings (Fig. 7.4) [23–25]. Economists attribute these gains to pandemic-era relief policies—expanded unemployment insurance, child tax credits,

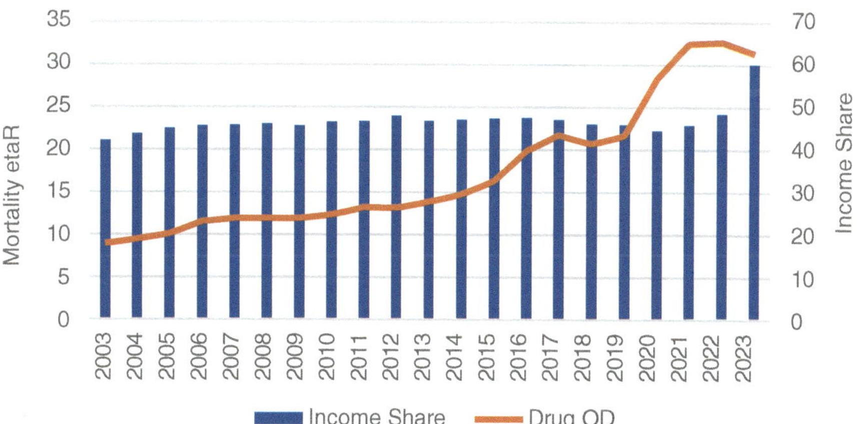

Fig. 7.2 Mortality rates are age-adjusted per 100,000 standard population. Income share data are based on pre-tax incomes. (Sources: Multiple Cause of Death Data at CDC Wonder; Income inequality (share of income to top 10%) data are from World Inequality Database. WID.world. http://wid.world/data)

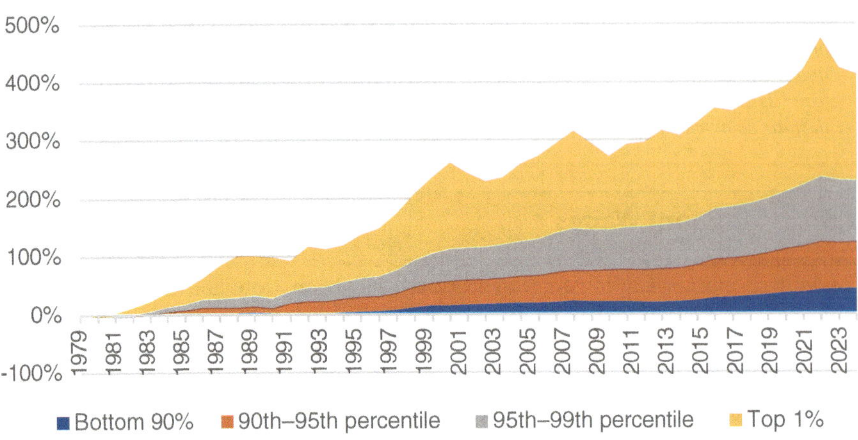

Fig. 7.3 Cumulative Percent Change in Real Annual Wages by Income Percentile, 1979–2023. The widening gap in U.S. wage growth over four decades, illustrating the disproportionate increase in real annual wages for the top 1% of earners relative to the bottom 90%. (Source: EPI analysis of Kopczuk et al. [19]; and Social Security Wage Statistics for 2023: https://www.ssa.gov/cgi-bin/netcomp.cgi?year=2023)

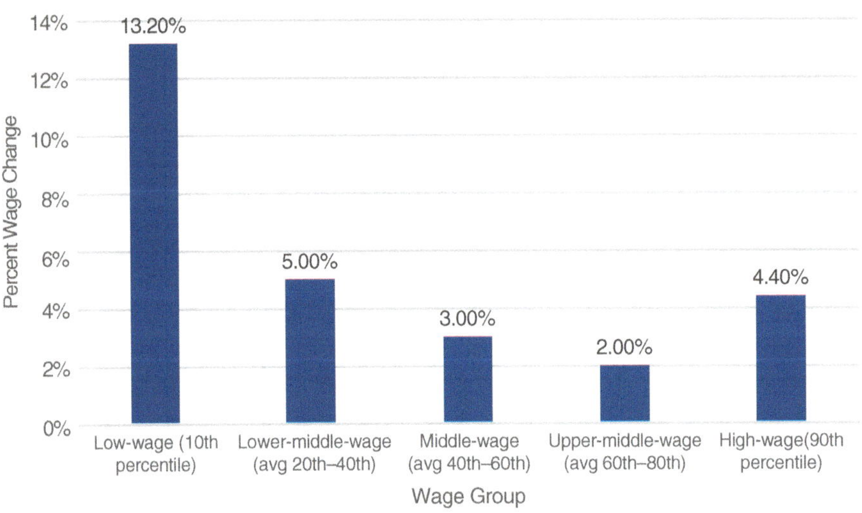

Fig. 7.4 Real Wage Growth Across the Wage Distribution, 2019–2023. Percentage change in real wages during the pandemic business cycle, showing historically high growth (13.20%) for low-wage workers (10th percentile) compared to higher earners. (Source: EPI analysis of the Current Population Survey Outgoing Rotation Group microdata, EPI Current Population Survey Extracts, Version 1.0.48 (2024a))

stimulus checks, and other measures—which reduced child poverty and helped buffer households against food insecurity, housing instability, and medical debt.

By mid-2025, real wage growth had largely returned to pre-pandemic patterns. Inflation fell from its 2022 peak by early 2024 and wage growth narrowly outpaced inflation, giving a modest boost to purchasing power for lower- and middle-income households. However, low-income workers experienced a sharp slowdown in gains, while higher income earners maintained steadier growth, and the expiration of key pandemic support programs erased improvements for low-income families with children, Black, Indigenous, and People of Color workers, and low-wage employees (Fig. 7.5). For example, the end of the expanded Child Tax Credit in January 2022 caused child poverty—which had nearly halved in 2021—to more than double within a year's time [26, 27].

The One Big Beautiful Bill Act, passed by Congress in July 2025, introduced fiscal measures that further risk exacerbating income disparities in the United States. It extends key provisions of the 2017 Tax Cuts and Jobs Act—such as lower marginal tax rates, a higher standard deduction, and expanded State and Local Tax deductions—that disproportionately benefit high-income earners and corporations [28, 29]. At the same time, the Act reduces funding for essential safety net programs such as Medicaid, the Affordable Care Act, and the Supplemental Nutrition Assistance Program. This retrenchment presents additional challenges for low-wage households, many of whom continue to struggle with withdrawal of pandemic-era supports, deteriorating the conditions that drive emotional distress and social division.

The decline of union power has further contributed to economic vulnerability as US workers lost protections. Over the past 50 years, unions' workplace influence has steadily declined, as corporations acquired greater power over workers. As a consequence, union membership has declined, and remaining members have suffered economic harm through income inequality and insufficient economic growth (Figs. 7.6 and 7.7) [30].

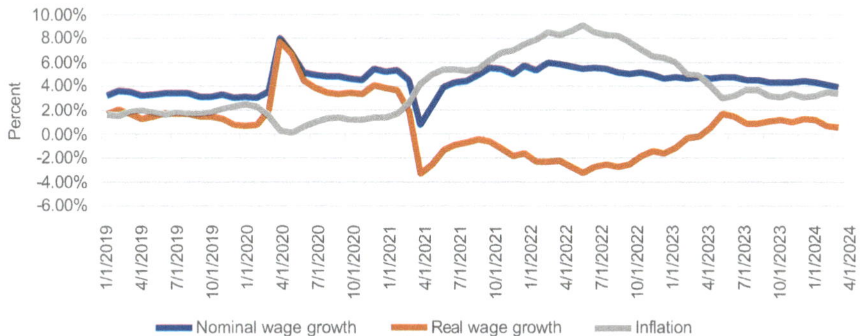

Fig. 7.5 Trends in Nominal Wages, Inflation, and Real Wages, 2019–2024. The relationship between wage growth and inflation, highlighting the 2022 period where surging inflation resulted in negative real wage growth for American households. (Source: Economic Policy Institute analysis of Bureau of Labor Statistics (BLS) Current Employment Statistics and Consumer Price Index public data series)

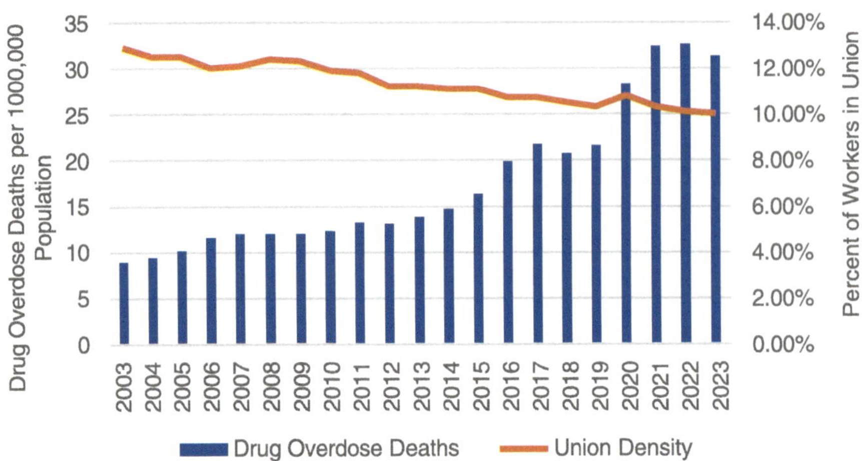

Fig. 7.6 The private and public sector labor union membership, coverage, and density estimates are compiled from the monthly household Current Population Survey (CPS) using Bureau of Labor Statistics methods. (Source: The Union Membership and Coverage Database: Unionstats.com)

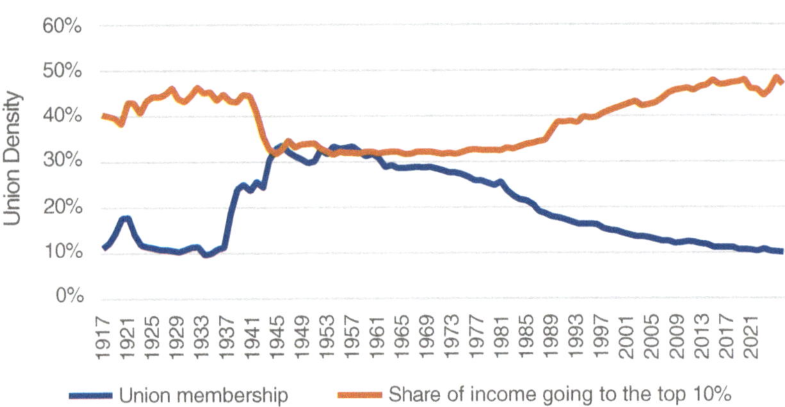

Fig. 7.7 Rates are age-adjusted per 100,000 Standard Population. (Source: Multiple Cause of Death data at CDC Wonder; The Union Membership and Coverage Database (unionstats.com))

Without strong unions, workers lost what is termed the "union advantage," which grants benefits to all workers, whether a specific worksite is unionized or not. These benefits include higher wages, smaller wage gaps, enhanced health and safety, and more expansive employer-sponsored benefits [30–38].

7.6 Democracy Deficit

As corporate power grows, many workers feel that their voices are no longer heard in the political process. This sense of political disempowerment can further fuel feelings of despair and alienation.

As numerous scholars have argued, free-market policies not only govern the global economy but exert powerful influence over politics and society. As Giroux writes [39]:

> Free-market fundamentalism rather than democratic idealism is now the driving force of economics and politics in most of the world. It is a market ideology driven not just by profits but by an ability to reproduce itself with such success that, to paraphrase Fredric Jameson (1994:xii), it is easier to imagine the end of the world than it is to imagine the end of capitalism, even as it creates vast inequalities and promotes human suffering throughout the globe. Wedded to the belief that the market should be the organizing principle for all political, social, and economic decisions, neoliberalism increasingly drives the meaning of citizenship and social life while waging an incessant attack on democracy, public goods, the welfare state, and noncommodified values (p. 495)

Perceiving a growing tension, social critics are raising important questions about whether free-market philosophy and democracy are compatible [40, 41]. Their concerns have emerged over the past 20 years as democratic governments worldwide faced intensifying income inequality, polarization, and populism [42, 43]. The difficulties stem from unchecked corporate power and a perception among the public that democratic institutions are no longer living up to core democratic ideals of equality and popular sovereignty, whether due to gridlock, ineptitude, or unscrupulousness. The end result is widespread dissatisfaction with politics and politicians [44].

Decline in democratic participation and growing distrust of corporate and democratic institutions, coupled with a lack of accountability on the part of those institutions, has been labeled the "democratic deficit," which increasingly affects the lives of ordinary people [45, 46]. Indeed, a political science study gained national prominence in 2014 after reporting that corporations and the mega rich have so much control over US policy that "the preferences of the average American appear to have only a minuscule, near-zero, statistically non-significant impact upon public policy" [47] (p. 21).

Evidence for a democratic deficit exists in polls showing that Americans' support for and belief in the legitimacy of governmental institutions is at its lowest point in decades. One national study found that just 4% of US adults think that the US political system is working extremely or very well, while 23% think it is working somewhat well [48]. A far larger share (63%) report not too much or no confidence at all in the future of the US political system.

When asked about the federal government specifically, just 16% of Americans express trust most of the time. Trust in the judicial branch has fallen sharply from 67% to 48% between 2020 and 2024 (Fig. 7.8). In 2022, for the first time since the 1980s, more Americans viewed the Supreme Court unfavorably than favorably—a historic shift in public opinion [49, 50].

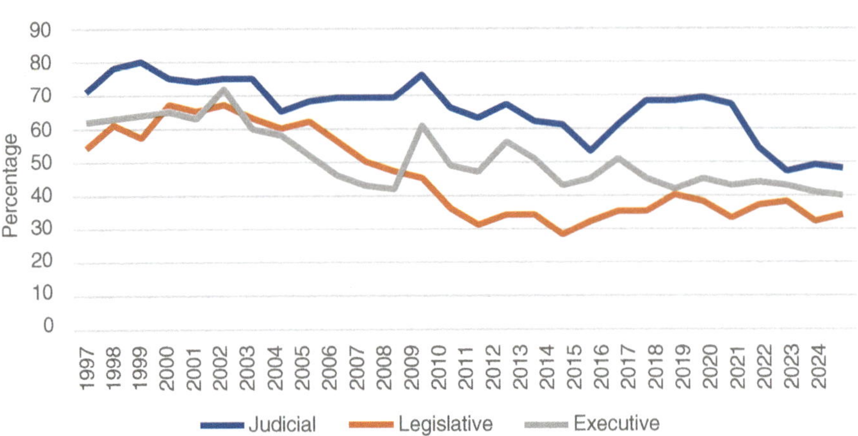

Fig. 7.8 Figures are the percentage who have a great deal or fair amount of trust in the institution or actor. (Source: Gallup. Trust in Government (2025): https://news.gallup.com/poll/5392/trust-government.aspx)

7.7 Polarization

The current economic and political landscape has also contributed to increased social polarization. The breakdown in social cohesion erodes the fabric of society and makes it harder to address pressing social problems.

Most Americans perceive their country as politically polarized. In one national survey, close to 90% of respondents viewed the country as ideologically divided [51]. In another, 70% said that America has become so polarized that it can no longer solve the key issues facing the country [52].

In fact, Americans' perceptions of a divided country are consistent with political reality. A study measuring affective polarization (the tendency to feel more negatively toward another political party than one's own) found that this sentiment has grown more rapidly in the United States in the past few decades than in European countries and other democracies [53, 54].

While political polarization can stem from many social and economic factors, it is strongly associated with (rising) income inequality. As income inequality increases, so does political intolerance and the inability to find common ground. At times, political polarization can benefit democratic societies, by clarifying policy choices and mobilizing political participation. However, severe polarization intensifies political intolerance, dilutes respect for social norms, and stymies effective governance [53, 55].

7.8 Social Cohesion and Social Connection

Social scientists link the issues discussed above—income inequality, globalization, polarization, and civic disengagement—with diminished social cohesion. They argue that for a democracy to function effectively, it must have a cohesive society, where the population shares certain attributes and behaviors, including a sense of belonging, solidarity, and a commitment to a common purpose or goal [56]. Instead, one could argue, contemporary society has given way to deep balkanization with individualistic and exclusionary policies that encourage unchecked free-market capitalism, promoting and upholding structural inequality.

Social cohesion describes the strength of community relationships that develop from trust and a sense of solidarity. It exists on a spectrum alongside other indicators of social connection, including social capital, isolation, loneliness, support, and networks. Social capital, discussed in detail later, refers to the resources people gain from their involvement in social or community networks. Both social cohesion and social capital are useful concepts for understanding the intermediate mechanisms linking social health determinants, such as income inequality, with physical health and mental wellbeing. For example, more income inequality weakens social cohesion, leading to poorer health outcomes.

The rise in drug overdose deaths cannot be fully understood without acknowledging the economic and ideological architecture that enabled it. Free-market capitalism, with its relentless pursuit of profit, deregulated power, and commodification of suffering, created fertile ground for pharmaceutical exploitation and systemic neglect. But more insidiously, it also hollowed out the conditions that make life livable—stable work, affordable housing, accessible health care, and social connection. In the vacuum left behind, despair took root. The same market logic that made opioids ubiquitous also stripped away the buffers that might have protected people from seeking solace in them. In this way, the opioid crisis is not just a public health failure—it is a predictable symptom of an economic system that prioritizes accumulation over care, and efficiency over empathy.

In this chapter, we have demonstrated how free-market capitalism has eroded economic stability, frayed social cohesion, and intensified despair, laying the groundwork for substance use and overdose. Yet, the response to this structural crisis has not been unified. Instead, it has unfolded through two competing and often contradictory frameworks: medicalization and criminalization. The next chapter examines how these responses are shaped by race, class, and political interests. These social factors have defined the nation's understanding of the opioid crisis and influenced who receives treatment, who is punished, and who profits. These institutional contradictions reveal much about the values embedded in our systems of health, justice, and commerce.

References

1. Friedman SR, Krawczyk N, Perlman DC, Mateu-Gelabert P, Ompad DC, Hamilton L, et al. The opioid/overdose crisis as a dialectics of pain, despair, and one-sided struggle. Front Public Health. 2020;8:540423.
2. Bloom P. The ethics of neoliberalism: the business of making capitalism moral. London: Routledge; 2017. 219 p.
3. Burtless G, Jencks C. American inequality and its consequences. LIS Working Paper Series. 2003. No.: 339.
4. Piketty T, Saez E. Inequality in the long run. Science. 2014;344(6186):838–43.
5. Harvey D. A brief history of neoliberalism. Oxford: Oxford University Press; 2007. 254 p.
6. Harvey D. Neoliberalism as creative destruction. Ann Am Acad Pol Soc Sci. 2007;610(1):21–44.
7. McNally D. Global slump: the economics and politics of crisis and resistance. Oakland, CA: PM Press; 2010. 176 p.
8. Moody K. Workers in a lean world: unions in the international economy. London: Verso Books; 1997. 350 p.
9. Andersen K. Evil geniuses: the unmaking of America: a recent history. New York: Random House; 2020. 464 p.
10. Brown R. Explaining the neoliberal turn: structural theories. In: The conservative counter-revolution in Britain and America 1980–2020. Cham: Springer International Publishing; 2022. p. 33–58.
11. Palley TI. From Keynesianism to neo-liberalism: shifting paradigms in economics. In: Saad-Filho A, Johnston D, editors. Neo-liberalism: a critical reader. London: Pluto Press; 2004.
12. Bockman J. Neoliberalism. Contexts. 2013;12(3):14–5.
13. Harvey D. The new imperialism. Oxford: Oxford University Press; 2005. 288 p.
14. Moody K. In solidarity: essays on working-class organization and strategy in the United States. Chicago, IL: Haymarket Books; 2014. 416 p.
15. Gills BK, Thompson W, editors. Globalization and global history. London: Routledge; 2006. 324 p.
16. Martin PL. Trade and migration: the case of NAFTA. Asian Pac Migr J. 1993;2(3):329–67.
17. van Neuss L. Globalization and deindustrialization in advanced countries. Struct Chang Econ Dyn. 2018;45:49–63.
18. Noguchi Y. The powerful pull of opioids leaves many 'missing' from U.S. workforce. NPR. 2017 Sep 8. Available from: https://www.capradio.org/news/npr/story?storyid=548867893.
19. Kopczuk W, Saez E, Song J. Uncovering the American Dream: inequality and mobility in social security earnings data since 1937. Cambridge (MA): National Bureau of Economic Research; 2007 Aug [cited 2025 Jul 14]. Working Paper 13345. Available from: https://www.nber.org/papers/w13345.
20. Office of the Chief Actuary, Social Security Administration. Wage statistics for 2023. In: Social security online [internet]. Washington (DC): Social Security Administration; [cited 2025 Jul 14]. Available from: https://www.ssa.gov/cgi-bin/netcomp.cgi?year=2023.
21. Congressional Research Service. Real wage trends, 1979 to 2019 [internet]. Washington: Congressional Research Service; 2020 Dec [cited 2025 Jul 11]. Report No.: R45090. Available from: https://sgp.fas.org/crs/misc/R45090.pdf.
22. Congressional Research Service. Average wage growth and related economic trends in 2022 [internet]. Washington: Congressional Research Service; 2023 Jan 11 [cited 2025 Jul 11]. Report No.: R47380. Available from: https://crsreports.congress.gov/product/pdf/R/R47380.
23. Gould E, deCourcy K. State of Working America Wages 2022: low-wage workers have seen historically fast real wage growth in the pandemic business cycle: policy investments translate into better opportunities for the lowest-paid workers [internet]. Washington, D.C.: Economic Policy Institute; 2023 Mar 23 [cited 2025 Oct 8]. Available from: https://www.epi.org/publication/swa-wages-2022/.

24. Gould E, Shierholz H. The economy is recovering fast. But we need to ensure it works for everyone [Internet]. CNN Business Perspectives. 2022 Mar 3 [cited 2025 Oct 8]. Available from: https://www.cnn.com/2022/03/03/perspectives/jobs-labor-market-stimulus-economy/index.html.
25. Gould E, deCourcy K. State of Working America Wages 2023: fastest wage growth over the last four years among historically disadvantaged groups: low-wage workers' wages surged after decades of slow growth [Internet]. Washington, D.C.: Economic Policy Institute; 2024 Mar 21 [cited 2025 Oct 8]. Available from: https://www.epi.org/publication/swa-wages-2023/.
26. Burns K, Fox L, Wilson D. Child poverty fell to record low 5.2% in 2021 [Internet]. Washington, D.C.: U.S. Census Bureau; 2022 Sep 13 [cited 2025 Oct 8]. Available from: https://www.census.gov/library/stories/2022/09/record-drop-in-child-poverty.html.
27. Schneider M. Child poverty in the US jumped and income declined in 2022 as coronavirus pandemic benefits ended [Internet]. AP News. 2023 Sep 12 [cited 2025 Oct 8]. Available from: https://apnews.com/article/poverty-income-health-insurance-census-623f928ddcceca2bc5e69948929d266c.
28. Piketty T, Saez E, Zucman G. Distributional National Accounts: methods and estimates for the United States*. Q J Econ. 2018;133(2):553–609.
29. Gale WG, Gelfond H, Krupkin A, Mazur MJ, Toder E. Effects of the tax cuts and jobs act: a preliminary analysis [Internet]. Washington, D.C.: Brookings Institution; 2018 Jun 13 [cited 2025 Oct 8]. Available from: https://www.brookings.edu/articles/effects-of-the-tax-cuts-and-jobs-act-a-preliminary-analysis/.
30. Shierholz H. Weakened labor movement leads to rising economic inequality [Internet]. Washington: Economic Policy Institute; 2020 Jan 27 [cited 2025 Jul 11]. Available from: https://www.epi.org/blog/weakened-labor-movement-leads-to-rising-economic-inequality/.
31. Card D. The effect of unions on the structure of wages: a longitudinal analysis. Econometrica. 1996;64(4):957–79. Available from: http://links.jstor.org/sici?sici=0012-9682%28199607%2964%3A4%3C957%3ATEOUOT%3E2.0.CO%3B2-F.
32. Ehrenberg RG, Smith RS. Modern labor economics: theory and public policy. 12th ed. New York: Routledge Publishers; 2015.
33. Mishel M. The enormous impact of eroded collective bargaining on wages [Internet]. 2021 Apr 8 [cited 2025 Jul 14]. p. 18. Available from: https://files.epi.org/uploads/225389.pdf.
34. US Department of Labor. The Union advantage [Internet]. Washington, DC: U.S. Department of Labor; [cited 2025 Jul 14]. Available from: https://www.dol.gov/general/workcenter/union-advantage#:~:text=According%20to%20the%20Center%20for,the%20course%20of%20their%20careers.
35. Card D, Mas A, Moretti E, Saez E. Inequality at work: the effect of peer salaries on job satisfaction. Am Econ Rev. 2012;102(6):2981–3003.
36. Donado A. Why do unionized workers have more nonfatal occupational injuries? ILR Rev. 2015;68(1):153–83.
37. Reynolds M, Brady D. Bringing you more than the weekend: union membership and self-rated health in the United States. Soc Forces. 2012;90:1023–49. https://doi.org/10.2307/41682687.
38. Sojourner A, Yang J. Effects of unionization on workplace-safety enforcement: regression-discontinuity evidence. IZA discussion paper 9610. Bonn, Germany: Institute of Labor Economics (IZA); 2015.
39. Giroux HA. Public pedagogy and the politics of neo-liberalism: making the political more pedagogical. Policy Futures Educ. 2004;2(3–4):494–503. Available from: https://eric.ed.gov/?id=EJ795548.
40. Streeck W. Buying time: the delayed crisis of democratic capitalism. Verso Books; 2014.
41. Warren ME, editor. Democracy and trust. Cambridge University Press; 1999.
42. Milner HV. Is global capitalism compatible with democracy? Inequality, insecurity, and interdependence. Int Stud Q. 2021;65(4):1097–110.
43. Boix C. Democratic capitalism at the crossroads. Princeton University Press; 2019.
44. Streeck W, Schäfer A, editors. Politics in the age of austerity. John Wiley & Sons; 2013.
45. Gould CC. Globalizing democracy and human rights. Cambridge University Press; 2004.

46. Levinson S. The democratic deficit in America. Harvard Law & Policy Review; 2006.
47. Gilens M, Page BI. Testing theories of American politics: elites, interest groups, and average citizens. Perspect Polit. 2014;12(3):564–81.
48. Pew Research Center. Americans' dismal views of the nation's politics [Internet]. 2023 [cited 2025 Jul 14]. Available from: https://www.pewresearch.org/politics/2023/09/19/americans-dismal-views-of-the-nations-politics/.
49. Jones M. Trust in Federal Government Branches Continues to falter [Internet]. Gallup; 2022 Oct 11 [cited 2025 Jul 14]. Available from: https://news.gallup.com/poll/402737/trust-federal-government-branches-continues-falter.aspx.
50. Jones M. Americans trust local government most [Internet]. Gallup; 2023 Oct 13 [cited 2025 Jul 14]. Available from: https://news.gallup.com/poll/512651/americans-trust-local-government-congress-least.aspx.
51. Silver L, Fetterolf J, Connaughton A. Diversity and division in advanced economies [Internet]. 2021 Oct 13 [cited 2025 Jul 14]. Available from: https://www.pewresearch.org/global/2021/10/13/diversity-and-division-in-advanced-economies/.
52. Murray M. 'Downhill,' 'divisive': Americans sour on nation's direction in new NBC News Poll [Internet]. Meet the Press. NBC News; 2022 Jan 23 [cited 2025 Jul 14]. Available from: https://www.nbcnews.com/politics/meet-the-press/downhill-divisive-americans-sour-nation-s-direction-new-nbc-news-n1287888.
53. Iyengar S, Lelkes Y, Levendusky M, Malhotra N, Westwood SJ. The origins and consequences of affective polarization in the United States. Annu Rev Polit Sci. 2019;22:129–46.
54. Boxell L, Gentzkow M, Shapiro JM. Cross-country trends in affective polarization. Rev Econ Stat. 2024;106(2):557–65.
55. Hetherington MJ, Rudolph TJ. Why Washington won't work: polarization, political trust, and the governing crisis. University of Chicago Press; 2020.
56. Moustakas L. Social cohesion: definitions, causes and consequences. Encyclopedia. 2023;3(3):1028–37.

8 Medicalization, Criminalization, and Contradictions

Every system is perfectly designed to get the results it gets.

—Paul Batalden (popularized; derived from concepts by W. Edwards Deming and Arthur Jones, as clarified by the Institute for Healthcare Improvement in "Like Magic? ['Every system is perfectly designed…']", August 21, 2015, which attributes specific phrasing to Batalden: https://www.ihi.org/library/blog/magic-every-system-perfectly-designed)

8.1 Introduction

This chapter explores the dual responses to the opioid crisis: medicalization and criminalization, highlighting how these approaches are shaped by racial biases. Medicalization frames drug use as an illness, individualizing the problem and downplaying systemic factors, while simultaneously commodifying addiction within a capitalist framework. In contrast, criminalization, historically exemplified by the punitive "War on Drugs," has disproportionately targeted Black communities, leading to mass incarceration and social devastation.

When crack cocaine ravaged Black communities, the response was predominantly punitive, marked by racialized media portrayals and severe sentencing. However, the prescription opioid epidemic, largely affecting white Americans, has been framed with sympathy, emphasizing treatment over incarceration. Racial disparities persist within the justice system: Black Americans are five times more likely to be incarcerated than white Americans, and are disproportionately arrested and imprisoned for drug offenses, even with similar usage rates. This chapter examines the inherent contradictions in a free-market system that prioritizes profit, leading to corporate misconduct, yet relies on reactive lawsuits rather than proactive regulation. It underscores the urgent need for systemic reform that not only prevents future crises but dismantles the structural inequities at the heart of America's drug policy failures.

L. R. Webster, S. Eichberg, *Deconstructing Toxic Narratives*,
https://doi.org/10.1007/978-3-032-23135-2_8

8.2 Racialized Framing of the Opioid Crisis: Medicalization Versus Criminalization

Experts have often applied medical language to opioid and other drug use, sometimes as part of a racially biased process. This tactic is central to the process of medicalization, which treats non-medical problems as an illness or pathology, centering the individual as the source of the problem while downplaying social factors [1]. This "othering" strategy functions as a form of social control over groups and their behaviors, especially against groups seen as threats [2–4]. In addition, in a capitalist society, medicalization commodifies addiction and its treatment. The mechanisms sustaining this process include consumerism, biotechnology, and managed care. Initially catalyzed by the pharmaceutical industry's claims that opioids could safely manage pain, the opioid problem bloomed as doctors unwittingly overprescribed medication, patient demand boosted sales, and the insurance industry's cost containment policies favored pills over other treatment modalities that form comprehensive, interdisciplinary care [5, 6].

Criminalization is another tactic, one infused with moral valence, that is used to control the threat of social instability. In recent US history, criminalization has often served as a response to public discontent with undesirable social conditions, stemming from free-market policies, such as rising income inequality, poorly paid wage labor, and dismantling of social welfare programs [7–10].

As previously discussed, race deeply influences how the opioid epidemic is understood and addressed, whether it is medicalized or criminalized. Media's portrayal of opioid users has long reflected racial bias. While white users were cast as victims of pharmaceutical greed, Black users were pathologized as criminal and dangerous—a dualism rooted in decades of racist drug policy [11–14]. Historians argue that the opioid epidemic itself would not have happened without the union of market capitalism and the long-standing racialized bifurcation of legal (prescription) and illegal drugs in America [15, 16].

In the past, when opioids and crack cocaine were ravaging Black communities, the federal response was not to medicalize the problem, but to launch the punitive "War on Drugs." These policies, which amplified tactics initiated in the 1970s, targeted Black communities and linked illicit drug use with poor parenting and personal irresponsibility, anathema to free-market capitalist principles [17]. In its coverage, the media dramatized the situation, distorted statistics, and emphasized criminality in ways that reflected and reinforced long-standing racial stereotypes [12, 18–22]. Across the country, mandatory sentencing and severe penalties for drug offenses fueled mass incarceration and inflicted deep harm in African American families and communities [23].

In contrast, the prescription opioid epidemic has been framed as a health emergency primarily affecting white Americans. Media coverage generally avoids narratives of criminality and presents addiction with a sympathetic tone, encouraging empathy [24–26]. Reports often explain the reason behind white individuals' opioid use [26, 27], portraying them not in terms of character flaws or neurochemical imbalances, but as victims of external forces, such as greedy corporations, reckless prescribers, or drug dealers infiltrating suburban spaces [28, 29]. When interventions are mentioned, the emphasis is on drug monitoring and therapeutic support rather than law enforcement [26, 30]. This coverage parallels reporting on powder cocaine, which linked the substance with white users and presented treatment, rather than punishment, as the appropriate response to addiction [31]. By disregarding the toll of opioids on wellbeing in Black communities, this disparity reinforces the historic marginalization of Black people, perpetuating the long-standing unsympathetic approaches to addiction in communities of color.

8.3 Persistent Racial Disparities in the Criminal Justice System

On top of this, Black Americans continue to be disproportionately sentenced and imprisoned for drug offenses under a criminal justice system that purports to be colorblind but, in reality, enacts widely differential treatment for people of color [32–36]. The system is also partially privatized, incentivized by funds acquired and saved by using incarcerated people—predominantly from Black, Indigenous, and People of Color (BIPOC) communities—as a cheap source of labor.

Although the prison population is down from its height in 2009, the system's decarceration rate has been slow, averaging only 2.3% annually [37]. Racial and ethnic disparities in the criminal justice system have narrowed due to more discretionary use of mandatory minimum laws in some jurisdictions. Yet, significant inequities persist: in 2022, Black Americans were twice as likely to be arrested as white Americans, while incarceration rates were five times higher for Black adults and 2.3 times higher for Hispanic adults than white adults—and even higher in some states [38, 39]. While Black and Hispanic Americans comprised 32% of the US population in 2022, they made up 55% of the adult US state and federal prison population [38]. By contrast, whites made up 59% of the total population but only 31% of the prison population. Jail populations reveal similar imbalances: at mid-year 2023, Black individuals were incarcerated at a rate of 552 per 100,000, compared to 152 per 100,000 for white individuals. Hispanic and white individuals were incarcerated at roughly the same rate (Figs. 8.1 and 8.2) [40].

Although racial and ethnic disparities are smaller among women than men, they remain observable when statistics are disaggregated by sex [38]. While the aforementioned statistics do not account for socioeconomic status or other confounding variables, public health studies using statistical methods have confirmed that racial disparities in imprisonment rates remain after controlling for other factors, including prior criminal histories, arrest offense, and demographic characteristics [41, 42]. Studies also have found residual racial incongruence in arrest and sentencing after controlling for relevant variables [42, 43].

Disparities are also present for people of color in drug offenses, the cause of incarceration for one out of five people in jails and prisons [44]. Although drug use rates are similar among Black and white populations and somewhat lower among Hispanics, and although people typically purchase drugs from sellers of the same

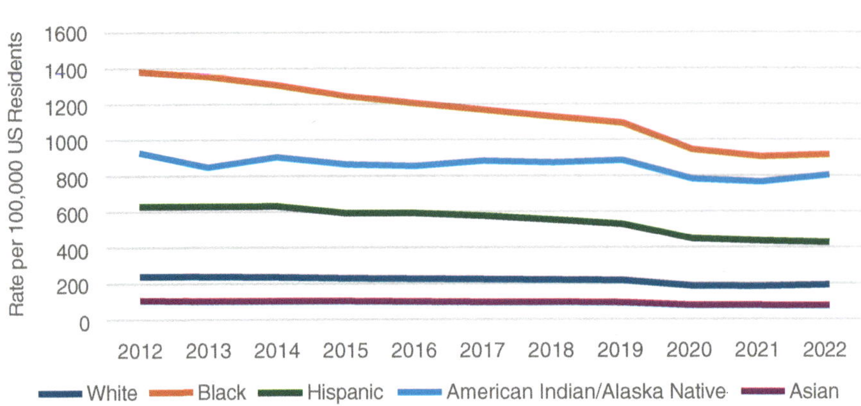

Fig. 8.1 Imprisonment rate is the number of sentenced prisoners per 100,000 US residents aged 18 or older in a given category. Rates are for December 31 of each year and are based on prisoners with a sentence of more than 1 year. (Source: Zeng [40])

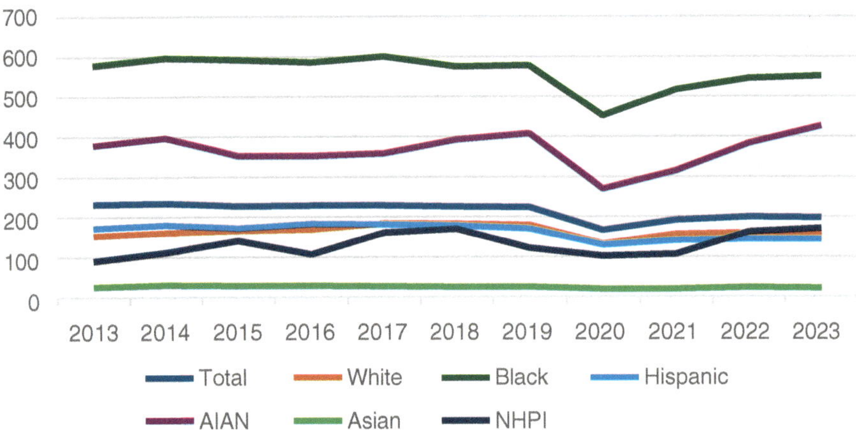

Fig. 8.2 Data are based on the last weekday in June. AIAN is an abbreviation for American Indian/Alaskan Native. NHPI Stands for Native Hawaiian/Other Pacific Islander. (Source: Zeng [40]; Census of Jails, 2019; and U.S. Census Bureau, Population Estimates by Age, Sex, Race, and Hispanic Origin for the United States: January 1, 2013 to January 1, 2024)

race, Black and Hispanic adults are disproportionately arrested, prosecuted, and imprisoned for drug offenses, most often for possession (Fig. 8.3) [45]. Their rate of incarceration for drug offenses is six times higher than that of white people [46]. Length of stay in prison for drug offenses is similarly imbalanced; in the last 20 years, length of stay increased from 1.5 years to 2.1 years for incarcerated Black people but decreased from 1.2. to 1.1 years for incarcerated white people [47]. Additionally, data on exonerations indicate that innocent Black people are 19 times more likely to be convicted of drug crimes than innocent white people [48].

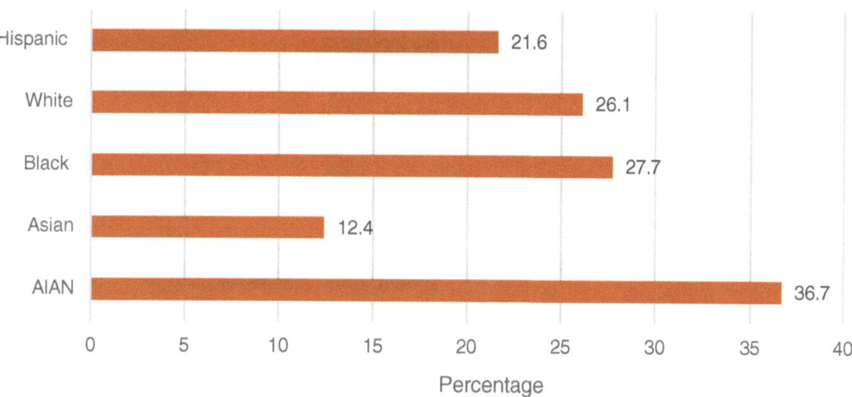

Fig. 8.3 AIAN refers to American Indian/Alaska Native. (Source: SAMSHA, National Survey on Drug Use and Health (NSDUH) 2023)

Various causal factors explain differential treatment in the criminal justice system based on race. Prior research indicates that racial differences in criminal histories and offending rates—which stem from inequality in risk, such as socioeconomic inequality and disparities in protective factors—contribute to harsher outcomes for BIPOC individuals in the criminal justice system. Multiple studies show that racial bias permeates the criminal justice system, whether as overt racism or implicit bias, producing disparate racial outcomes that vary by jurisdiction and type of crime committed [35, 49–51].

Disparities are also common for possession of the same illegal substance. The American Civil Liberties Union found that in 2018, Black people were 3.7 times more likely to be arrested for marijuana possession than white people, despite comparable rates of use [52].

Disparities extend to the treatment for opioid use disorder. Nearly half (47%) of people in state and federal prisons have a substance use disorder (SUD); yet, access to comprehensive, evidence-based care remains limited [53, 54]. Formerly incarcerated individuals face an overdose risk more than 100 times that of the general population [55], despite robust evidence that medication-assisted treatment (MAT) reduces mortality, improves recidivism, and supports continuity of care [53, 56–58]. Yet, MAT is the least commonly available treatment: in 2021, only 1% of incarcerated individuals with SUD in federal prisons reported receiving MAT at any point during incarceration, leaving most at heightened risk of relapse, re-incarceration, and fatal overdose (Fig. 8.4) [53, 56, 57, 59].

In the correctional settings where effective substance misuse treatment is available, there are striking racial discrepancies among the individuals receiving appropriate MAT (methadone, buprenorphine, and naltrexone) and therapeutic treatments. A study conducted in 2024 in New York, just one in 10 MAT recipients in the state's prisons were Black, even though Black people comprised half of the state's prison population [60]. Another study found that nearly half of jails (49.8%) cited a shortage of licensed staff as the primary barrier to providing MAT. Facilities that were

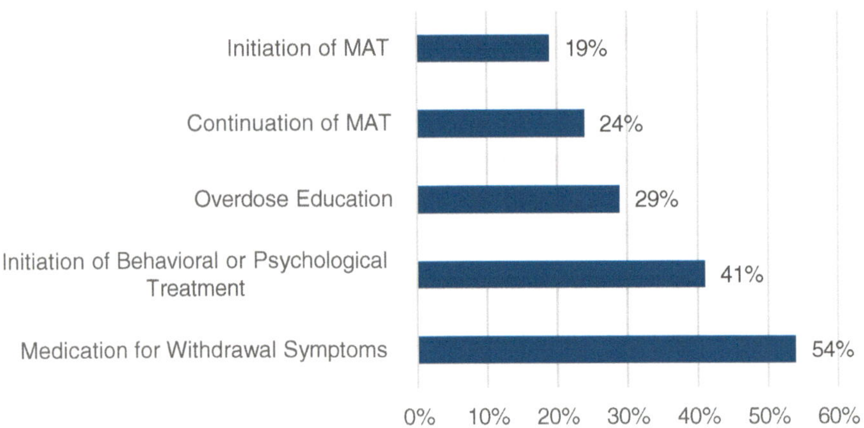

Fig. 8.4 Source: Maruschak et al. [59]. Bulletin, Table 5

larger, located in areas with lower social vulnerability, and situated near community MAT providers were more likely to offer treatment [61].

Black and Hispanic offenders are also not as likely to be redirected to drug courts as white offenders, despite similar arrest details and criminal histories [62]. Studies show that these programs benefit non-violent drug users who are less likely to relapse when referred to drug courts and placed in community-based settings as alternatives to prison [63–65].

8.4 Legal Recourse and the Contradictions of Free-Market Accountability

Having examined how race and criminalization shaped perceptions of opioid use, we now turn to the role of free-market capitalism in enabling pharmaceutical exploitation. A free-market system that eschews significant government oversight runs into obvious tensions when it comes to regulating drugs or holding corporations accountable for unscrupulous practices. Despite this conflict, states like Oklahoma have pursued lawsuits against pharmaceutical giants, including Purdue Pharma, on behalf of their citizens. These legal battles are difficult to win, given the high evidentiary standards required to prove that state and federal laws regulating controlled substances were violated. Nevertheless, as of March 2024, opioid retailers, manufacturers, and distributors, including national pharmacy chains, have been ordered to pay out over $54 billion to settle these claims [66, 67].

The paradox of suing pharmaceutical companies is vividly illustrated by Oklahoma's Attorney General Mike Hunter's comments at the Bipartisan Policy Center on May 13, 2019, following the state's initial $270 million settlement with Purdue Pharma [68]. The purpose of the event was to discuss how to allocate funds from a Purdue settlement (approximately one-fifth of which went to legal fees) and anticipated funds from other pharmaceutical companies [69]. Hunter openly acknowledged his initial hesitation in going after Purdue for damages, citing his Republican principles against suing Fortune 500 companies, but ultimately justified the action by stating that sometimes "businesses do bad things" [69]. This underscores a deeper flaw: when profit eclipses public welfare, the system not only fails but becomes complicit in the crises it claims to solve. Furthermore, the terms stipulate that the monies awarded will involve "future profits and the value of drugs currently in development," actually allowing Oklahoma to profit from sales of OxyContin [70]. These contradictions underscore a broader pattern in which free-market principles are championed until corporate misconduct leads to public harm—at which point litigation is used as a remedy, often after irreparable damage has been done. This highlights the inherent tensions within a free-market system that prioritizes profit over public health.

8.4.1 Corporate Accountability and Free-Market Paradoxes

The legal accountability and massive settlements extended far beyond Purdue Pharma, showing how the broader pharmaceutical and distribution ecosystem contributed to the opioid crisis. For example, Insys Therapeutics was a specialty pharmaceutical company known for marketing *Subsys*, a fentanyl-based pain medication—even off-label—and aggressively targeting prescribers. Their tactics included bribing doctors and misleading insurers. In 2019, the Department of Justice and state authorities prosecuted Insys executives for racketeering [71]. The company pled guilty and paid over $225 million in criminal and civil settlements. Multiple executives faced prison time, including founder John Kapoor, who was convicted in May 2019.

This case illustrates that the same tactics used by Purdue, scheming to profit from addictive medications, weren't unique to them. Insys leveraged similar mechanisms: deceptive marketing, targeting vulnerable populations, and evading clinical safety standards.

Not only manufacturers but also drug distributors have been held accountable for fueling opioid oversupply. In a 2021 nationwide agreement, AmerisourceBergen, McKesson, and Cardinal Health, three of the largest pharmaceutical distributors, committed to paying over $26 billion to resolve lawsuits that accused them of shipping an equivalent of 144 hydrocodone pills per adult in certain counties, without adequate controls on suspicious orders [72].

These distributors were essential links in the supply chain, literally moving massive volumes of opioids into high-risk areas; yet, they faced legal scrutiny only after the magnitude of the crisis became undeniable.

Even consulting firms face legal consequences for their role. McKinsey & Company advised Purdue and other opioid manufacturers over a decade, including recommending sales strategies tied to overdose and addiction metrics. In 2024, McKinsey agreed to pay $650 million to settle criminal and civil investigations alleging they helped "turbocharge" opioid sales by incentivizing doctors and pharmacies using crisis-linked metrics [73]. This represents a broader market logic at play, not just marketing via pharmaceutical companies, but behind-the-scenes advisory that prioritized profit over public safety.

These cases reinforce that the opioid crisis was not just the result of one company's missteps, but a reflection of systemic corporate behavior across manufacturers, distributors, and consultants. Regulation can create a form of corporate accountability, particularly when companies make business decisions that destabilize entire communities. When corporations shut down factories and relocate operations overseas (or elsewhere) to capitalize on cheaper labor, they often leave economic devastation in their wake—unemployment, poverty, and the collapse of local economies. While globalization may have benefits, the problem lies in the absence of safeguards to help the communities that are left behind.

A useful analogy is strip mining: companies that extract minerals from the land are typically required to restore the environment to a usable state once mining operations cease. Similarly, corporations that extract economic value from a community should bear some responsibility for mitigating the damage they leave behind. This could take the form of mandatory reinvestment in workforce retraining programs, direct contributions to local economic development initiatives, or tax incentives that encourage businesses to assist in transitioning displaced workers into new industries.

The goal is not to punish corporations for seeking efficiency but to ensure that economic progress does not come at the cost of widespread social and economic harm. Free markets function best when they account for both profit motives and the long-term wellbeing of the communities they impact. Otherwise, the burden of corporate decisions falls squarely on workers and local economies, perpetuating cycles of economic distress that could have been mitigated with responsible corporate policies and sensible regulations.

The political and economic frameworks that prioritize deregulation can inadvertently create the very conditions that enable such crises. Ultimately, relying on reactive lawsuits and the pursuit of financial settlements should not obscure the need for systemic change to prevent future crises.

Taken together, these paradoxes illustrate how both medical and criminal justice systems, rooted in structural racism and market logic, have failed to respond adequately to the opioid crisis. Instead of offering healing or justice, they have reinforced inequity and deepened suffering. This sets the stage for the next chapter's discussion of more holistic and equitable solutions.

References

1. Conrad P. Medicalization and social control. Annu Rev Sociol. 1992;18(1):209–32.
2. Esposito L, Perez FM. Neoliberalism and the commodification of mental health. Humanity Soc. 2014;38(4):414–42.
3. Freidson E. Professional dominance: the structure of medical care. New Brunswick (NJ): Transaction Publishers; 1970. 242 p.
4. Zola IK. Medicine as an institution of social control. Sociol Rev. 1972;20(4):487–504.
5. Schatman ME, Webster LR. The health insurance industry: perpetuating the opioid crisis through policies of cost-containment and profitability. J Pain Res. 2015;8:153–8.

6. Smith DE. Medicalizing the opioid epidemic in the U.S. in the era of health care reform. J Psychoactive Drugs. 2017;49(2):95–101.
7. Aviram H. Are private prisons to blame for mass incarceration and its evils: prison conditions, neoliberalism, and public choice. Fordham Urb LJ. 2014;42:411.
8. Dollar C. Criminalization and drug "wars" or medicalization and health "epidemics": how race, class, and neoliberal politics influence drug laws. Crit Criminol. 2019;27:305. https://doi.org/10.1007/s10612-018-9398-7.
9. Wacquant L. Punishing the poor: the neoliberal government of social insecurity. Durham NC: Duke University Press; 2009.
10. Wacquant L. Crafting the neoliberal state: workfare, prisonfare, and social insecurity 1. Sociol Forum. 2010;25(2):197–220.
11. Chong D, Druckman JN. Framing theory. Annu Rev Pol Sci. 2007;10:103–26.
12. Hartman DM, Golub A. The social construction of the crack epidemic in the print media. J Psychoactive Drugs. 1999;31(4):423–33.
13. Iyengar S, Kinder D. News that matters. Chicago: University of Chicago Press; 1987.
14. McCombs ME, Shaw DL. The agenda-setting function of mass media. Public Opinion Q. 1972;36(2):176–87.
15. Herzberg D. White market drugs: big pharma and the hidden history of addiction in America. First Edition. Chicago: University of Chicago Press; 2020. p. 400.
16. Murch D. Racist logic: markets, drugs, sex. Boston Review / MIT Press; 2019.
17. Baum D. Legalize it all: how to win the war on drugs. Harper's Magazine. 2016 Apr 1.
18. Cobbina JE. Race and class differences in print media portrayals of crack cocaine and methamphetamine. J Crim Justice Popular Culture. 2008;15(2):145–67.
19. Orcutt JD, Turner JB. Shocking numbers and graphic accounts: quantified images of drug problems in the print media. Soc Probl. 1993;40(2):190–206.
20. Reeves JL, Campbell R. Coloring the crack crisis. In: The Media in Black and White. Routledge; 1996. p. 7.
21. Reinarman C, Levine HG. Crack in the rearview mirror: deconstructing drug war mythology. Social Justice. 2004;31(1/2):182–99.
22. Taylor S. Outside the outsiders: media representations of drug use. Probat J. 2008;55:369–87. https://doi.org/10.1177/0264550508096493.
23. James K, Jordan A. The opioid crisis in black communities. J Law Med Ethics. 2018;46(2):404–21.
24. Brown L, Tucker-Seeley R. Commentary: will 'deaths of despair' among whites change how we talk about racial/ethnic health disparities? Ethn Dis. 2018;28(2):123–8.
25. Cohen A. How white users made heroin a public-health problem. The Atlantic. 2015 Aug [cited 2025 Jul 15]. Available from: https://www.theatlantic.com/politics/archive/2015/08/crack-heroin-and-race/401015.
26. Netherland J, Hansen HB. The war on drugs that wasn't: wasted whiteness, "dirty doctors," and race in media coverage of prescription opioid misuse. Cult Med Psychiatry. 2016;40(4):664–86.
27. Murakawa N. Toothless: the methamphetamine "epidemic," "meth mouth," and the racial construction of drug scares. Du Bois Rev. 2011;8(1):219–28. https://doi.org/10.1017/S1742058X11000208.
28. Mendoza S, Rivera-Cabrero AS, Hansen H. Shifting blame: buprenorphine prescribers, addiction treatment, and prescription monitoring in middle-class America. Transcult Psychiatry. 2016;53(4):465–87.
29. Richards C. The role of race and class in local media coverage of Utah's opioid epidemic. Hinckley J Polit. 2018 Aug [cited 2025 Jul 15];19(1). Available from: https://epubs.utah.edu/index.php/HJP/article/view/4127.
30. Lindsay SL, Vuolo M. Criminalized or medicalized? Examining the role of race in responses to drug use. Soc Probl. 2021;68(4):942–63.
31. Reeves JL, Campbell R. Cracked coverage: television news, the anti-cocaine crusade, and the Reagan legacy. Duke University Press; 1994.

32. Alexander M. The new Jim Crow: mass incarceration in the age of colorblindness. The New Press; 2012.
33. Foreman J Jr. Racial critiques of mass incarceration: beyond the new Jim Crow. Faculty Scholarship Series. 2012 Feb 26; Paper 3599.
34. Hinton E. From the carceral to the welfare state: America's failed response to social inequality, 1965–2000. Harvard University Press; 2016.
35. Tonry M, Melewski M. The malign effects of drug and crime control policies on black Americans. Crime Justice. 2008;37(1):1–44.
36. Wacquant L. From slavery to mass incarceration: rethinking the 'race question' in the US. In: Race, Law and Society. Routledge; 2017. p. 277–96.
37. Ghandnoosh N. Ending 50 years of mass incarceration: urgent reform needed to protect future generations. Washington, D.C.: The Sentencing Project; 2023. Feb 8 [cited 2025 Jul 15]
38. Carson EA. Prisoners in 2022–statistical tables. NCJ 307149. 2023 Nov.
39. U.S. Census Bureau. Quick facts United States. Population Estimates, July 1, 2023. [cited 2025 Jul 15]. Available from: https://www.census.gov/quickfacts/fact/table/US/PST045223.
40. Zeng Z. Jail Inmates in 2023—Statistical Tables. Washington (DC): Bureau of Justice Statistics (US); 2025 Apr. Report No.: NCJ 309965. Available from: https://bjs.ojp.gov/library/publications/jail-inmates-2023-statistical-tables/web-report.
41. Bales WD, Piquero AR. Racial/ethnic differentials in sentencing to incarceration. Justice Q. 2012;29(5):742–73.
42. Durante KA. Racial and ethnic disparities in prison admissions across counties: an evaluation of racial/ethnic threat, socioeconomic inequality, and political climate explanations. Race Justice. 2020;10(2):176–202.
43. Rehavi MM, Starr SB. Racial disparity in federal criminal sentences. J Polit Econ. 2014;122(6):1320–54.
44. Prison Policy Initiative. Mass Incarceration: The Whole Pie 2024. 2024 Mar 14 [cited 2025 Jul 15].
45. SAMHSA, Center for Behavioral Health Statistics and Quality. National Survey on Drug Use and Health, 2015–2019. [cited 2025 Jul 15]. Available from: [https://www.samhsa.gov/data/sites/default/files/reports/rpt35326/2021NSDUHSUChartbook102221B.pdf].
46. NAACP. Criminal Justice Fact Sheet. NAACP. 2023 [cited 2025 Jul 15]. Available from: https://naacp.org/resources/criminal-justice-fact-sheet.
47. Council on Criminal Justice. Pushing toward parity. Justice system disparities Black-White National Imprisonment Trends, 2000 to 2020. Council on Criminal Justice. 2022 Sep [cited 2025 Jul 15]. Available from: https://counciloncj.foleon.com/reports/racial-disparities.
48. Gross S, Possley M, Otterbourg K, Stephens K, Paredes J. Race and wrongful convictions in the United States 2022. University of Michigan Law School; 2022. [cited 2025 Jul 15]. Available from: https://papers.ssrn.com/sol3/papers.cfm?abstract_id=4245863.
49. Spohn C. Race, crime, and punishment in the twentieth and twenty-first centuries. Crime Justice. 2015;44(1):49–97.
50. Hetey RC, Eberhardt JL. The numbers don't speak for themselves: racial disparities and the persistence of inequality in the criminal justice system. Curr Dir Psychol Sci. 2018;27(3):183–7.
51. DeLisi M, Piquero AR. New frontiers in criminal careers research, 2000–2011: a state-of-the-art review. J Crim Just. 2011;39(4):289–301.
52. American Civil Liberties Union. A tale of two countries: racially targeted arrests in the era of marijuana reform. American Civil Liberties Union. 2020 [cited 2025 Jul 15].
53. Homans M, Allen D, Mazariegos Y. A review of medication assisted treatment (MAT) in United States jails and prisons. Sacramento, CA: California Department of Corrections & Rehabilitation; 2023. Available from: https://cchcs.ca.gov/wp-content/uploads/sites/60/MAT-in-United-States-Jails-and-Prisons-Final.pdf.

54. Widra E. Addicted to punishment: jails and prisons punish drug use far more than they treat it. Prison Policy Initiative. 2024 Jan 30 [cited 2025 Jul 15]. Available from: https://www.prisonpolicy.org/blog/2024/01/30/punishing-drug-use/.
55. Binswanger IA, Blatchford PJ, Mueller SR, Stern MF. Mortality after prison release: opioid overdose and other causes of death, risk factors, and time trends from 1999 to 2009. Ann Intern Med. 2013;159(9):592–600.
56. Bird SM, Fischbacher CM, Graham L, Fraser A. Impact of opioid substitution therapy for Scotland's prisoners on drug-related deaths soon after prisoner release. Addiction. 2015;110:1617–24.
57. Gisev N, Larney S, Kimber J, Burns L, Weatherburn D, Gibson A, et al. Determining the impact of opioid substitution therapy upon mortality and recidivism among prisoners: a 22-year data linkage study. Trends Issues Crime Criminal Justice [Internet]. 2015 [cited 2025 Jul 15];(498). Available from: https://www.aic.gov.au/publications/tandi/tandi498.
58. Rich JD, McKenzie M, Larney S, Wong JB, Tran L, Clarke J, et al. Methadone continuation versus forced withdrawal on incarceration in a combined US prison and jail: a randomised, open-label trial. Lancet. 2015;386(9991):350–9.
59. Maruschak LM, Minton TD, Zeng Z. Opioid use disorder screening and treatment in local jails, 2019. Washington (DC): U.S. Department of Justice, Office of Justice Programs, Bureau of Justice Statistics; 2023 Apr. 12 p. Report No.: NCJ 305179. Available from: https://bjs.ojp.gov/document/oudstlj19.pdf.
60. Norris S. In these state prisons, addiction treatment is out of reach. New York Focus [Internet]. 2024 Mar 22 [cited 2025 Jul 15]. Available from: https://nysfocus.com/2024/03/22/opioid-addiction-treatment-prisons-racial-gap.
61. Flanagan Balawajder E, Ducharme L, Taylor BG, Lamuda PA, Kolak M, Friedmann PD, et al. Factors associated with the availability of medications for opioid use disorder in US jails. JAMA Netw Open. 2024;7(9):e2434704.
62. Nicosia N, Macdonald JM, Arkes J. Disparities in criminal court referrals to drug treatment and prison for minority men. Am J Public Health. 2013;103(6):e77–84.
63. Csete J. Drug courts in the United States: punishment for 'patients.' In: Rethinking drug courts: International experience of a US export. 2019. p. 1–20.
64. Latessa EJ, Reitler AK. What works in reducing recidivism and how does it relate to drug courts. Ohio NUL Rev. 2014;41:757.
65. Polenberg S. Factors affecting success and failure among drug court participants in the United States: an examination of program completion and post-program outcomes [Doctoral dissertation]. University of Miami; 2015.
66. Kaiser Family Foundation. Payback: tracking the opioid cash settlement. KFF Health News [Internet]. 2024 [cited 2025 Jul 15]. Available from: https://kffhealthnews.org/payback/.
67. Hoffman J. Opioid distributors cleared of liability to Georgia families ravaged by addiction. New York Times. 2023 Mar 1.
68. Bebinger M. Purdue pharma agrees to $270 million opioid settlement with Oklahoma. NPR [Internet]. 2019 Mar 26 [cited 2025 Jul 15]. Available from: https://www.npr.org/sections/health-shots/2019/03/26/706848006/purdue-pharma-agrees-to-270-million-opioid-settlement-with-oklahoma.
69. The role of litigation in response to the opioid epidemic. Washington: Bipartisan Policy Center [Internet]. 2019 May 13 [cited 2025 Jul 15]. Available from: https://bipartisanpolicy.org/event/the-role-of-litigation-in-response-to-the-opioid-epidemic/.
70. American Bar Association. Opioid lawsuits generate payouts, controversy. 2019. Available from: https://www.americanbar.org/news/abanews/aba-news-archives/2019/09/opioid-lawsuits-generate-payouts-controversy.
71. U.S. Attorney's Office, District of Massachusetts. Insys therapeutics agrees to enter into $225 million global resolution of criminal and civil investigations [Internet]. Washington: U.S. Department of Justice; 2019 Jun 5 [cited 2025 Jul 30]. Available from: https://www.justice.gov/usao-ma/pr/insys-therapeutics-agrees-enter-225-million-global-resolution-criminal-and-civil.

72. AmerisourceBergen, Cardinal Health, McKesson. Distributors announce proposed opioid settlement agreement [Internet]. Conshohocken, PA: AmerisourceBergen; 2021 Jul 21 [cited 2025 Jul 30]. Available from: https://investor.amerisourcebergen.com/news/news-details/2021/Distributors-Announce-Proposed-Opioid-Settlement-Agreement/default.aspx.
73. NPR. McKinsey and DOJ reach settlement in opioid prosecution [Internet]. Washington, D.C.: NPR; 2024 Dec 13 [cited 2025 Jul 30]. Available from: https://www.npr.org/2024/12/13/nx-s1-5155962/mckinsey-purdue-opioid-prosecution-doj.

Econometric Studies 9

People are not dying from mysterious forces. They are dying from the failure of economic and social institutions.

—Anne Case and Angus Deaton (Deaths of Despair and the Future of Capitalism, 2020)

9.1 Introduction

This chapter examines the intricate relationship between economic conditions and the opioid crisis, highlighting how various econometric studies have explored the impact of factors like unemployment, plant closures, and trade policies on opioid use and mortality. While some research indicates an association between economic downturns and increased opioid-related harms, the findings are often mixed, suggesting that a simple causal link is insufficient to explain the epidemic's scale.

A critical review of this research reveals that most utilize panel data and quantitative methods, which can show associations but not direct causation. Furthermore, the majority focus on the era of prescription opioid deaths, leaving a research gap regarding the later rise of synthetic opioids and their disproportionate impact on Black, Indigenous, and People of Color (BIPOC) communities.

The chapter also explores how opioid supply can influence labor force participation. Overall, the evidence suggests that economic decline contributes to opioid misuse through complex, indirect pathways, with more robust effects observed in specific demographics, particularly white, rural, male workers in manufacturing or resource extraction industries. Understanding these nuances is crucial for developing effective interventions and addressing the evolving nature of the crisis.

L. R. Webster, S. Eichberg, *Deconstructing Toxic Narratives*,
https://doi.org/10.1007/978-3-032-23135-2_9

9.2 Initial Assessment of Economic–Opioid Links

In Lordstown, Ohio, the closure of a General Motors plant left not just economic ruin but a trail of lost lives. Within three years, overdose deaths in the county nearly doubled, as despair met the easy availability of painkillers [1].

Early econometric studies of the opioid crisis often focused narrowly on predominantly white, rural, or post-industrial communities, inadvertently reinforcing the misconception that opioid misuse is a "white problem." This exclusion of Black, Indigenous, and other communities of color from analytic models has perpetuated a racial blind spot in both academic research and policy response. By failing to capture the structural racism embedded in housing, employment, health care, and criminal justice systems, these studies have overlooked critical drivers of opioid vulnerability in BIPOC populations and contributed to inequitable interventions. If we only look where the data is easiest to collect, we miss where the damage is deepest.

Assessing the relationship between opioid-related health outcomes and economic trends is integral to uncovering the epidemic's root causes. Over the last decade, a growing body of research on this topic has explored how general economic conditions (e.g., plant closures, employment swings, and trade/import strain) affect opioid use or opioid-related mortality in various social groups. Results have been mixed, suggesting that there is no simple causal relationship between economic conditions and opioid use [2].

While several studies have identified an association between macroeconomic conditions and opioid-related behavior, findings are often nominal or weak. MacLean et al. contend that these empirical findings are unconvincing, stating that "the magnitudes of the predicted effects are small relative to the overall increases in opioid prescribing and overdoses and are therefore unlikely to be key determinants of the crisis" [3] (p. 10). They suggest incorporating mediating factors, such as the level of social cohesion (as discussed in the previous chapter), to better understand how structural determinants affect opioid misuse across multiple disease pathways. Similarly, Currie and Schwandt argue that short- and long-term economic measures show only limited associations with opioid outcomes and are insufficient to explain the epidemic's scale [4]. While noting that economic decline appears to increase drug mortality, Ruhm observes that the relationship is significantly reduced (sometimes to zero) by controlling for confounding factors [5].

There are two key points to keep in mind about the econometric studies discussed below. First, most are panel studies (cross-section time series), which merge multiple longitudinal datasets from different sources. The data are analyzed using conventional quantitative methods, such as multivariate regression. Regression in the studies typically involves fixed effects. Fixed-effects models are applied to panel data to control for variables that do not vary across time, thus solely estimating effects for those variables that change across observations. Fixed effects offer advantages over cross-sectional analysis by limiting bias to time-varying variables that correlate with the treatment as well as with the outcome over time. Limitations include limited external validity, reverse causality, lack of suitability for estimating absolute group differences, and unobserved heterogeneity [6]. This type of statistical analysis cannot engender causal claims about relationships between variables but can indicate significant associations.

In a few studies, more robust methods are applied to assess drug policy impacts, typically quasi-experiments to account for confounding variables. As quasi-experiments, the studies rely on a difference-in-difference approach, which combines insights from cross-sectional treatment–control comparisons and before–after studies [7]. This approach is applied to estimate causal effect of an intervention by comparing changes in outcomes over time between the treatment group and the comparison group. It is used when randomization on the individual level is not possible. Still, because temporal and geographic contexts vary, it is not possible to completely isolate health impacts without conducting randomized, controlled experiments.

The second key point about most econometric research is that it concentrates on a time period marked by prescription opioid deaths rather than overdose fatalities from synthetic drugs, which occurred as the racial composition of fatalities transitioned from predominantly white to increasingly BIPOC. Thus, there is little analysis of how the economic factors influencing overdose risk may have changed over time, indicating a significant research gap [8].

As the crisis evolves, so too must econometric methods. The synthetic opioid era—with its rapid fluctuations in drug supply and shifting racial demographics—demands more adaptive models. Time-series analyses with finer temporal granularity, integration of qualitative inputs, and structural equation modeling may help capture the interplay between economic shocks, drug market volatility, and race-based policy impacts (Fig. 9.1). Furthermore, models that account for intersecting vulnerabilities such as race, geography, and health status can better predict where future harms may concentrate.

9.3 Labor Market Disruptions and Opioid Outcomes

Here, we turn to some key findings on opioid use and labor markets, keeping in mind the limitations of the research discussed previously. One strategy to separate out the effects of economic conditions on opioid-related overdose deaths (OODs) is to examine the intended and unintended impacts from specific types of economic shocks, such as unemployment, plant closures, and trade liberalization. The majority of studies show an association between OODs and these kinds of economic conditions. However, the evidence is not always robust (e.g., observable effects are minor), making it difficult to draw definitive conclusions.

Some studies have found a link between unemployment and increased opioid use, as well as opioid-related emergency department visits and/or fatalities [1, 9–14]. However, it is not clear from this work how short-term economic changes, like unemployment, are related to longer term fluctuations in the economy, which offer a more protracted span of time for socioeconomic decline to influence mortality [15]. Still, Hollingsworth, Ruhm and Simon determined that from 2002 to 2014,

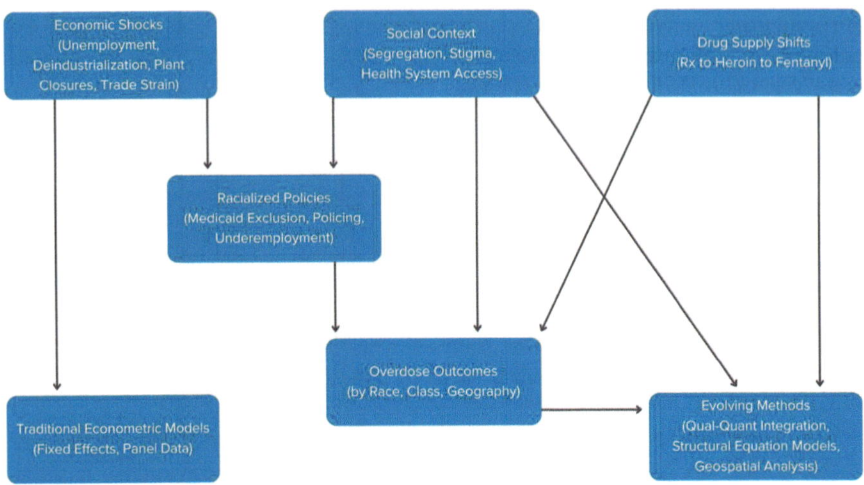

Fig. 9.1 This conceptual diagram illustrates how economic conditions, racialized social structures, drug supply transitions, and modeling approaches interact to shape opioid overdose risk. It highlights the limitations of conventional econometric methods and the need for more inclusive, context-aware approaches that integrate structural racism, geographic vulnerability, and the changing nature of drug supply

a one percentage point increase in the county unemployment rate predicted opioid fatalities by a statistically significant 0.19 per 100,000 (3.6%) [14]. Betz and Jones observed that job loss (and wage declines) in lower skilled industries were associated with higher opioid overdose mortality rates from 2001 to 2014 [11]. Using a quasi-experimental method, Carpenter, McClellan, and Rees found a significant relationship between substance use disorders involving analgesics (both opioid and non-opioid versions) and unemployment for 2002–2013, with robust effects concentrated in non-elderly adult white men with low levels of education [9].

However, other research reveals ambiguous results or an inverse relationship between unemployment and opioid-related harms. For example, Maclean, Horn, and Cantor showed a significant inverse association between heroin and admissions to substance abuse treatment in which a one percentage point increase in the state unemployment rate led to a 5.9% reduction in admissions [16].

Several studies have indicated a strong association between plant closures and increased opioid misuse and deaths. Most of the studies on plant closures and trade policy employ a quasi-experimental approach, lending greater rigor to their analysis. Each study discussed below detected an association between plant closings or (free) trade policies and a rise in opioid misuse and OOD [1, 10, 12, 13]. Examining data from 1999 to 2016, Venkataramani et al. found that in counties exposed to plant closures, mortality rates increased by 8.6 OODs per 100,000 individuals over 5 years, an 85% increase relative to the mortality rate before closure [1]. Pierce and Schott found that counties with greater exposure to Permanent Normal Trade Relations with China displayed relative increases in deaths of despair, including opioid fatalities, with the effects mainly observed in the white working-age population [13]. Declining manufacturing appears to negatively affect wages and labor force participation, which may be the mechanism through which plant closings and trade policies influence opioid misuse and death [12, 13].

There is some evidence that employment expansion increases the consumption of opioids because of increased rates of on-the-job injury [17, 18]. This finding complements the body of literature that has found that health and longevity improve during recessions and worsen during periods of economic expansion [19]. Metcalf and Wang determined that lower dependence on coal mining is associated with lower opioid death rates [17]. In particular, from 2010 to 2015, a 1% increase among the coal-producing counties in the share of coal miners in the workforce increased the opioid mortality rate by 0.192%. Metcalf and Wang posit that one possible reason for this finding is that increasing coal mining activity results in more workplace injuries and more opioid prescriptions leading to overdose deaths.

Musse proposed two potential pathways by which employment could influence opioid use [18]. First, as employment improves, workers may experience increased physical pain from on-the-job injuries, elevating demand for opioids. Second, better economic conditions could reduce workers' mental distress, reducing opioid consumption. To test these hypotheses, Musse analyzed the distinct effects of employment changes on opioid and over-the-counter (OTC) painkiller use, recognizing that OTC painkillers primarily target physical pain, not mental wellbeing. Musse found that a 1% increase in the employment-to-population ratio resulted in a 0.20% decrease in per-capita opioid demand and a 0.14% increase in per capita OTC painkiller demand [18]. Further analysis showed that the significant reduction in opioid use was largely driven by employment gains in low-injury-rate industries, while the increase in OTC painkiller use was primarily associated with high-injury-rate industries. Additionally, Musse examined the effect of a law to restrict opioid prescribing, calculating the substitution between opioids and OTC painkillers. Results indicated that a 1% increase in the employment-to-population ratio led to a 0.27% decrease in opioid use for substance abuse and to an increase of 0.08% in opioid use for physical pain [18].

The impact of opioid supply on labor force participation has been a subject of considerable research, focusing on the effects of policy changes and prescribing practices. Some of these factors include the reformulation of OxyContin and increases in practitioner prescribing. There is some evidence that the supply of prescription opioids in an area depresses labor force participation rates, although findings exhibit some variation. An examination of county data from state-level prescription drug monitoring programs found that a 10% increase in opioid prescriptions led to a 0.56% point reduction in labor force participation [20]. However, it is not clear if the reduction in labor force participation due to injuries was the reason for the increase in opioid prescriptions. Laird and Nielsen found that additional opioid prescribing was associated with a decreased labor force participation and income in Denmark [21]. Likewise, Savych et al. showed that long-term opioid prescribing expands the length of temporary disability episodes among individuals receiving Workers' Compensation benefits [22]. Again, is it the chicken or egg? Were workers receiving benefits because of injuries requiring long-term opioid prescribing, or was the prescribing a barrier to return to work? This is not clear from the studies.

In a review of five sets of state laws to control prescribing, Deiana and Giua observed an improvement in labor market participation as well as a rise in crime after implementation, suggesting that regulatory control of prescription drugs may come with undesirable outcomes [23]. In a slightly different approach, Park and Powell found reduced state-level labor market engagement and increased disability applications and enrollment for 2001–2015 after the reformulation of OxyContin induced transition from prescription opioids to illicit opioids [24]. Using county-level data from 2006 to 2014, Currie, Jin, and Schnell aimed to determine the direction of causality between per capita opioid prescription rates and employment-to-population ratios [2]. Specifically, they sought to understand whether opioid prescriptions influenced employment, or vice versa. They found a small, positive effect of opioid prescriptions on female employment-to-population ratios, implying that increased prescription rates might lead to a marginal increase in female employment. However, this effect was not observed for men. Conversely, when they analyzed the impact of employment-to-population ratios on opioid prescription rates, the results proved to be ambiguous, failing to establish a clear causal link.

9.4 Implications of Econometric Studies

Overall, studies examining the link between economic conditions and opioid-related issues offer mixed and nuanced results. The effects in studies often differ by population group and economic sector, suggesting a diversity of experience for populations touched by the opioid epidemic. Generally, more robust effects are found for white male workers in rural areas and/or those in manufacturing and resource extraction. Most of this research focuses on the prescription opioid period, potentially missing the evolving nature of the crisis, particularly the rise of synthetic opioids and their disproportionate impact on BIPOC communities. This highlights the complex interplay of economic and social factors at play.

Taken together, these findings suggest that while economic decline contributes to opioid misuse and mortality, it does so through complex, indirect pathways shaped by social context, policy choices, and health system infrastructure. Future research must examine how these relationships evolved in the era of fentanyl and rising BIPOC overdose mortality. In the end, econometric models can reveal patterns, but without integrating lived experience and social context, they risk flattening a crisis rooted in both economic despair and systemic neglect. The numbers tell us where the crisis spreads, but not how it feels. That requires listening, not just modeling.

Appendix A summarizes each econometric study, highlighting data sources, methods, foci and results.

References

1. Venkataramani AS, Bair EF, O'Brien RL, Tsai AC. Association between automotive assembly plant closures and opioid overdose mortality in the United States: a difference-in-differences analysis. JAMA Intern Med. 2020;180(2):254–62.
2. Currie J, Jin J, Schnell M. US employment and opioids: is there a connection? Res Labor Econ. 2019;47:253–80.
3. Maclean JC, Mallatt J, Ruhm CJ, Simon K. Economic studies on the opioid crisis: a review. NBER Working Paper No. 28067 [Internet]. Cambridge, MA: National Bureau of Economic Research; 2020 [cited 2025 July 15]. Available from: http://www.nber.org/papers/w28067.
4. Currie J, Schwandt H. The opioid epidemic was not caused by economic distress but by factors that could be more rapidly addressed. NBER Working Paper No. 27544 [Internet]. Cambridge, MA: National Bureau of Economic Research; 2020 [cited 2025 July 15]. Available from: http://www.nber.org/papers/w27544.
5. Ruhm CJ. Drivers of the fatal drug epidemic. J Health Econ. 2019;64:25–42.
6. Hill TD, Davis AP, Roos JM, French MT. Limitations of fixed-effects models for panel data. Sociol Perspect. 2020;63(3):357–69.
7. Lechner M. The estimation of causal effects by difference-in-difference methods. Found Trends Econom. 2011;4(3):165–224.
8. Cerdá M, Krawczyk N, Hamilton L, Rudolph KE, Friedman SR, Keyes KM. A critical review of the social and behavioral contributions to the overdose epidemic. Annu Rev Public Health. 2021;42:95–114.
9. Carpenter CS, McClellan CB, Rees DI. Economic conditions, illicit drug use, and substance use disorders in the United States. J Health Econ. 2017;52:63–73.
10. Autor DH, Dorn D, Hanson GH. The China syndrome: local labor market effects of import competition in the United States. Am Econ Rev. 2013;103(6):2121–68.
11. Betz MR, Jones LE. Wage and employment growth in America's drug epidemic: is all growth created equal? Am J Agric Econ. 2018;100(5):1357–74.
12. Charles KK, Hurst E, Schwartz M. The transformation of manufacturing and the decline in US employment. NBER Macroecon Annu. 2019;33(1):307–72.
13. Pierce JR, Schott PK. Trade liberalization and mortality: evidence from US counties. Am Econ Rev Insights. 2020;2(1):47–64.
14. Hollingsworth A, Ruhm CJ, Simon K. Macroeconomic conditions and opioid abuse. J Health Econ. 2017;56:222–33.
15. Becker T, Majmundar MK, Harris KM. The relationship between economic factors and mortality. In: National Academies of sciences, engineering, and medicine, committee on population. High and rising mortality rates among working-age adults. Washington (DC): National Academies Press (US); 2021.
16. Maclean JC, Horn BP, Cantor JH. Business cycles and admissions to substance abuse treatment. Contemp Econ Policy. 2020;38(1):139–54.
17. Metcalf GE, Wang Q. Abandoned by coal, swallowed by opioids? (no. w26551). Cambridge, MA: National Bureau of Economic Research; 2019.
18. Musse I. Employment shocks and demand for pain medication. 2020. Available from: https://ssrn.com/abstract=3646543.
19. Ruhm CJ. Are recessions good for your health? Q J Econ. 2000;115(2):617–50.
20. Harris MC, Kessler LM, Murray MN, Glenn B. Prescription opioids and labor market pains: the effect of schedule II opioids on labor force participation and unemployment. J Hum Resour. 2020;55(4):1319–64.
21. Laird J, Nielsen T. The effects of physician prescribing behaviors on prescription drug use and labor supply: evidence from movers in Denmark [Job Market Paper]; 2016. Available from: https://scholar.harvard.edu/files/lairdja/files/Laird_JMP.pdf, https://scholar.harvard.edu/files/lairdja/files/Laird_JMP.pdf.

22. Savych B, Neumark D, Lea R. The impact of opioid prescriptions on duration of temporary disability. Cambridge, MA: Workers Compensation Research Institute; 2018. Report No.: WC-18-18. Available from: https://www.wcrinet.org/reports/the-impact-of-opioid-prescriptions-on-duration-of-temporary-disability.
23. Deiana C, Giua L. The US opidemic: prescription opioids, labour market conditions and crime. Munich: University Library of Munich; 2018. MPRA Paper 85712.
24. Park S, Powell D. Is the rise in illicit opioids affecting labor supply and disability claiming rates? Cambridge, MA: National Bureau of Economic Research; 2020. Working Paper 27804. Available from: http://www.nber.org/papers/w27804.

Place-Based and Contextual Factors 10

The ability to see the world from another's point of view is essential to justice.

—Martha C. Nussbaum (Frontiers of Justice, Harvard University Press, 2006)

10.1 Introduction

The opioid crisis, initially understood as a singular national issue, is increasingly recognized as a collection of distinct sub-epidemics shaped by geographic and contextual factors. This chapter explores how place (rural vs. urban settings) influences patterns of opioid use disorder (OUD) and opioid-related overdose deaths (OOD). Rural areas often see prescription opioid misuse among younger, white males, linked to chronic pain from manual labor and limited access to health care and treatment. Urban environments, conversely, experience a greater diversity of substances, including illicit opioids, affecting older, more racially and ethnically diverse populations, and present barriers to care, despite often having more robust overall healthcare infrastructures.

Spatial analysis[1]—a set of methods used to examine patterns, relationships, and trends across physical space—reveals uneven distributions of OUD and OOD in the United States, with varying correlations to socioeconomic indicators. While

[1] *Spatial analysis* refers to a set of methods used to examine patterns, relationships, and trends across physical space. In public health and social science, spatial analysis helps researchers understand how geographic factors—such as location, proximity, and distribution—affect outcomes like disease rates, healthcare access, or environmental exposure. In the context of the opioid crisis, spatial analysis is used to identify geographic hotspots for overdose deaths, examine how socioeconomic conditions (e.g., poverty and unemployment) cluster in certain areas, and understand how factors like rural isolation or urban segregation shape vulnerability to addiction and barriers to treatment. For example, a spatial analysis might show that overdose rates are highest in counties with high job loss and limited treatment facilities—revealing place-based disparities that are invisible in aggregate national data.

L. R. Webster, S. Eichberg, *Deconstructing Toxic Narratives*,
https://doi.org/10.1007/978-3-032-23135-2_10

economic disadvantage is a common thread, its impact differs regionally, suggesting mediating factors like social cohesion. The emergence of polysubstance use further complicates the landscape. Understanding these localized dynamics is crucial for developing targeted, effective interventions that acknowledge the multifaceted nature of the crisis beyond a single narrative.

10.2 Rural Versus Urban Differences

Over the past 20–25 years, place has become a prominent topic in health outcomes research. Although initial research focused on drug use in urban environments, the explosion of OOD and other deaths of despair in rural communities drew attention to this new setting [1–4]. An emerging question in the literature asks: to what degree do supply and demand factors drive geographic differences in drug mortality rates?

Spatial analysis helps to address these concerns by exploring the relative contribution of supply- and demand-side factors across different geographic scales and by identifying spatial determinants of the uneven distribution of social and health inequalities [5]. These include structural factors and the unequal distribution of individuals in geographic space [6]. As opposed to large national studies, which tend to obscure geographic diversity in drug-related behavior, spatial analysis of rural health highlights regional variation in OUD and OOD [7]. However, definitions and measurement parameters (e.g., how is rural or urban measured? What is the spatial unit of analysis?) differ across studies, resulting in patterns that are not always consistent. Even when spatial patterns are clear, questions remain about the specific risk factors and pathways shaping regional drug use patterns and the social groups most vulnerable to addiction.

What begins to emerge is the realization that where one lives matters when it comes to the opioid crisis. While the crisis affects both rural and urban areas, the specific challenges and patterns of substance misuse differ, as the context of place shapes the experience. There are important differences in risk factors for OUD and OOD between rural and urban settings [8]. People who misuse opioids (PWMO) in rural locations are more likely to misuse prescription opioids rather than heroin, in contrast to PWMO residing in urban settings [9–11].

In rural areas, substance misuse occurs most often among young, white males with lower educational attainment [12]. Chronic pain and injury are more common in rural than in urban places, due, in part, to greater prevalence of manual and injury-prone jobs [13, 14]. Thus, in rural areas, prescription opioid misuse has been more prevalent. Rural communities often have more limited access to health care, including primary and emergency health facilities and drug prevention, detoxification, and treatment programs [15, 16]. Medication-assisted treatments, such as buprenorphine and methadone, are scarce in rural settings: 90.4% of physicians who are authorized to prescribe buprenorphine are located in urban areas compared to just 1.3% in rural locations [17]. Harm reduction interventions are also less prevalent in rural environments [18]. Hospitals, clinics, and drug treatment specialists are dispersed across large geographic areas, making it harder for PWMO to access these services and eliminating a possible buffer against overdose [19]. And finally, with limited primary healthcare options, rural residents rely on emergency departments more often, where doctors are more likely to prescribe opioids [20, 21].

By contrast, in urban locations, people who misuse substances are older and more racially and ethnically diverse. Urban and rural environments differ also in the onset of substance misuse. One study found that rural drug users initiate drug use at earlier ages using oxycodone, hydrocodone, benzodiazepines, cocaine, and crack. Urban drug users are more likely to have recently used crack. They also have higher odds of lifetime and recent use of methadone, OxyContin, oxycodone, cocaine, and crack [22]. Another study found that urban residents had earlier first regular use of methamphetamine and earlier presentation for treatment [23].

Therefore, urban areas tend to see a broader range of substances, including heroin, synthetic opioids, and street drug combinations, concentrated among an older and more racially and ethnically diverse population compared to rural counterparts. While urban areas may have more readily available healthcare facilities, access can still be an issue due to factors like cost, insurance coverage, and social stigma.

10.3 Spatial Literature Insights

An evolving literature details spatial and spatiotemporal trends in opioid misuse and overdose mortality. This body of work, building on econometric studies that emphasize regional factors (as discussed in the previous chapter), reveals distinct regional disparities. The studies highlighted below demonstrate a progression toward greater analytical complexity, culminating in an exploration of how specific types of drug use and mortality rates vary by place. These studies primarily use panel data—collected from the same subjects (such as counties or individuals) at multiple points in time—to investigate the spatial distribution of opioid use and mortality over time, while controlling for unobserved differences across subjects. Data analysis techniques include spatial analysis or geographic information science combined with statistical inference through spatial statistics and spatial regression models that account for geographic relationships between data points, adjusting for the fact that nearby areas often influence each other. These methods aim to identify factors driving disease distribution and opioid-related harm, but they cannot establish causal relationships.

In general, opioid misuse and overdose mortality are spread unevenly across vast sections of the country. Mortality rates for prescription opioids are high in rural Appalachia, New England, the Midwest, and the Mountain West, but are comparatively low in other rural areas, such as the Delta South and Great Plains (Fig. 10.1) [24–26]. Deaths involving illicit synthetic opioids and street mixtures are increasingly prevalent in more racially diverse urban areas [5, 27, 28]. While deaths involving synthetic opioids were originally concentrated on the East Coast and other eastern regions, the COVID-19 pandemic heightened these fatalities in most states, although the magnitude varies [29].

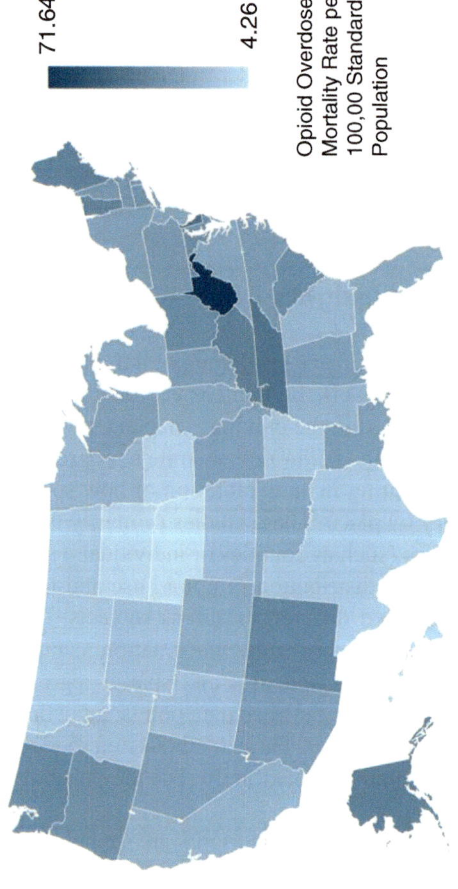

Fig. 10.1 Rates are age-adjusted and per 100,000 standard population. Drug overdose deaths were identified using International Classification of Diseases, Tenth Revision underlying cause-of-death codes X40–X44, X60–X64, X85, and Y10–Y14. (Source: Centers for Disease Control and Prevention, National Center for Health Statistics via CDC WONDER Database)

Spatial epidemiology research examining the distribution of OOD and OUD aims to determine how social and economic indicators relate to opioid prevalence measures across different geographic locations. Commonly, counties or ZIP codes serve as the units of analysis. Several studies indicate that higher rates of opioid use and mortality are concentrated in economically disadvantaged areas across the urban–rural continuum [25, 30, 31]. However, this pattern is not universally observed. For instance, Ghertner and Groves found that while higher rates of hospitalization and OOD were concentrated in economically distressed counties in specific rural regions, these effects were not consistent across other economically distressed areas, suggesting that some locations may have protective factors against the opioid epidemic [25]. Wilkes et al. found that opioid-related hospital inpatient stays and emergency department visits in the northwestern United States seemed to decrease with increasing rurality; however, this trend was not seen in other geographic regions of the country [24].

What to make of these (and other) anomalous findings?

In Mingo County, West Virginia—once a coal-mining stronghold—communities saw opioid prescription rates skyrocket as jobs disappeared, and poverty deepened. Even churches stepped in as informal support networks. The human toll was staggering, overdose death rates surpassed 52 per 100,000 residents, more than ten times the national average, in a county flooded with prescription pain pills [32].

In addition to potential discrepancies in methodology or timeframe, other variables—such as social cohesion or collective trauma—may be mediating the relationship between socioeconomic indicators and substance use measures, contributing to regional variation [25]. Identifying which variables take on moderating roles within different spatial contexts and socioeconomic conditions is vital for producing more robust research in the field.

The strength of relationships between variables may also depend on which socioeconomic indicators or drug classes are considered in spatial and statistical analysis. In a ZIP code-level study, Pear et al. found a positive relationship between prescription opioid overdoses and rates of poverty and lower educational attainment levels (less than high school), regardless of a place's urbanicity [31]. However, the same study revealed that heroin overdose is correlated with low educational attainment only in rural areas.

A related strand of research focuses on identifying the specific types of opioids or drug classes that cluster in different geographic areas. These studies examine the relationship between opioid-related metrics and factors like population density, economic conditions, and labor market characteristics. Over a roughly 20-year period, these studies document an increase in drug deaths [5, 27, 28]. Notably, deaths from illicit opioids have risen sharply, especially in large urban areas. However, increases in prescription opioid deaths have also been observed in counties with smaller cities and in rural areas (where deaths from methamphetamines were also common) [27].

10.4 Mapping the Opioid Sub-Epidemics

Overall, the findings support the idea that the opioid epidemic is not a single phenomenon but rather a collection of "sub-epidemics," as proposed by Jalal et al. and mentioned at the start of this book [33]. These sub-epidemics vary over time by drug combinations, social groups affected, and geographic location. Addressing this complex situation will require innovative policy solutions that move beyond previous approaches.

Among these findings, Monnat et al. identified six "opioid mortality classes" reflecting low-to-high mortality levels and growth rates from 2002–2004 to 2014–2016, based on four types of opioids: prescription opioids, synthetic opioids, heroin, and all opioid combinations, called a syndemic [5]. A syndemic occurs when two or more health problems interact in ways that worsen their effects in social, temporal, or geographic contexts, especially under conditions of social inequality [34]. The study found that higher overall drug mortality rates existed in counties characterized by greater economic disadvantage, more blue-collar and service employment, and higher opioid prescription rates. Yet, each of the six mortality classes exhibited unique demographic characteristics and opioid-prevalence patterns. For example, high rates of prescription opioid overdoses were clustered in economically distressed counties with a history of agricultural or manufacturing employment, now dominated by the service sector.

Examining county-level data for the periods 2002–2004, 2008–2012, and 2014–2016, Peters et al. identified three distinct epidemics (prescription opioids, heroin, and prescription-synthetic opioid mixtures) and one syndemic involving all opioids [28]. Again, each sub-epidemic and the syndemic was linked to distinct economic and population characteristics. Heroin sub-epidemic and opioid syndemic counties were more urban, economically advantaged, and racially diverse. Prescription opioid epidemic counties were less populated, whiter, had a history of drug misuse, and were former agricultural and manufacturing communities, aligning with Case and Deaton's "deaths of despair" scenario.

Table 10.1 and Fig. 10.2 summarize the key characteristics associated with each identified opioid epidemic and the overall syndemic, as described by Peters et al.

Table 10.1 Characteristics of opioid epidemics and syndemic

Epidemic type	Population type	Race/ Demographics	Economic characteristics	Historical context
Prescription opioids	Rural, less populated	Majority white	Economically disadvantaged	Former agricultural, manufacturing
Heroin	Urban, more populated	Racially diverse	Economically advantaged	Not specified
Prescription-Synthetic Mixture	Mixed	Mixed	Varied	Mixed
Opioid Syndemic	Urban, more populated	Racially diverse	Economically advantaged	Not specified

Source: Adapted from concepts presented in Peters et al. [28]

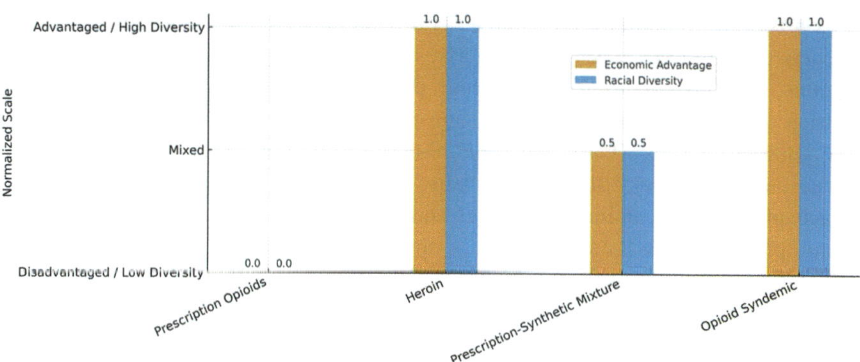

Fig. 10.2 This bar chart presents a simplified, visual comparison of the relative economic advantage and racial diversity associated with each major opioid epidemic type, based on Peters et al.'s county-level analysis. Numeric labels indicate the normalized scale (0 = disadvantaged/low diversity, 0.5 = mixed, 1 = advantaged/high diversity). For example, counties experiencing the prescription opioid epidemic tend to be rural, economically disadvantaged, and majority white, while those with heroin and opioid syndemics are more urban, economically advantaged, and racially diverse. This visualization clarifies the socio-demographic distinctions across sub-epidemics that are often obscured by national-level narratives. Graph: Economic and Demographic Context by Opioid Epidemic Type. (Source: Peters et al. [28])

[28]. Each epidemic shows distinct geographic, racial, economic, and historical patterns, reflecting the multifaceted nature of the crisis.

Hochstetler and Peters expanded prior research by analyzing the spatial distribution of the emerging polysubstance drug problem [5, 27, 28]. Counties were categorized by syndemic composition, and their geographic location was predicted using 2000–2002 and 2017–2019 mortality rates, including all deaths with a drug as a contributing cause rather than just overdoses (drug poisonings). The analysis identified seven classes of drug mortality clusters or sub-epidemics, each distinguished by geography, population, and labor market characteristics [27]. In general, the findings supported insights from the authors' previous articles while providing more detail of current sub-epidemics, including the following:

- A *polysubstance* problem that includes prescription and illicit opioids, heroin, sedatives, methamphetamine, antidepressants, and hallucinogens in places that were home to the prescription opioid problem in prior decades. The affected areas are located along the Ohio River in Kentucky, Ohio, and West Virginia, the Great Lakes, the Northeast, and New Mexico. The communities are characterized by high poverty, unemployment, prescription dispensing, and disability rates, above-average mining employment, and low percentages employed in manufacturing industries. These areas are somewhat more urban and less remote than places still experiencing a prescription opioid problem, which has allowed the communities to easily transition to heroin, synthetic opioids, and other illicit drugs [27].

- A *prescription opioid* (and sedatives) problem clustered in predominantly white rural communities with high poverty, unemployment, prescription dispensing rates, and disability claims, and a high percentage of jobs in injury-prone industries, such as agriculture, mining, and manufacturing [5, 27, 28]. Again, these communities typify Case and Deaton's notion of "deaths of despair." Possible reasons why prescription opioid misuse endures in these places may be cultural acceptance of medicinal painkillers and disapproval of illicit drugs, as well as comparatively lax state regulation of pharmaceutical opioids. Prior to increased scrutiny in the 2010s, few safeguards or guidelines were in place to monitor opioid prescribing patterns, dosage amounts, or the appropriateness of prescriptions for certain conditions. This lack of oversight, which appropriately resides with state medical boards rather than through Drug Enforcement Administration (DEA) enforcement or federal restrictions, contributed to the widespread availability of prescription opioids in some communities, particularly those with high rates of workplace injuries and chronic pain.
- An *illicit opioid* (and cocaine) problem clustered in urban areas, which are less remote and have more professionals, fewer injury-prone jobs, low prescription dispensing rates, and more racial and ethnic minorities. The opioid problem in these metropolitan settings affects a small, underserved, and disadvantaged Black subpopulation rather than the entire population [5, 27, 28]. These are the kinds of substances and communities typically associated with narratives about drug use and illegal drug trafficking.
- A *methamphetamine* problem in West Virginia, Oklahoma, and the Southwestern states in communities that are rural and remote, have high rates of disability, greater racial diversity, specifically "other" (e.g., Asian, Native American, and Pacific Islander) or multiple races, and are positioned near Native American reservations. Reasons why prescription opioids play a minor role in these areas may be low dispensing rates and a lack of pharmacies in remote areas. Geographic isolation may also help to explain why illicit opioids do not have a major presence, as drug traffickers have been hindered from making significant inroads [27].

Appendix B summarizes each spatial analysis study, highlighting data sources, methods, foci, and results.

10.5 Policy and Research Implications

The findings presented here highlight several crucial implications for both policy development and future research. First, the recognition of distinct "sub-epidemics" underscores the need for region-specific, tailored interventions rather than a one-size-fits-all national strategy. For instance, rural communities grappling with prescription opioid and polysubstance issues require enhanced access to specialized medication-assisted treatments and comprehensive harm reduction services, given their current scarcity. In contrast, urban areas facing illicit opioid and polysubstance challenges may benefit from different approaches that address factors like racial disparities, housing instability, and targeted outreach to vulnerable, underserved populations, particularly within the Black community. Policymakers should allocate resources and design programs with these unique geographical and demographic contexts in mind.

Second, the evolving nature of the opioid crisis, particularly the rise of synthetic opioids like fentanyl, demands that treatment protocols and public health campaigns be continuously updated. The traditional focus on OUD alone is insufficient when polysubstance misuse becomes increasingly widespread. Healthcare systems, especially in rural areas, must be equipped to handle complex polysubstance use, integrating care for multiple substance dependencies and co-occurring mental health conditions. There are significant barriers to opioid treatment in rural areas, and the addition of polysubstance misuse compounds pre-existing service gaps [35].

Finally, future research should continue to employ spatial analysis and mixed-methods approaches to identify the mediating roles of social cohesion, collective trauma, and other contextual variables in shaping regional drug use patterns. There is a particular need to explore how the relationships between economic conditions and opioid-related harms are evolving in the current fentanyl era, and how these shifts disproportionately affect Black, Indigenous, and People of Color (BIPOC) communities, whose experiences have been less thoroughly examined in the earlier research primarily focused on prescription opioid deaths. Understanding these nuances will be critical for developing equitable and effective responses to the ongoing crisis.

However, no discussion of spatial trends is complete without addressing a critical omission in early research. Despite the spatial and contextual sophistication of many recent studies, research on the opioid crisis has too often treated BIPOC communities as statistical afterthoughts. Much of the early scholarship focused on predominantly white rural areas and post-industrial towns, reinforcing the false narrative that the crisis is primarily a "white problem." This limited framing has contributed to a racialized policy response—public health for some, criminalization for others.

Yet, overdose mortality has surged among Black and Native American populations in recent years, often outpacing that of white populations. In many urban settings, long-standing structural inequities—underinvestment in health care, discriminatory policing, residential segregation, and disproportionate exposure to trauma—have heightened vulnerability to substance use and fatal overdose. Native communities face unique barriers including geographic isolation, historical trauma, and chronically underfunded Indian Health Services.

Place-based research must do more than map rural decline; it must interrogate how structural and environmental factors shape the geography of risk. This includes examining surveillance and access gaps in harm reduction, medication-assisted treatment, and culturally competent care. Moreover, BIPOC communities are often left out of localized interventions and research designs, perpetuating cycles of exclusion and inadequate response. Taken together, these studies make clear that opioid use and overdose deaths are not evenly distributed across space or time, and they are certainly not the result of a singular, homogeneous crisis. Instead, the data reveal a patchwork of overlapping sub-epidemics, each shaped by geography, economic precarity, industry-specific injury patterns, racial inequality, and uneven access to care. These spatial insights dismantle the dominant narrative that the opioid crisis can be traced to a singular villain or a simple failure of medical ethics. Instead, they compel us to recognize how structural, historical, and place-based forces shape vulnerability and drug-related harm. Geography doesn't just describe where people live. It helps explain why despair takes root there. Any serious solution must be as nuanced as the problem itself.

References

1. Cooper HL, Tempalski B. Integrating place into research on drug use, drug users' health, and drug policy. Int J Drug Policy. 2014;25(3):503–7.
2. Cooper HL, Des Jarlais DC, Tempalski B, Bossak BH, Ross Z, Friedman SR. Drug-related arrest rates and spatial access to syringe exchange programs in New York City health districts: combined effects on the risk of injection-related infections among injectors. Health Place. 2012;18(2):218–28.
3. Knight KR, Lopez AM, Comfort M, Shumway M, Cohen J, Riley ED. Single room occupancy (SRO) hotels as mental health risk environments among impoverished women: the intersection of policy, drug use, trauma, and urban space. Int J Drug Policy. 2014;25(3):556–61.
4. Strathdee SA, Hallett TB, Bobrova N, Rhodes T, Booth R, Abdool R, et al. HIV and risk environment for injecting drug users: the past, present, and future. Lancet. 2010;376(9737):268–84.
5. Monnat SM, Peters DJ, Berg MT, Hochstetler A. Using census data to understand county-level differences in overall drug mortality and opioid-related mortality by opioid type. Am J Public Health. 2019;109(8):1084–91.
6. Lobao LM, Hooks G, Tickamyer AR. Introduction: advancing the sociology of spatial inequality. In: Lobao LM, Hooks G, Tickamyer AR, editors. The sociology of spatial inequality. Albany: State University of New York Press; 2007. p. 1–25.
7. Buchanich JM, Balmert LC, Pringle JL, Williams KE, Burke DS, Marsh GM. Patterns and trends in accidental poisoning death rates in the US, 1979-2014. Prev Med. 2016;89:317–23.
8. Keyes KM, Cerdá M, Brady JE, Havens JR, Galea S. Understanding the rural-urban differences in nonmedical prescription opioid use and abuse in the United States. Am J Public Health. 2014;104(2):e52–9.
9. Cicero TJ, Surratt H, Inciardi JA, Munoz A. Relationship between therapeutic use and abuse of opioid analgesics in rural, suburban, and urban locations in the United States. Pharmacoepidemiol Drug Saf. 2007;16(8):827–40.
10. Rigg KK, Monnat SM. Urban vs. rural differences in prescription opioid misuse among adults in the United States: informing region specific drug policies and interventions. Int J Drug Policy. 2015;26(5):484–91.
11. Wang KH, Fiellin DA, Becker WC. Source of prescription drugs used nonmedically in rural and urban populations. Am J Drug Alcohol Abuse. 2014;40(4):292–303.
12. Schalkoff CA, Richard EL, Piscalko HM, Sibley AL, Brook DL, Lancaster KE, et al. "Now We Are Seeing the Tides Wash In": trauma and the opioid epidemic in rural Appalachian Ohio. Subst Use Misuse. 2021;56(5):650–9.
13. Hoffman PK, Meier BP, Council JR. A comparison of chronic pain between an urban and rural population. J Community Health Nurs. 2002;19(4):213–24.
14. McGranahan DA. How people make a living in rural America. In: Brown DL, Swanson LE, editors. Challenges for rural America in the twenty-first century. University Park: Penn State University Press; 2003. p. 135–51.

15. Heil SH, Sigmon SC, Jones HE, Wagner M. Comparison of characteristics of opioid-using pregnant women in rural and urban settings. Am J Drug Alcohol Abuse. 2008;34(4):463–71.
16. Paulozzi LJ, Xi Y. Recent changes in drug poisoning mortality in the United States by urban-rural status and by drug type. Pharmacoepidemiol Drug Saf. 2008;17(10):997–1005.
17. Rosenblatt RA, Andrilla CH, Catlin M, Larson EH. Geographic and specialty distribution of US physicians trained to treat opioid use disorder. Ann Fam Med. 2015;13(1):23–6.
18. Taylor M. Few needle exchanges in small towns, suburbs hit by surge in heroin use. Al Jazeera [Internet]. 2015 Dec [cited 2024 Jul 16]. Available from: http://america.aljazeera.com/articles/2015/12/10/needle-exchanges-lacking-in-suburban-rural-areas.html.
19. Benavides-Vaello S, Strode A, Sheeran BC. Using technology in the delivery of mental health and substance abuse treatment in rural communities: a review. J Behav Health Serv Res. 2013;40(1):111–20.
20. Haggerty JL, Roberge D, Lévesque JF, Gauthier J, Loignon C. An exploration of rural-urban differences in healthcare-seeking trajectories: implications for measures of accessibility. Health Place. 2014;28:92–8.
21. Hoppe JA, Nelson LS, Perrone J, Weiner SG. Opioid prescribing in a cross section of US emergency departments. Ann Emerg Med. 2015;66(3):253–9.e1.
22. Young AM, Havens JR, Leukefeld CG. A comparison of rural and urban nonmedical prescription opioid users' lifetime and recent drug use. Am J Drug Alcohol Abuse. 2012;38(3):220–7.
23. Grant KM, Kelley SS, Agrawal S, Meza JL, Meyer JR, Romberger DJ. Methamphetamine use in rural Midwesterners. Am J Addict. 2007;16(2):79–84.
24. Wilkes JL, Montalban JN, Pringle BD, Monroe D, Miller A, Zapata I, et al. A demographic and regional comparison of opioid-related hospital visits within community type in the United States. J Clin Med. 2021;10(16)
25. Ghertner R, Groves L. The opioid crisis and economic opportunity: geographic and economic trends. ASPE Res Brief. 2018:1–22.
26. Rigg KK, Monnat SM, Chavez MN. Opioid-related mortality in rural America: geographic heterogeneity and intervention strategies. Int J Drug Policy. 2018;57:119–29.
27. Hochstetler A, Peters DJ. Geography of poly-substance drug mortality. J Crim Just. 2023;86:102044.
28. Peters DJ, Monnat SM, Hochstetler AL, Berg MT. The opioid hydra: understanding overdose mortality epidemics and syndemics across the rural-urban continuum. Rural Sociol. 2020;85(3):589–622.
29. Brown KG, Chen CY, Dong D, Lake KJ, Butelman ER. Has the United States reached a plateau in overdoses caused by synthetic opioids after the onset of the COVID-19 pandemic? Examination of Centers for Disease Control and Prevention Data to November 2021. Front Psych. 2022;13:947603.
30. Monnat SM. The contributions of socioeconomic and opioid supply factors to U.S. drug mortality rates: urban-rural and within-rural differences. J Rural Stud. 2019;68:319–35.
31. Pear VA, Ponicki WR, Gaidus A, Keyes KM, Martins SS, Fink DS, et al. Urban-rural variation in the socioeconomic determinants of opioid overdose. Drug Alcohol Depend. 2019;195:66–73.
32. Horwitz S, Rich S, Higham S. Opioid death rates soared in communities where pain pills flowed. The Washington Post; 2019.
33. Jalal H, Buchanich JM, Roberts MS, Balmert LC, Zhang K, Burke DS. Changing dynamics of the drug overdose epidemic in the United States from 1979 through 2016. Science. 2018;361(6408)
34. Singer M, Clair S. Syndemics and public health: reconceptualizing disease in bio-social context. Med Anthropol Q. 2003;17(4):423–41.
35. Jenkins RA. The fourth wave of the US opioid epidemic and its implications for the rural US: a federal perspective. Prev Med. 2021;152(Pt 2):106541.

11 Errors in Fentanyl and Media Reporting

It isn't what we don't know that gives us trouble; it's what we know that ain't so.

—Will Rogers (The Wit and Wisdom of Will Rogers, Dover Publications)

11.1 Introduction

Official reporting on opioid-related overdose deaths (OODs), particularly involving fentanyl, has been critically flawed with devastating consequences. The years-long narrative of a prescription opioid crisis largely driven by overprescribing was incomplete, even misleading, giving rise to misdirected efforts that ultimately failed to address the true nature of the evolving crisis.

The Centers for Disease Control and Prevention (CDC), the primary data source for OODs, inflated prescription opioid death counts for nearly a decade due to an outdated coding method. While the CDC adjusted its calculations in 2015, revealing that prescription opioid deaths remained stable as synthetic opioid fatalities surged, the initial narrative was already deeply ingrained. Critics suggest the CDC may have been aware of these issues much earlier. Media outlets amplified these inaccuracies, prioritizing engagement and emotional resonance over factual precision, ultimately shaping public perception and policy while overshadowing accurate data.

11.2 Official Misreporting on Fentanyl and Other Opioid Overdose Deaths

As this book has repeatedly stressed (and shown with empirical evidence), the opioid crisis is at a stage where the predominant public health dilemma has shifted from prescription opioid use to synthetic opioid and increasing polysubstance use.

L. R. Webster, S. Eichberg, *Deconstructing Toxic Narratives*,
https://doi.org/10.1007/978-3-032-23135-2_11

Official statistics have lagged in reflecting this crucial transition, leading to misinterpretations and misdirected public health efforts.

The CDC has several limitations in the methods of reporting overdose fatalities, particularly fentanyl deaths, as already discussed in this book. In 2018, four analysts at the CDC published an editorial in the *American Journal of Public Health,* acknowledging that the agency had inflated counts of prescription opioid deaths for nearly a decade [1]. They blamed the error on the long-time CDC coding method for calculating underlying causes of OOD. Under the *International Classification of Diseases (ICD)* program, only heroin, methadone, and opium were given individual program codes. Other opioids were classified under just two codes: In the case of prescription opioid overdose deaths, estimates were traditionally obtained by adding together T40.4, *Synthetic Opioid Analgesics Other than Methadone;* T40.2, *Natural and Semi-synthetic Opioids*; and T40.3, *Methadone* (Table 11.1) [1]. By grouping various opioids together, the coding system made it difficult to distinguish deaths caused by prescription opioids from those involving illicitly manufactured synthetic opioids like fentanyl.

According to the CDC analysts, it was not until 2015 that the CDC noticed an unusually high number of overdose deaths involving illicitly manufactured synthetic opioids. After recognizing the error, the agency addressed *ICD* limitations by adopting a more "conservative" approach that tabulated deaths involving synthetic opioids separately from estimates for prescription opioid deaths. Using this conservative method, the newly tabulated number of prescription opioid deaths reported in 2016 fell from 32,445 to 17,087, a 47.3% decline. This change can be seen retroactively, in that 2015 numbers dropped from 22,598 to 15,281, and in 2014, they declined from 18,893 to 14,838, around the same amount originally (and erroneously) reported for prescription opioid overdoses in 2007.

What the adjustment in calculations exposed was that death rates involving prescription (natural and semi-synthetic) opioids stayed relatively stable (unchanged) from 2009 to 2016 (with an annual change of 3.4%), while deaths from synthetic opioids markedly increased from 2013 to 2016 [1].[1] By this time, however, the

Table 11.1 Drugs and International Classification of Diseases-10 codes

Drug category	ICD-10 code	Drugs
Natural and semi-synthetic analgesics	T40.2	Oxycodone, Hydrocodone, Hydromorphone
Methadone	T40.3	Methadone
Synthetic opioid analgesics, excluding methadone	T40.4	Fentanyl, Meperidine
Heroin	T40.1	Heroin
Cocaine	T40.5	Cocaine

Source: CDC

[1] This correction may also have produced an undercount of deaths from synthetic opioid analgesics (e.g., meperidine, pentazocine, propoxyphene, tapentadol, buprenorphine, and tramadol) coded under T40.4 that were removed from the prescription opioid overdose death tally.

national narrative that the opioid crisis was a prescription opioid crisis was embedded in the psyche of the media and most Americans.

Despite the CDC's claim that they only noticed the high proportion of illegally manufactured fentanyl deaths in 2015, it is possible that the agency was aware of this problem a decade earlier. Critics, such as Peppin and Coleman, point as proof to a 2008 CDC report that documented an outbreak of illicitly manufactured fentanyl-related deaths between April 2005 and March 2007 that was responsible for the deaths of 1013 people [2]. Such evidence suggests that the CDC could have corrected its reporting methods sooner than it did.

The CDC's traditional coding system also struggles to differentiate between licit and illicit forms of other controlled substances. Following its recognition of the fentanyl problem, the CDC again scrutinized their data and discovered similar single-code classification problems for benzodiazepines, cocaine, and methadone, which have licit and illicit forms. For example, methadone, which has dual indications for treating pain and treating opioid use disorder (OUD), is mainly administered at narcotic treatment facilities for OUD. Staff at these facilities are authorized to dispense methadone but prohibited by federal law from prescribing it. Despite this, even now, the CDC codes all methadone-related overdose deaths as pain-related, raising doubts about the integrity of the data; as of 2017, the volume of methadone prescribed to treat OUD was more than four-fold the volume prescribed for pain [2]. Moreover, the agency has not fully remedied the original coding issue, namely the difficulty distinguishing between licit and illicit fentanyl. While the CDC has established an enhanced data collection program to obtain more detailed mortality data, fewer than half of US states participate, limiting the accuracy of current reporting [2]. Moreover, the current *ICD*-based system remains inadequate for capturing racial and ethnic disparities in opioid-related mortality. Without consistent, disaggregated data, the full burden of fentanyl-related deaths in historically marginalized communities remains underrecognized.

The consequences of the CDC's miscalculations have been tremendous. For 10 years, the agency's inaccurate estimates were taken as fact by federal and state governments and relied upon to inform public policy. The CDC's controversial *Guideline for Prescribing Opioids for Chronic Pain,* issued in 2016, profoundly altered the practice of pain management in the United States, encouraging strict rules on how and when physicians could prescribe opioids for pain [3]. The heavy restrictions sometimes came with unintended consequences, such as forced tapers and pushing patients toward the illicit market [4–6].

The general fuzziness in the way the CDC reported deaths also shaped public perception. Inaccurate reporting found its way into mainstream media reports, which were nearly always skewed toward overstating the role of prescribed opioids.

11.3 News Media Misrepresentation of Prescription Opioids

The media played a central role in cementing the perception that the volume of prescription opioids issued was the primary driver of the overdose crisis, often drawing from and amplifying flawed or outdated data. Several high-profile examples illustrate how this narrative gained traction and persisted, even as the actual causes of opioid-related mortality shifted. There are good reasons why this happened.

In *Nexus*, published in 2024, Yuval Noah Harari argues that in today's information environment, accuracy is no longer the principal standard by which information is judged [7]. Instead, information is valued for its ability to attract attention, affirm group identity, and generate emotional impact. "The question is no longer 'Is it true?' but 'Does it spread?'" Harari observes, pointing to a fundamental shift away from truth-seeking toward virality. Stories that are emotionally resonant, morally straightforward, and aligned with institutional or ideological interests are more likely to gain traction, regardless of their factual accuracy. In such an environment, what Harari describes as "engagement-first" storytelling becomes the norm: media narratives succeed not because they are nuanced or empirically grounded, but because they are simple, shareable, and symbolically powerful. This helps explain why the media so strongly embraced a narrative in which prescription opioids, and the physicians and companies linked to them, were cast as the central villains of the overdose crisis. The story was not just easy to tell; it was easy to believe, quick to spread, and emotionally satisfying.

Media outlets like *Time*, *60 Minutes*, *The Washington Post*, and *The New York Times* amplified these narratives, not necessarily because they reflected the evolving epidemiology of opioid-related deaths, but because they conformed to a dominant storyline that generated outrage, political pressure, and public engagement. These narratives conformed to Harari's model: they were not constructed for accuracy, but for maximum impact and uptake. They became durable, not through their empirical fidelity, but through their emotional and symbolic power.

11.3.1 *Time Magazine* 2001: "The Potent Perils of a Miracle Drug"

In January 2001, *Time* ran a widely read feature, "The Potent Perils of a Miracle Drug," casting OxyContin as a menace poised to "succeed crack cocaine on the street [8]." The piece spotlighted dramatic anecdotes and law-enforcement fears but gave scant attention to structural drivers of drug harm or to the distinction between medically supervised use and diversion. By conflating clinical prescribing with illicit consumption, the article reinforced a simple villains-and-victims frame that would shape policy discourse for years—undermined by later evidence that the steepest mortality increases were driven by illicitly manufactured fentanyl and polysubstance use, not by prescribed opioids alone.

11.3.2 *The Washington Post's* "76 Billion Pills" Investigation

In July 2019, *The Washington Post* published an investigative piece titled "76 Billion Opioid Pills: Newly Released Federal Data Uncovers the Scale of the Opioid Epidemic," based on Drug Enforcement Administration (DEA) shipment records from its Automated Reports and Consolidated Ordering System from 2006 to 2012 [9]. The report highlighted massive volumes of oxycodone and hydrocodone pills distributed across the United States, focusing public outrage on pharmaceutical manufacturers and chain pharmacies.

Although grounded in real data, the article failed to contextualize these figures within broader epidemiological trends. It offered little acknowledgment that the sharpest rise in overdose deaths occurred only after 2013, driven by illicit fentanyl and heroin, not prescription opioids. Moreover, the reporting did not question the CDC's flawed mortality coding, which at the time conflated illicit synthetic opioids with prescription opioids. By emphasizing volume without distinguishing between legitimate prescribing and diversion, the piece reinforced the misleading notion that prescription opioids alone were to blame.

11.3.3 *60 Minutes* and the "Whistleblower" DEA Narrative

In October 2017, *60 Minutes* aired an episode titled "The Whistleblower," centered on former DEA official Joe Rannazzisi's allegations that pharmaceutical companies and distributors were fueling the opioid epidemic through unchecked pill dumping [10]. The program presented prescription opioids as the sole driver of rising overdose deaths, largely ignoring the concurrent and accelerating role of illicitly manufactured fentanyl and heroin.

Crucially, the broadcast did not interrogate the CDC's flawed classification system, which had overstated prescription opioid involvement for nearly a decade. The narrative it promoted aligned with and reinforced punitive prescribing restrictions already underway while sidelining calls for investment in treatment infrastructure or harm reduction services. It also helped enshrine a simplistic villain-versus-victim framing that failed to account for the multifactorial and evolving nature of the crisis.

11.3.4 *The New York Times*, CNN, and the *Los Angeles Times* Distorted Public Understanding of Overdose Deaths

In October 2017, *New York Times* columnist Nicholas Kristof published a provocative op-ed titled "Drug Dealers in Lab Coats," in which he criticized the pharmaceutical industry for aggressively promoting opioid prescribing and accused drug executives of fueling the overdose epidemic through profit-driven deception [11]. Physicians, in his account, were largely unwitting accomplices, misled by a coordinated campaign of marketing, lobbying, and industry-funded education.

Kristof's central claim that *"The industry systematically manipulated the entire country for 25 years, and its executives are responsible for many of the 64,000 deaths of Americans last year from drugs"* dramatically overstated the role of prescription opioids in the crisis. While there were indisputable instances of pharmaceutical misconduct, CDC data corrected for classification errors show that approximately 17,000 overdose deaths in 2016 involved prescription opioids, a number that had remained essentially stable over the previous decade. This stability undermines the idea that prescription volume is strongly correlated with overdose deaths. In contrast, the majority of fatalities that year, and in every year since, have been linked to illicitly manufactured fentanyl, heroin, and polysubstance use involving methamphetamine, benzodiazepines, and alcohol.

Kristof also asserted, *"In the 1960s, for example, 80 percent of Americans hooked on opioids began with heroin. That has completely changed. Today, 75 percent of people with opioid addictions began with prescription painkillers."* This widely repeated claim is highly misleading. Although many individuals with OUD report having used prescription opioids at some point, it remains unclear how many began with medications obtained through a legitimate prescription versus those accessed illicitly. More importantly, research shows that most people who develop substance use disorders initiate use in adolescence, typically with alcohol, cannabis, or stimulants, well before they encounter prescription opioids, whether legally or illegally obtained. The use of prescription opioids for non-medical purposes is usually the result of a trajectory of drug use that begins with other substances well before being exposed to a prescription opioid.

Kristof's article is not an anomaly but rather a reflection of a broader pattern in media coverage during this period. His framing echoed the dominant narrative that overprescribing was the primary cause of the opioid crisis. While this view contains elements of truth, it failed to capture the crisis' full complexity and obscured the structural, economic, and social conditions that created widespread vulnerability to addiction.

Kristof is a respected journalist and an impassioned advocate for social justice. Yet, in this case, his oversimplified account exemplifies how much of the media helped entrench a misleading narrative, one that profoundly influenced public perception and policymaking. The result was widespread dissemination of misinformation that hindered effective responses to the true drivers of overdose deaths. By focusing on "drug dealers in lab coats," the media stigmatized pain patients, constrained legitimate medical practice, and diverted attention from urgent considerations such as expanded access to substance use disorder treatment, harm reduction, and upstream socioecological factors described in this book.

Other media outlets reinforced this narrative. The *Los Angeles Times* unabashedly claimed that the opioid crisis "killed more than 64,000 Americans" in 2016 [12]. That too is inaccurate. The implication is that those deaths were due to prescription opioids. In reality, the majority involved illicit drugs. CNN made a similar error, initially reporting that 64,000 overdose deaths in 2016 were due to opioids. Although CNN later corrected the headline to refer to "drug overdoses" and added a clarifying statement that most involved opioids, the initial misrepresentation had already been widely disseminated [13]. The important point is that the media consistently conflated harm from prescription opioids with illicit drugs.

Not all media coverage fell into this trap. Maia Szalavitz's *Columbia Journalism Review* article, "What the Media Gets Wrong About Opioids," critiques how news outlets prioritized "accidental-addict" stories that exclude broader structural drivers [14]. Similarly, Sally Satel's *National Affairs* essay, "The Truth about Painkillers," challenges the trope that most addictions begin with a medically prescribed pill, showing instead that most people with OUDs had preexisting substance use or mental health conditions [15]. These examples demonstrate that rigorous journalism can both inform and engage the public without resorting to oversimplification or scapegoating.

To be clear, pharmaceutical companies played a role in shaping prescribing practices and public perceptions of opioid safety, and some physicians overprescribed, often under the influence of flawed, biased, or incomplete information. But the opioid crisis cannot be reduced to a morality tale of corporate greed and physician gullibility. More accurate and nuanced analyses reveal a crisis driven by deteriorating social conditions, untreated mental illness, inadequate access to addiction care, and a dangerously evolving illicit drug market.

11.4 How TV Fiction Spreads Misinformation

While news media outlets helped cement a misleading public understanding of the opioid crisis, television dramas have further embedded misinformation into public consciousness through repeated, emotionally charged misrepresentations of what causes addiction and those allegedly responsible for the crisis. Though packaged as entertainment, these depictions have had real-world consequences for policy, clinical practice, and public perception.

For at least two decades, television dramas have misrepresented fentanyl exposure, overdose, and addiction risks [16]. One of the most pernicious examples is the trope that merely touching fentanyl can cause a fatal overdose. Shows like *NCIS*, *9-1-1*, *Blue Bloods*, and *Chicago Med* have depicted law enforcement officers or paramedics collapsing after incidental contact with fentanyl, sometimes simply by inhaling powder that becomes airborne during a bust [16].

In reality, such exposure scenarios are medically implausible. Transdermal absorption of fentanyl requires sustained contact with a transdermal patch or an environment conducive to dermal penetration, not momentary skin contact with powder. Inhalation overdose also requires a quantity and purity level far beyond what is typically airborne in routine scenarios.

These same dramatizations also distort public understanding of addiction by asserting that fentanyl is 50 to 100 times more addictive than heroin or morphine. While it is true that fentanyl and its analogues are more potent—meaning a smaller amount can produce a physiological effect—potency is not equivalent to addictive potential. Higher potency drugs can be more lethal due to dose sensitivity but are not necessarily more reinforcing or addiction-forming. Such scientific distinction is often lost in dramatized narratives and contributes to misinformation.

Numerous professional organizations, including the American College of Medical Toxicology and the American Academy of Clinical Toxicology, have issued position statements to debunk these myths [17]. Yet, these and similar scenes have contributed to widespread public fear and distorted emergency response practices. Multiple police departments have issued protocols based on these fictionalized risks, advising hazmat-style precautions and calling for naloxone deployment on officers exposed to powder, even when no overdose symptoms are present. In some cases, these misinterpretations have delayed aid to actual overdose victims for fear of secondary exposure [18].

Television also misrepresents fentanyl as a bioweapon. In episodes of *FBI: Most Wanted* and *S.W.A.T.*, fentanyl is shown being aerosolized and deployed in terrorist attacks or criminal plots, killing multiple people instantly [16]. This framing has influenced legislation and security protocols by dramatizing a threat that, while theoretically possible, is logistically improbable and unsupported by real-world events [19]. These portrayals encourage panic-driven policymaking rather than evidence-based harm reduction.

Beyond emergency exposure myths, television often simplifies addiction itself. Shows like *House*, *The Good Doctor*, and *Euphoria* frame opioid addiction as an immediate and inevitable outcome of a single prescription or dose and as a binary state (either fully addicted or fully recovered) that can be resolved within a short plot arc [16]. This narrative obscures the complexity of addiction as a chronic, relapsing condition shaped by social, psychological, and biological variables [20]. The effect is to reinforce stigma and misunderstanding, suggesting that addiction is a personal failing or the consequence of medical recklessness rather than a multifactorial health issue.

Perhaps most insidious is the way these media reinforce the notion that the opioid crisis is primarily a crisis of prescription volume and medical malfeasance. These themes echo the narratives presented in documentaries like *Dopesick*, where the crisis is largely attributed to Purdue Pharma and irresponsible physicians. While corporate misconduct and overprescribing were important contributors during the early phase of the crisis, these portrayals obscure the role of illicit fentanyl, social instability, and untreated mental illness that now drive the epidemic [21].

Taken together, these media portrayals act as what Harari might call "attention-maximizing distortions": dramatic, visually arresting, and emotionally charged, but empirically unsound [7]. Their reach, amplified through syndication, streaming, and social media, has solidified false understandings of fentanyl risk and opioid addiction in the public mind. By promoting fear over nuance, these shows have inadvertently shaped policing protocols, emergency medical responses, and public attitudes toward people who use drugs. As with news media, these fictions succeeded not because they were accurate, but because they were transmissible. The consequences continue to reverberate across public health and policy domains. These fictional narratives, when layered atop already flawed data reporting and sensationalized journalism, reinforce a distorted view of addiction—one that narrows public understanding and supports reactive rather than restorative responses to a complex health crisis.

11.5 Implications of Reporting Through a Distorted Lens

These stories, shaped and reinforced by media, distorted the public's understanding of the opioid crisis. Prescription opioids became synonymous with the opioid crisis and ingrained in the collective consciousness, overshadowing the growing role of illicitly manufactured fentanyl and other synthetic opioids. By anchoring blame in prescription practices, they deflected attention from the illicit drug supply and broader structural inequities. As fentanyl reporting errors reveal, these distortions were not simply journalistic oversights. They were compounded by data misclassification, delayed institutional corrections, and a persistent reluctance to revise deeply embedded storylines.

Valid questions around the fentanyl reporting errors should be addressed. Were inaccuracies simply the result of an inadequate coding system, or was there something more deliberate at play? If inaccurate figures were knowingly reported, why was this done? Some critics have raised the possibility that these data limitations persisted not only due to bureaucratic inertia but also because correcting them might have undermined dominant narratives or threatened institutional credibility. While definitive evidence of intentional obfuscation is lacking, the delay in addressing known issues raises important questions about accountability and transparency in public health communication.

Harari would argue that in an environment where information competes for attention, the media's influence depends not on its accuracy but on its emotional resonance. To be heard, the media had to amplify anger, anxiety, or fear—often at the expense of truth. This observation ties back to the chapter's opening: narratives about the opioid crisis succeeded not because they were the most accurate, but because they were the most transmissible.

The questions raised in this chapter are not about assigning blame but about understanding how and why these errors occurred. By understanding the flaws in our approach to data collection and reporting, we can begin to correct courses and develop more effective strategies to address the complex and evolving opioid crisis.

Keeping these concerns in mind is important when reading the next chapter. It will shift away from abstract statistics to a focus on people's stories about how the proliferation of opioids and other drugs has affected their individual, family, and community wellbeing. These excerpts, shared from qualitative research, vividly spotlight the social devastation worsened by the failure to match an accurate timeline and portrayal of opioid mortality with fitting policy solutions.

The dominant focus on prescription opioids also diverted attention away from communities disproportionately affected by the illicit drug supply. As Hansen and Netherland have argued, the framing of the crisis as a "white, middle-class" problem contributed to more empathetic portrayals of people who use opioids—so long as they were seen as patients, not criminals [21]. In contrast, Black and Latinx communities experiencing fentanyl-related harms often received far less attention, and when they did, the coverage was more likely to invoke criminality than compassion.

This asymmetry in narrative framing shaped not only public perception but also the allocation of resources, leaving many Black, Indigenous, and People of Color communities underserved by harm reduction, treatment, and prevention programs.

References

1. Seth P, Rudd RA, Noonan RK, Haegerich TM. Quantifying the epidemic of prescription opioid overdose deaths. Am J Public Health. 2018;108(4):500–2.
2. Peppin JF, Coleman JJ. CDC's efforts to quantify prescription opioid overdose deaths fall short. Pain Ther. 2021;10(1):25–38.
3. Dowell D, Haegerich TM, Chou R. CDC guideline for prescribing opioids for chronic pain - United States, 2016. MMWR Recomm Rep. 2016;65(1):1–49.
4. Dowell D, Ragan KR, Jones CM, Baldwin GT, Chou R. CDC clinical practice guideline for prescribing opioids for pain - United States, 2022. MMWR Recomm Rep. 2022;71(3):1–95.
5. Dowell D, Haegerich T, Chou R. No shortcuts to safer opioid prescribing. N Engl J Med. 2019;380(24):2285–7.
6. Kertesz SG, Gordon AJ. A crisis of opioids and the limits of prescription control: United States. Addiction. 2019;114(1):169–80.
7. Harari YN. Nexus: a brief history of information networks from the stone age to AI. New York: Random House; 2024.
8. Roche T. The potent perils of a miracle drug: OxyContin is a leading treatment for chronic pain, but officials fear it may succeed crack cocaine on the street. Time. 2001;
9. Higham S, Horwitz S. 76 billion opioid pills: newly released federal data unmasks the epidemic. Washington Post. 2019 Jul 16. Available from: https://www.washingtonpost.com/investigations/76-billion-opioid-pills-newly-released-federal-data-unmasks-the-epidemic/2019/07/16/5f29fd62-a73e-11e9-86dd-d7f0e60391e9_story.html.
10. The whistleblower/redemption. 60 minutes. CBS; 2017 Oct 15.
11. Kristof N. Drug dealers in lab coats. New York Times. 2017 Oct 18. Available from: https://www.nytimes.com/2017/10/18/opinion/opioid-pharmaceutical-addiction-pain.html.
12. Levey NN. Trump calls opioid epidemic an 'emergency' but offers few new resources to combat it. Los Angeles Times. 2017 Oct 26 [cited 2025 Jul 17]. Available from: https://www.latimes.com/politics/la-na-pol-trump-opioids-20171026-story.html.
13. Webster LR. We have a drug overdose crisis, not a prescription opioid crisis. The Hill. 2017 Nov 16 [cited 2025 Jul 17]. Available from: https://thehill.com/opinion/healthcare/360781-we-have-a-drug-overdose-crisis-not-a-prescription-opioid-crisis/.
14. Szalavitz M. What the media gets wrong about opioids. Columbia Journalism Review. 2018 Aug 15. Retrieved from https://www.cjr.org on August 8, 2025.
15. Satel S. The truth about painkillers. National Affairs. 2021; (64, Summer). Retrieved from https://nationalaffairs.com/publications/detail/the-truth-about-painkillers on August 8, 2025.
16. Marino R, Gilbert BD. What Cop Shows get WRONG about FENTANYL [Video]. 2023 May 3 [cited 2025 Jul 22]. Available from: http://www.youtube.com/watch?v=_7OBdD7zubg.
17. Moss MJ, Warrick BJ, Nelson LS, McKay CA, Dubé PA, Gosselin S, et al. ACMT and AACT position statement: preventing occupational fentanyl and fentanyl analog exposure to emergency responders. J Med Toxicol. 2017;13(4):347–51.
18. Beletsky L, Seymour S, Kang S, Siegel Z, Sinha MS, Marino R, et al. Fentanyl panic goes viral: the spread of misinformation about overdose risk from casual contact with fentanyl in mainstream and social media. Int J Drug Policy. 2020;86:102951.
19. Beletsky L, Davis CS. Today's fentanyl crisis: prohibition's iron law, revisited. Int J Drug Policy. 2017;46:156–9.
20. Volkow ND, Koob G. Brain disease model of addiction: why is it so controversial? Lancet Psychiatry. 2015;2(8):677–9.
21. Hansen H, Netherland J. Is the prescription opioid epidemic a white problem? Am J Public Health. 2016;106(12):2127–9.

Mapping the Risk Environment: Socioeconomic Dimensions of the Crisis

12

The idea that some lives matter less is the root of all that is wrong with the world.

—Paul Farmer (quoted in Kidder, T. Mountains Beyond Mountains, Random House, 2003)

12.1 Introduction

The opioid crisis is not merely the result of individual choices; it is rooted in interconnected forces that constrain opportunities and shape lives. This chapter applies Rhodes' Risk Environment Framework (REF) to examine how such factors drive drug-related harms [1]. Drawing on qualitative studies, primarily in rural and Appalachian settings, we highlight the economic dimensions of the crisis. Deindustrialization, economic decline, and job market stagnation fuel opioid use in rural and urban contexts. High poverty, unemployment, and housing insecurity limit access to health care and essential resources, fostering despair that leads many to use drugs as a coping mechanism. This desperation encourages riskier drug practices and sustains informal economies.

Ultimately, this chapter reveals that the opioid crisis is not merely about personal failings but reflects deep structural vulnerabilities and collective suffering. Addressing it means dismantling the underlying risk environments.

While much of the research cited here focuses on rural, predominantly white communities, Black, Indigenous, and other People of Color experience distinct, structurally embedded risk environments. Factors like systemic racism, residential segregation, over-policing, and underinvestment in urban infrastructure create pathways to drug risk. Future research and policy must address these racialized contexts to avoid perpetuating a white-centered understanding of the crisis.

L. R. Webster, S. Eichberg, *Deconstructing Toxic Narratives*,
https://doi.org/10.1007/978-3-032-23135-2_12

12.2 Understanding the "Why": Rhodes' Risk Environment Framework

Throughout this book, we have worked to deconstruct toxic narratives and uncover the social and economic roots of the crisis. We now seek to build on that foundation by widening the lens to examine the broader environment in which drug use occurs. Rhodes' REF offers a valuable tool, facilitating analysis of how economic conditions, social dynamics, physical surroundings, and public policies interact to produce or mitigate drug-related harms. While the qualitative insights presented here may not be statistically generalizable, they offer a rich, grounded understanding of the complex contexts in which substance use unfolds.

Rhodes' REF fits with newer conceptual frameworks of substance misuse research that highlight the broad role of environmental factors in shaping health outcomes for people who misuse drugs (PWMD). It was introduced as an alternative to harm reduction models, which are primarily focused on individual behavioral change. Instead, Rhodes' model maps how individual dynamic interactions with environmental and structural factors produce and reduce drug harm.

Rhodes' model is a useful heuristic for qualitative and quantitative sociological and epidemiological studies on opioid use and overdose in any geographic context. While quantitative studies can detect relationships between variables, acting as the standard source for policy recommendations, they are not suitable for addressing the "why" questions underpinning these relationships. Qualitative research illuminates this missing element through in-depth exploration of people's experiences with phenomena and the meanings they assign to them. This type of narrative analysis is valuable because it captures the complexity present in the social world and provides insights necessary to develop more targeted prevention and treatment strategies.

Qualitative claims, derived from comparatively small sample sizes, are not meant to be generalized to the entire population. However, they are produced through strict standards for rigor and quality, and data analysis is theory-driven and systematic. Qualitative research's greatest strength is its rich descriptions of social processes, including drug use, which allow researchers to identify the mechanisms or mediating variables, such as mental health or social cohesion, through which economic or geographic conditions influence opioid-related harms.

This chapter, together with the following one, utilizes a narrative review to synthesize evidence and address the research topic or question in a holistic manner. Peer-reviewed studies and systematic reviews have been evaluated to identify principal themes and patterns, accompanied by detailed descriptions that highlight participants' lived experiences and give voice to individuals represented in the sample. This approach is particularly appropriate for examining environmental risk factors related to opioid use and overdose fatalities, where the objective is to generate an integrated understanding of risk rather than assessing all available empirical research.

Through a thematic and interpretive analysis of findings, the review systematically identifies context and nuance in the findings, highlighting the influence of environmental factors on opioid use and overdose fatalities. This approach allows for a structured analysis of data, yielding detailed findings. The reviewed articles were published over the last two decades, with most focusing on remote or rural environments, including over a third in Appalachia. Several, however, examine substance use disorder (SUD) and opioid use disorder (OUD) in large and small cities and suburbs. Reflecting the predominantly rural focus, most participants are white, whereas studies conducted in urban locations (e.g., Baltimore; Dane County, WI; St. Louis) include entirely BIPOC participants.

The studies used semi-structured or in-depth interviews and focus groups as part of a standalone or larger mixed-methods research project. Sample sizes ranged from 18 to 90, yielding over 460 participants. Local stakeholders represented in the studies included community residents, active and recovering drug users, business owners, law enforcement officials, health and social services providers, and community leaders. Drug use typically involved prescription opioids and/or heroin, but street fentanyl, cocaine/crack, methamphetamines, buprenorphine, benzodiazepines, and barbiturates were also mentioned as drugs of choice.

Rhodes' framework explores four types of environmental influences: economic, social, physical, and policy. While these factors are discussed separately, it is crucial to remember that they are interconnected and mutually influential (Fig. 12.1) [1]. The processes within each category overlap to affect the risk environment, illustrating some of the complex dynamics that are hinted at by quantitative studies but not yet captured in econometric and spatial analysis/geographic systems modeling. Appendix C provides an overview of the studies, their methods, community sites, and themes.

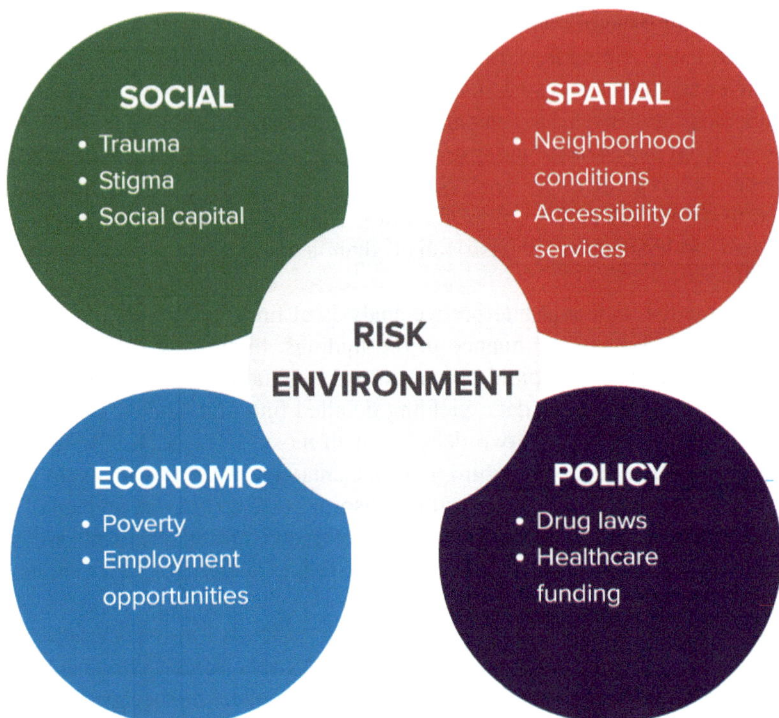

Fig. 12.1 This diagram illustrates the interaction of four domains—social, spatial, economic, and policy—that together constitute the broader risk environment influencing opioid use disorder (OUD) and overdose vulnerability. Each domain contributes distinct yet interrelated structural forces. *Social*: Includes trauma, stigma, and social capital. These interpersonal and cultural dynamics shape vulnerability, resilience, and care-seeking behavior. *Spatial*: Refers to neighborhood conditions, geographic isolation, and service accessibility. Spatial disinvestment can restrict treatment access and reinforce marginalization. *Economic*: Encompasses poverty and employment opportunities. Economic distress is a key upstream driver of substance use initiation and barriers to recovery. *Policy*: Includes drug laws and healthcare funding structures. These shape criminalization, treatment availability, and equity in access to care. Together, these domains form the risk environment—a multidimensional context in which structural, social, and spatial inequities compound to elevate risk and hinder recovery. (Source: Adapted to support the Risk Environment Framework as applied to the opioid crisis from concepts in Rhodes [1])

12.3 Economic Factors and Cycles of Despair

Economic conditions are central to shaping risk in the lives of participants in rural and urban communities. In rural towns, the uncertain economic transitions linked to deindustrialization, economic decline, and labor market stagnation were frequently mentioned as contributors to opioid use [2–13]. McLean interviewed 18 clients at a substance misuse center in the city of McKeesport in the Monongahela Valley region of Pennsylvania [6]. Participants reported that deindustrialization of the city's once flourishing steel industry had left behind an environment conducive to drug misuse and overdose, as jobs vanished, people moved away, and economic disadvantages took root. In her ethnography of Weymouth, Massachusetts, a working-class commuter town, Sered notes that plant closures in the 2000s eliminated secure blue-collar union jobs, leaving only temporary and low-wage employment options, which in turned fueled substance misuse [8].

A current drug user in a study by Thompson et al., set in an Appalachian coal mining community, commented on the allure of drugs following loss of manufacturing jobs and economic security [11]:

> I think as the mill was closed, and everything closes, other businesses leave, opportunities leave, things for people to do because they don't have the money to do it no more, everything leaves. When the drugs come in, the education doesn't come with it. So, it all goes together.

Economic hardship in general, not necessarily tied to deindustrialization, was highlighted in urban and rural environments alike. High rates of poverty were present in most research settings; in the cluster of five rural Appalachian counties studied by Cloud et al., 23–32% of residents lived below the federal poverty level [3]. Unemployment and/or housing insecurity also were common in communities in economic distress [11, 14, 15]. In George et al.'s study on hotspots for diseases of despair in Central Pennsylvania, a member of a community focus group observed [4]:

> Over the last 30 years there's been a great increase in economic disparity. Especially in rural communities where there already weren't a lot of economic opportunities to begin with … you start chipping away at them, people start not going to the dentist or getting mental health care they need because maybe they can't afford [and] access it. It's families choosing to see a therapist or buy their groceries (p. 5).

Within economically depressed communities, community resources were scarce, and services were chronically underfunded, leaving residents with limited health services or none at all [3, 6, 10, 11, 14]. When available, health care, including harm reduction, medical treatment for OUD, and prescriptions for hepatitis C virus or other medical conditions, was financially out of reach for many on low incomes, who had little or no insurance [6, 10, 13]. A participant in Walters et al.'s study, set in rural southern Illinois, commented [13]:

> I had pneumonia in late December, went to the ER...It was horrible…I couldn't even come up with $17.00 for the pills. I don't have healthcare, you know what I mean, public aid assistance, so I pretty [much] didn't even get the script.

Within each of the REF's domains, upstream forces help shape the downstream environment of hazardous behaviors, played out in interpersonal relationships as well as through the influence of community norms and practices (See Table 12.1). In the economic sphere, rampant poverty, unemployment, and lack of opportunity, brought on by deindustrialization, have led to psychosocial distress, disillusionment, and depression over bleak or uncertain futures [3, 5–7, 11, 16, 17]. This

Table 12.1 Micro and macro risk environment factors (economic)

Microenvironment	Macroenvironment
Unaffordable costs for living and health-related expenses Unemployment and labor market stagnation Housing insecurity Riskier drug activities to cut costs Informal economies/illicit drug market	Poverty Income inequality Deindustrialization Healthcare/insurance policies and access Devolution of government funding (lack of federal and state funding for services)

Source: Adapted from concepts in Rhodes [1]

pervasive despair, arising from lack of opportunity, is a barrier to community recovery and triggers disengagement from civic life [7, 12]. To suppress these feelings of pain and emotional trauma, participants use drugs as a mechanism for relief. (This is more extensively discussed in the Sect. 13.2 in the next chapter.)

A service provider in Thompson et al.'s Appalachia-based study further articulated the connection between economic decline, depression, and drug use [11]:

> Because if you know anything about [this area] and you went around here, you would think it's almost like in a war zone. You see all these abandoned houses in the community. You see lots with grass growing six feet high. You just see trash in the community. It's just a depressing area. And when people live in a depressed area, they have a tendency to become depressed themselves. And depression leads to something to anesthetize themselves, something like a drug or alcohol just to get through a day, you know (p. 11)?

12.3.1 Life After the Mill Closure in Ironton, Ohio

The vignette in the text box is a composite based on recurring themes in qualitative studies and journalistic reports of post-industrial communities [18, 19]. It serves to humanize structural patterns rather than to represent a specific individual.

When the steel mill shut down in Ironton, Ohio, it wasn't just the loss of 400 jobs—it was the unraveling of an entire support system. Tommy, a former millwright, now delivers groceries part-time. With chronic back pain and no insurance, he began using opioids after borrowing pills from a neighbor. Now, 5 years later, he's one of hundreds in his town who cycle in and out of treatment and housing instability. "The pills weren't the start," he says. "They just made the pain quiet for a while."

A participant in McLean's study echoed these sentiments when discussing the city of McKeesport [6]:

> It's just a depressing area, there's nothing.. .I mean people come to McKeesport to get drugs, from other areas. . .because that's what is here. . .McKeesport, I just think there's nothing- . . .all the good people have kind of moved out and moved away because of all the

> drug addiction and all the mental health here and, I mean, I think it's just depressing, there's really no good jobs here, no good, you know, anything (p. 25).

Economic distress motivated some participants to engage in riskier drug-related practices to economize use, including injecting or sharing needles [3, 11, 13, 16]. In interviews with self-described injectors in rural Ohio, Draus and Carlson noted that participants switched from snorting heroin to injecting it to cut costs: *Well, I started shootin' it, ya know, to save money 'cause I didn't, so I wouldn't have to spend as much, and I'd get twice as high off [half as much]* [16].

Economic desperation can also drive the emergence of informal economies that provide participants with vital earnings for survival [2, 5, 6, 20]. In rural often deindustrialized settings, it was common for individuals to sell prescription opioids on the black market to supplement low incomes [2, 5]. One of the participants in McLean's research explained why selling drugs was an inevitable outcome of living in blighted surroundings [6]:

> Well, I think a lot of it is the, the income rate of people around here. It's so low income. The people don't have, like, stuff, so they turn to drugs easier when you're poor. At least for me it was easier for me to turn to drugs, because I didn't really have anything in my life to lose. . .And then, I think the problem is with, whenever you have low income like that, people start selling drugs, people's mothers and fathers start selling drugs, so people grow up in that environment, and then they become drug sellers themselves…(p. 24).

A microenvironment refers to the immediate, small-scale social and physical contexts that directly shape an individual's risk of drug-related harms. Essentially, it's about the local, day-to-day settings where people live, interact, and use drugs, as opposed to broader societal or structural factors. The macroenvironment refers to the broad, large-scale social, economic, political, and cultural forces that shape drug-related risks at the population level. These are the structural conditions that influence entire communities or societies, rather than individual behavior or immediate local surroundings.

12.4 Beyond Interdiction: Fostering Resilience and Rebuilding Communities

The economic findings presented in this chapter underscore the urgent need to move beyond simplistic explanations of drug use rooted in moral failing or personal weakness. What emerges instead is a portrait of communities shaped by industrial abandonment, structural poverty, and psychological despair, conditions that incubate risk and strip away the scaffolding of health and resilience. Drug use, in such environments, becomes less a choice than a symptom of disconnection, survival, and unaddressed pain. This structural vulnerability is a core element in understanding the overdose crisis.

Too often, public discourse has focused narrowly on the supply of drugs as if restricting access alone could prevent addiction. But as this chapter illustrates, and the next will further elaborate, the roots of the opioid crisis lie not simply in the presence of drugs, but in the absence of opportunity, belonging, and basic supports that make life bearable. Reducing overdose deaths and preventing future harm demand more than interdiction; it requires dismantling the risk environments that perpetuate despair. Mapping the social risk environment reveals not only the architecture of despair but also the systemic choices that have produced and prolonged this crisis. Despair didn't arrive with the drugs, it was already here. The overdose crisis simply made it visible.

As we turn to the next chapter, we widen the aperture again—exploring how social dynamics, built environments, and policy structures work together to deepen vulnerability or, alternatively, offer pathways to healing. By continuing to apply Rhodes' REF, we move closer to a more complete and humane understanding of how drug-related harm is produced and how it might be prevented.

References

1. Rhodes T. The 'risk environment': a framework for understanding and reducing drug-related harm. Int J Drug Policy. 2002;13(2):85–94.
2. Buer LM, Leukefeld CG, Havens JR. "I'm stuck": women's navigations of social networks and prescription drug misuse in central Appalachia. North Am Dialogue. 2016;19(2):70–84.
3. Cloud DH, Ibragimov U, Prood N, Young AM, Cooper HLF. Rural risk environments for hepatitis c among young adults in appalachian kentucky. Int J Drug Policy. 2019;72:47–54.
4. George DR, Snyder B, Van Scoy LJ, Brignone E, Sinoway L, Sauder C, et al. Perceptions of diseases of despair by members of rural and urban high-prevalence communities: a qualitative study. JAMA Netw Open. 2021;4(7):e2118134.
5. Leukefeld C, Walker R, Havens J, Leedham CA, Tolbert V. What does the community say: key informant perceptions of rural prescription drug use. J Drug Issues. 2007;37(3):503–24.
6. McLean K. "There's nothing here": deindustrialization as risk environment for overdose. Int J Drug Policy. 2016;29:19–26.
7. Schalkoff CA, Lancaster KE, Gaynes BN, Wang V, Pence BW, Miller WC, et al. The opioid and related drug epidemics in rural Appalachia: a systematic review of populations affected, risk factors, and infectious diseases. Subst Abus. 2020;41(1):35–69.
8. Sered SS. The opioid crisis and the infrastructure of social capital. Int J Drug Policy. 2019;71:47–55.
9. Nolte K, Drew AL, Friedmann PD, Romo E, Kinney LM, Stopka TJ. Opioid initiation and injection transition in rural northern New England: a mixed-methods approach. Drug Alcohol Depend. 2020;217:108256.
10. Thomas N, van de Ven K, Mulrooney KJD. The impact of rurality on opioid-related harms: a systematic review of qualitative research. Int J Drug Policy. 2020;85:102607.
11. Thompson JR, Creasy SL, Mair CF, Burke JG. Drivers of opioid use in Appalachian Pennsylvania: cross-cutting social and community-level factors. Int J Drug Policy. 2020;78:102706.
12. Trappen SL, McLean KJ. Policing pain: a qualitative study of non-criminal justice approaches to managing opioid overdose during the COVID-19 pandemic. J Prev Interv Community. 2021;49(2):136–51.
13. Walters SM, Frank D, Felsher M, Jaiswal J, Fletcher S, Bennett AS, et al. How the rural risk environment underpins hepatitis C risk: qualitative findings from rural southern Illinois, United States. Int J Drug Policy. 2023;112:103930.

14. Linton SL, Winiker A, Tormohlen KN, Schneider KE, McLain G, Sherman SG, et al. "People Don't just start shooting heroin on their 18(th) birthday": a qualitative study of community stakeholders' perspectives on adolescent opioid use and opportunities for intervention in Baltimore, Maryland. Prev Sci. 2021;22(5):621–32.
15. Rigg KK, Murphy JW. Understanding the etiology of prescription opioid abuse: implications for prevention and treatment. Qual Health Res. 2013;23(7):963–75.
16. Draus PJ, Carlson RG. Needles in the haystacks: the social context of initiation to heroin injection in rural Ohio. Subst Use Misuse. 2006;41(8):1111–24.
17. Redican KJ, Marek LI, Brock DJ, McCance-Katz EF. Exploring the etiologic factors and dynamics of prescription drug abuse in Southwest Virginia. Health Promot Perspect. 2012;2(2):153–65.
18. Dasgupta N, Beletsky L, Ciccarone D. Opioid crisis: no easy fix to its social and economic determinants. Am J Public Health. 2018;108(2):182–6.
19. Quinones S. Dreamland: the true tale of America's opiate epidemic. 1st ed. New York: Bloomsbury Press; 2015.
20. Smith BD, Lewis Q, Offiong A, Willis K, Prioleau M, Powell TW. "It's on every corner": assessing risk environments in Baltimore, MD using a racialized risk environment model. J Ethn Subst Abus. 2024;23(1):95–109.

Risk and Resilience: The Social Ecology of Addiction

13

Inequalities in health are not randomly distributed: they follow the contours of power.

—Nancy Krieger (Epidemiology and the People's Health, Oxford University Press, 2011)

13.1 Introduction

The previous chapter described how structural economic conditions, job loss, disinvestment, and community abandonment, create the groundwork for substance use and overdose risk. Here, we continue that trajectory by examining the broader social ecology of addiction. As in the last chapter, we draw on Rhodes' Risk Environment Framework (REF) to explore how stigma, geography, and policy converge to shape both vulnerability and survival [1]. Addiction, in this view, is not simply a response to pain or pleasure, but a reflection of environments that constrain opportunity and isolate individuals from care and connection. Understanding these dynamics is critical to constructing interventions that address the roots of harm rather than their symptoms (Fig. 13.1) [1].

L. R. Webster, S. Eichberg, *Deconstructing Toxic Narratives*,
https://doi.org/10.1007/978-3-032-23135-2_13

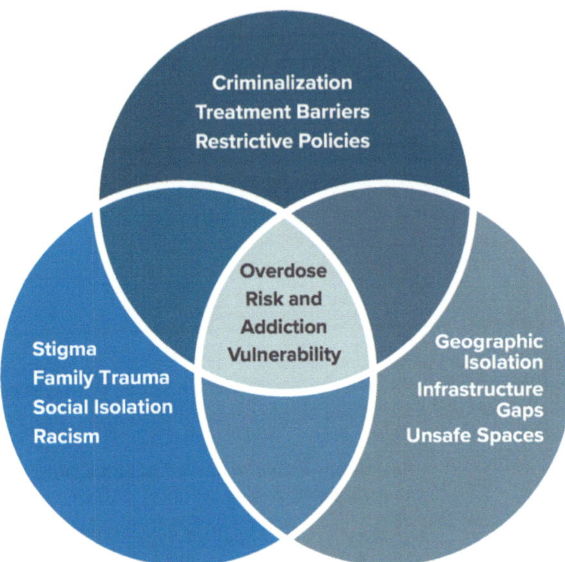

Fig. 13.1 This Venn diagram illustrates the intersecting social, spatial, and policy factors that shape vulnerability to opioid use and overdose. The model demonstrates how overlapping structural conditions amplify individual risk. *Social Environment*: Stigma, family trauma, social isolation, and structural racism contribute to diminished social capital and deter people who use drugs from seeking care. *Physical/Spatial Environment*: Geographic isolation, inadequate transportation, and unsafe or surveilled spaces restrict access to harm reduction and health care. *Policy Environment*: Criminalization, restrictive prescribing rules, treatment access barriers, and systemic discrimination often worsen outcomes. *Intersection*: The convergence of all three domains produces the most acute vulnerability—where exclusion, neglect, and constrained environments coalesce to increase the likelihood of substance-related harm. (Source: Adapted to support the Risk Environment Framework as applied to the opioid crisis from concepts in Rhodes [1])

13.2 Social Factors

Social, cultural, and psychological factors operate in tandem with economic determinants to shape the risk environment and a community's outlook on life. Many participants discussed the social stigma attached to opioid use, attributing the stigma to the conservative beliefs that are common in small towns and recognizing it as a major contributor to the marginalization of people who misuse opioids (PWMO). A resident of Appalachia in Cloud et al.'s study noted [2]:

> Everybody's judgmental, and it just keeps you from reaching out. The only other person you're going to reach out to is the guy that can get you a needle or the drugs you're trying to score (p. 6).

In Williams and Dodge Francis's study in Dane County, WI, Black community members reported avoiding community-based programs in what were termed "third" (or neutral) spaces because of disapproving staff who had the power to disrupt their lives—through arrest, eviction, or intervention by protective services—if they were honest about drug use or other non-normative behaviors [3]. Third spaces were defined as places where Black people gather and socialize away from home, school, and work to receive emotional and psychological support [4]. Commenting on the quality of supportive spaces in her neighborhood, a woman stated [3]:

> First of all, believe me, I got my ... what is it called, it's called a support system. I know where to go for mines. It would be nowhere in Wisconsin. Trust me (p. 344).

These narratives highlight how stigma—rooted in cultural conservatism, racialized surveillance, and systemic discrimination—acts as a structural barrier to care. In both rural Appalachia and urban Black communities, fear of judgment or punitive consequences discourages people from seeking help. This aligns with the *social environment* dimension of the REF where stigma creates exclusionary spaces and increases health vulnerability by discouraging harm reduction and healthcare engagement.

Stigma also kept PWMO from accessing harm reduction and mental health as well as more routine medical attention in conventional healthcare settings [2, 5–8]. This avoidance was based on the belief, accumulated through past experience, that providers were judgmental, unresponsive, and unlikely to offer beneficial aid: A participant in Walters et al. observed [9]:

> In my experience with doctors...after you admit to drug use... they have really no use for you...You're nothing but a drug seeker, and you can have some legitimate issues, concerns and they just don't care.

Nationally, an estimated 86.6% of individuals with opioid use disorder received no treatment between 2010 and 2019, underscoring how stigma is compounded by systemic inaccessibility—even when individuals are willing to seek help [10].

Motivated by stigma avoidance, individuals who injected drugs were especially unlikely to access services or make use of other opportunities to minimize risky behavior [5, 9]. A participant who injected drugs in Walters et al.'s study explained why they put off purchasing sterile syringes at local pharmacies [9]:

> I don't like to ask [for sterile syringes]...I'm ashamed of it...It makes me feel this small to go there and ask.

These negative sentiments were amplified when pharmacy staff refused to provide service because they suspected that the syringes would be used to inject drugs.

Thompson et al. identified "acceptance and denial of use" as an important theme in their participants' narratives, creating a "duality of experience" for residents in the study's Appalachian community [11]. On the one hand, opioid use was common among families and peers. On the other hand, the social acceptance of opioid use often existed alongside people's unwillingness to accept the reality of drug use in their own households or communities. Media messages stigmatizing certain racial groups or other neighborhoods exacerbated residents' denial about the pervasive use of opioids in their own town. Lack of anonymity in close-knit communities prevented individuals from using drug treatment or other services out of fear of being identified as a user by staff or neighbors.

Social relationships and social networks played a role in either aggravating or minimizing risk. Some people leaned on families and friends for support with managing stigma, shielding themselves from potential risky behaviors or negative outcomes. In research in Appalachia, Roberson et al. noted that social networks improved resiliency to opioids, such as when relatives cared for users' children [12].

Indeed, initial exposure to drugs often began in family homes. In a study in western Virginia, Redican et al. observed that youth were frequently initiated into prescription drug use by accessing pills in their family's medicine cabinets [13]. Sered found that cultural patterns in Weymouth, especially refusal to seek help from others, exacerbated the community's drug issues and its structural challenges [14]. Finally, many participants reported intrafamilial drug use, serving to offset buffering effects of strong family ties and, instead, reinforcing an intergenerational cycle of poverty and addiction.

A participant in Cloud et al.'s study commented on his history shooting heroin with his father [2]:

> All three of our dads were drug dealers. So, we'd seen junkies and stuff. [My cousins and I] never wanted to be that. My dad… my life is like his… and my whole life he tried to get me to go on a different path. Somehow I got brought into it (p. 7).

A current drug user in Thompson et al. offered another example of intergeneration drug use [11]:

> I was in and out of the county jail. I was staying at a friend's house, back and forth with my mom. My mom uses too, my mom, my brother, my sister, and it's like it runs in my family (p. 3).

The examples of intrafamilial drug use, drawn largely from rural Appalachia, illustrate how the social environment becomes a conduit for both risk and normalization. Exposure to opioid use in family settings—often shaped by poverty, trauma, and lack of mental health services—contributes to a cycle of intergenerational substance use. In REF terms, the *micro-social environment* reinforces behaviors and limits exit pathways for youth who grow up in these constrained conditions (See Table 13.1).

In several studies, family fragmentation from divorce, conflict, or estrangement was mentioned as a risk factor for impaired psychosocial development. Family disintegration was also viewed as another source of the mounting despair contributing to drug use in many rural, often deindustrialized, communities [15, 16].

High levels of interpersonal violence and emotional trauma were pervasive throughout the study settings; women and children were frequently victims of physical and sexual assault in rural communities [3, 13, 16–18]. Redican et al. noted that in Southwestern Virginia, child abuse and neglect exceeded state averages by up to

Table 13.1 Micro and macro risk environment factors (social, physical, and policy)

	Micro factors	Macro factors
Social	Avoidance of harm reduction/treatment, preventive and specialty healthcare and community-based emotional/financial support programs Riskier drug activities (e.g., avoiding purchasing clean needles) Intergenerational drug use Social networks or family ties as coping mechanisms Family distress Interpersonal violence Emotional trauma and despair Racist interactions with health and service providers and law enforcement Social isolation and eroded trust—Low social capital	Societal stigma against people who use drugs Structural racism Diminished social capital/cohesion/polarization Strong intersection with economic domain (poverty, unemployment, devolution of funding, income inequality, etc.) to create microenvironment effects
Physical	Limited community infrastructure funding Drug use settings ("trap houses") and behaviors such as sharing or reusing equipment due to fear of police Lack of safe physical spaces to congregate Geographic isolation and large distances between population centers Limited public transportation Long wait times for treatment Lack of access to prevention resources Clinician and staff shortages	Economic policies reducing federal or state support of programs (devolution of funding) Healthcare and drug treatment policies/shortages Law enforcement
Policy	Lack of access to treatment Lack of access to new injecting equipment Discrimination from police, pharmacy, healthcare providers and social services Use of illicit opioids and other underground drugs as substitutes for pharmaceutical opioids Dependency on prescription opioids for pain management	Criminalization/law enforcement policies Political opposition to harm reduction drug policies Regulations to control prescription opioid access Disability program requirements

Source: Adapted from concepts in Rhodes [1]

52% [13]. Buer, Leukefeld, and Havens discussed prescription opioid use among women in Central Appalachia and observed that geographic isolation interacted with gender roles to increase the risk of opioid-related harm [17]. Specifically, women often reported that their opioid use was influenced by a male partner in an intimate relationship; when these relationships involved physical violence, the violent behavior and residential isolation converged to make it difficult to leave the partnership.

Those affected by trauma turned to drugs to cope with unwanted memories and emotional pain or to self-medicate against mood and anxiety disorders [3, 16, 18].

In addition to social stigma, the scarcity of available mental health services and lack of resources for travel deterred participants from accessing services to address harm from drug use, as well as physical, sexual, and emotional trauma.

Social and peer groups also developed their own "risk norms," determining what information about drug use was shared among group members and what risk behaviors were accepted [16]. In many studies, networks composed of friends or family introduced individuals to drug use, and continued group interaction was a socialization process that normalized the practice [7, 19, 20]. In certain social networks, risky behaviors, such as sharing needles, were commonplace [2, 21]. Using drugs as a part of a social group also provided a sense of belonging for some individuals [21].

Despite these risks, some communities and individuals demonstrated remarkable resilience. Family members' assumption of caregiving roles, peer-led support networks, and informal community efforts to reduce harm all played a part in mitigating risk. These instances suggest that interventions leveraging existing social capital—however limited—can be effective in transforming risk environments into spaces of support and recovery.

In a few studies, participants directly connected economic decline with a loss of community life that increased social isolation, fostered social alienation, and eroded civic trust [14, 15, 18, 22]. A community resident in George et al.'s 2021 study remarked [15]:

> If you'd ask my next-door neighbor my son's name, what he wanted to do, where he wanted to go, they'd have no idea. Because we don't talk to each other or help each other like we used to. And if we think decades back, we hung out with neighbors every night…. It [isolation] impedes people asking for help (p.7).

In her ethnography of Weymouth, MA, Sered discussed long-term structural, political, and cultural patterns that came together with the easy availability of prescription opioids during the 1990s and 2000s to create the town's opioid crisis [14]. These included job and opportunity loss, the Catholic Church's sexual abuse scandal, and weakening community cohesion, all of which left residents feeling betrayed by institutions—economic, religious, municipal, and national. Similar sentiments were expressed in George et al. [15]:

> Right now, not just the community, but just the generation, no one trusts anyone…that promotes isolation (p. 7).

The deterioration of these institutions over recent decades led to loss of social capital among residents, meaning they lost the benefits derived from strong social networks [23, 24]. Sered links Weymouth residents' loss of social capital with a loss of cultural capital, described as "the available repertoire of ideas and practices that facilitate the ability to make sense out of the world, manage suffering, and imagine and work with like-minded others towards a better future" [14]. Without meaningful life scripts, people in Weymouth were predisposed to misuse substances to manage their pain, disappointments, and restlessness. This decay in life scripts stemmed from several sources, including labor market shifts that weakened social ties and collective power associated with union jobs. Additionally, changes in the local school system, transitioning from vocational education to a purely college-preparatory track, further contributed to this decline. This shift emphasized material success over the bonds and identity formed by blue-collar jobs, effectively setting up students for failure who were uninterested in college.

Participants in Black communities described living in a "racialized risk society," characterized by increased vulnerability [20]. In Dane County, WI, Black residents attributed drug use in their communities to cumulative trauma stemming from daily negative interactions with interlocking systems of oppression that offered little social support and failed to improve their material circumstances [3]. Participants specifically pointed to racism and power imbalances within social service agencies, law enforcement agencies, hospitals, schools, and other community structures. Hostile and unsupportive staff in these institutions often discouraged participants from accessing vital services, including addiction recovery programs. This left residents feeling isolated, trapped, and anti-social, contributing to diminished social capital in the neighborhood and hindering hope for social or economic mobility. As one male focus group member commented [3]:

> There are external things that people who are coming here are encountering with the system here in Dane County…they face racism and discrimination. So, they're facing, you know, those internal traumas, and then they're trying to manage or deal with the external social traumas that are being placed upon them every day (p. 340).

These inequities are evident in opioid-involved overdose outcomes: In 2023, American Indian and Alaska Native individuals experienced the highest opioid overdose death rate at 49.4 per 100,000, followed by Black individuals at 37.6, compared to 25.5 for white individuals—a stark illustration of the intersection between racialized trauma and policy neglect [25].

13.3 Physical Factors

A common concern among participants in urban and rural environments was lack of funding for local infrastructure. In several articles set in rural communities, the lack of infrastructure manifested in a lack of recreational options for young people (e.g., a youth center) and older people; as a result, residents used opioids to offset their boredom [2, 5, 11, 13, 19]. One participant from Cloud et al. connected a community's economic decline with shrinking resources for social enrichment, as follows [2]:

> They used to have a bowling alley. They shut that down. They took the city pool out. There's nothing. There's no events to take the kids to – no concerts – You sit at home, or … maybe get to go to McDonald's or something (p. 5).

A community resident with a history of drug use in Thompson et al.'s study made a similar observation, noting that substance use became normalized in a community with poor infrastructure and little to do [11]:

> There is no activities, not only for the kids, I mean there's playgrounds and what-not, but there is no activities for the younger kids and the older kids. We are talking about the 18-year-olds, the 7 to 18-year-olds... then you talk about the 30-year-olds. And there is nothing to do but get high. I've always seen that as normal, so to speak (p. 5).

Focus group discussions in Dane County, WI, as reported by Williams and Dodge Francis, highlighted the important role of physical space in promoting community health. Participants identified the absence of safe physical spaces to gather in their neighborhoods as a barrier to social networking, relationship building, and community wellbeing [3]. These difficulties forming social bonds and receiving emotional sustenance hindered addiction recovery and resulted in more drug use to manage the pain. As a male participant commented [3]:

> We don't have those connections; those resources, the people who are in the city who say they can connect them to the resources ... They're not seen. Our churches, the Black church, derelict in its duties when it comes to the community's safety and health, or providing that safe space, just providing a safe space, will not even open the church to have a group (p. 344).

In certain regions (Appalachia in particular), prescription opioid dependence often originated with physician-prescribed opioids used to treat pain from workplace injuries associated with manual labor [2, 7, 13, 26]. Leukefeld et al. identified two primary pathways to prescription opioid misuse as reported by their key informants, represented by educators, community leaders, healthcare providers, and law enforcement officials: recreational use and physical pain [26]. While physical pain was generally cited as a more common pathway than recreational use, perspectives differed across informant groups. Community leaders were more likely to attribute opioid use to recreational activity (89%) than to physical pain (84%), whereas healthcare providers more often pointed to pain (93%) over recreational use (60%). Educators also emphasized physical pain (95%) more than law enforcement officials did (76%).

Spatial inequalities were often perceived by study participants as risk factors for opioid use, particularly in rural environments. These populations are widely dispersed with significant geographic distances between destinations. Remoteness and long travel distances to services compound existing local shortages, further complicating access to overdose prevention education and harm reduction services [2, 5, 6, 8, 15, 16]. Limited and costly public transportation options, difficulties with retaining specialists and staff at treatment facilities, and poor access to the remaining manufacturing jobs in the region also contributed to this risk environment [6, 8, 15, 17]. Even in study settings where treatment programs or harm reduction services were available, transportation barriers (e.g., no private car) prevented clients from reaching them. As one participant in Nolte et al.'s study in rural New England observed [7]:

> If you take limited hours and then you take limited transportation, you put the two things together, you have a serious access problem… And sometimes you might have to hang out for hours just finding something to do before you can make it back to your home.

Various aspects of the physical environment also influenced where individuals used drugs, whether in public or in private. In several studies, participants explained that fear of law enforcement shaped the physical spaces and social environments in which young adults (in urban or rural places) elected to use drugs [2, 5, 7, 20]. In Cloud et al.'s study, most drug users preferred injecting drugs in the privacy of their homes, where they could control safety and hygiene (e.g., personal syringes and cookers, sanitized counter tops) [2]. However, to evade arrest, they often resorted to using drugs in "trap houses," which were private homes, apartments, trailers, or motel rooms where groups of people gathered to buy and inject drugs. These environments fostered common proximal risk behaviors, such as sharing drug equipment.

13.4 Policy Factors

The policy dimension of the risk environment for drug users contains multiple barriers, including limited access to harm reduction and drug treatment services, lack of accessible mental health services, and a dearth of program-level policies. Risk of harm is magnified accordingly. Participants commonly mentioned that lack of harm reduction services resulted in inadequate access to clean needles and syringes, increasing the unsafe practice of sharing injecting equipment [2, 5, 6, 21].

Political factors further compound these issues. Fear of arrest follows policies like restrictive policing practices or opposition to sterile needle programs, driving potentially riskier injecting behaviors [2, 5]. As one drug user in Cloud et al. suggested, his firsthand encounters with the police posed a dilemma: admit to carrying syringes, leading to paraphernalia charges, or deny it, risking "wanton endangerment" charges for an accidental needle stick [2]:

> And the cop, the first thing they ask is there anything that will stick me or poke me? If you say no, and hope they don't find it, then you're going to get like wanton endangerment and do a long time [in prison], you know. Nobody is going to say, 'I've got a needle in my back pocket.' because then you're getting paraphernalia or whatever, and still wanton endangerment. They still might charge you with it (p. 10).

Treatment center policies can also contribute to the risk environment. Participants in Linton et al. criticized rigid, zero-tolerance policies and one-size-fits-all drug programs that discouraged seeking treatment [5]. Additionally, Buer, Leukefeld, and Havens observed that excessive paperwork prevented women from accessing buprenorphine and methadone at local clinics [17].

These program-level challenges intersected with physical factors and spatial inequalities in the rural risk environment. The shortage of treatment programs, coupled with high clinician caseloads at existing sites and vast geographic service areas, limited the time staff could spend with clients and resulted in lengthy appointment wait times [16, 17]. As a participant in George et al. commented, mental healthcare access is hampered by these excessive wait times [15]:

> Some people do need access to mental health care because I know, people among work and my own family, … if they want to schedule appointments with mental health providers, it's like, well, this is 2 months in advance. So, really disheartening to wanna reach out and you're willing to get help, but just can't get it (p. 6).

State and federal policies also contribute to the possibility of opioid-related harms, according to study participants. For example, to qualify for government disability after a workplace injury, individuals were required to submit evidence of medication use, thereby increasing their exposure to prescription opioids. A participant in Redican et al. expanded on this inadvertent promotion of opioid use [13]:

> If you worked in the coal mines and you didn't have a college education and you got a back injury, you weren't likely to go to the college and get a degree and get a different job. You were going on disability. And if you go on disability … one of the things that they look at is your medication. So if you're trying to get disability and you've got a back problem, then your doctor's going to say, well you need these medications. So a lot of people get addicted to pain medications not because they choose to or because they want to, but because the system has kind of set it up…. Because if you want your disability, you better be showing that you're disabled (p. 160).

Additional policy challenges are often linked to gender and family roles. As Buer, Leukefeld, and Havens note, child protective services (CPS) tend to target mothers rather than fathers for intervention [17]. As a result, men were able to prevent their female partners from leaving drug-centered relationships by threatening to contact CPS and have their children taken away. Racialized surveillance also extends to child welfare systems: By age 18, 53% of Black children will have experienced a CPS investigation, compared to 37.4% among all children, reinforcing a cycle where addiction and parenting are more harshly scrutinized for families of color [27].

Newly implemented policies limiting opioid prescriptions for chronic pain also led to frustration and reduced quality of life [12, 13]. In Roberson et al., participants with pain complained that systemwide changes to address the opioid epidemic had negatively impacted their daily lives in several ways [12]:

> Without opioids, I wouldn't be able to do things for my family. They work. However, I live in an area where they are abused. Because of this, I can't get them anymore. I have severe sciatic nerve pain. It's the only thing that had worked for me (Literature Supplement).

Without access to prescribed opioids, some people chose another route to manage ongoing pain and withdrawal symptoms: They substituted street drugs—black market pharmaceuticals, heroin, fentanyl, or other substances—for legal painkillers. A participant in Nolte et al.'s study described the path that took her from prescription opioids to heroin [7]:

> And then the doctor took them [prescription opioids] away from me, and I was in pain. I was sick, throwing up…physically sick from not having it. And where did I go? I went to the streets to find them. And then that became too expensive. And then I went to heroin (p. 4).

All of the risks described above, in both rural and urban places, were exacerbated by COVID-19 and the rising misuse of synthetic opioids and polysubstances. Disturbingly, a study by Trappen and McLean that revisited the city of McKeesport during the pandemic found that these negative impacts were compounded by long-time social isolation and physical distancing already present in the area [22]. Future qualitative research should delve deeper into these interconnected factors to enhance understanding of community experiences and to aid development of more effective interventions.

13.5 Addressing the Roots of Harm

This chapter has illustrated how economic dislocation, social disintegration, geographic isolation, and punitive policy frameworks combine to produce environments saturated with risk and despair. Rather than viewing opioid-related harms as the inevitable outcome of drug availability, it is more accurate and more productive to examine how the conditions outlined here predispose individuals to seek solace in substances. The persistent policy focus on supply-side enforcement, while politically expedient, fails to address the environmental roots of substance use and often exacerbates harm.

To meaningfully reduce drug-related suffering, policymakers must stop treating addiction as a matter of individual failure or illicit supply and instead address the societal fractures that fuel demand. This means building recovery-oriented systems of care, investing in social infrastructure, and creating environments of inclusion and dignity. In the next chapter, we further explore how to redesign communities and policies to reduce demand by meeting people's basic social, psychological, and economic needs—thereby confronting the crisis at its foundation.

References

1. Rhodes T. The 'risk environment': a framework for understanding and reducing drug-related harm. Int J Drug Policy. 2002;13(2):85–94.
2. Cloud DH, Ibragimov U, Prood N, Young AM, Cooper HLF. Rural risk environments for hepatitis c among young adults in Appalachian Kentucky. Int J Drug Policy. 2019;72:47–54.
3. Williams TM, Dodge FC. Third spaces and opioid use within Black communities of Dane County: a qualitative secondary data analysis. J Community Pract. 2022;30(3):332–50.

4. Oldenburg R. The great good place: cafes, coffee shops, community centers, beauty parlors, general stores, bars, hangouts and how they get you through the day. 1st ed. New York: Paragon House; 1989. p. 338.
5. Linton SL, Winiker A, Tormohlen KN, Schneider KE, McLain G, Sherman SG, et al. "People don't just start shooting heroin on their 18(th) birthday": a qualitative study of community stakeholders' perspectives on adolescent opioid use and opportunities for intervention in Baltimore, Maryland. Prev Sci. 2021;22(5):621–32.
6. McLean K. "There's nothing here": deindustrialization as risk environment for overdose. Int J Drug Policy. 2016;29:19–26.
7. Nolte K, Drew AL, Friedmann PD, Romo E, Kinney LM, Stopka TJ. Opioid initiation and injection transition in rural northern New England: a mixed-methods approach. Drug Alcohol Depend. 2020;217:108256.
8. Cody SL, Newman S, Bui C, Sharp-Marbury R, Scott L. Substance use and opioid-related stigma among Black communities in the rural South. Arch Psychiatr Nurs. 2023;46:127–32.
9. Walters SM, Frank D, Felsher M, Jaiswal J, Fletcher S, Bennett AS, et al. How the rural risk environment underpins hepatitis C risk: Qualitative findings from rural southern Illinois, United States. Int J Drug Policy. 2023;112:103930.
10. Substance Abuse and Mental Health Services Administration. Key substance use and mental health indicators in the United States: results from the 2020 National Survey on Drug Use and Health, HHS Publication No. PEP21-07-01-003, NSDUH Series H-56. Rockville: Center for Behavioral Health Statistics and Quality, Substance Abuse and Mental Health Services Administration; 2021. Available from: https://www.samhsa.gov/data/.
11. Thompson JR, Creasy SL, Mair CF, Burke JG. Drivers of opioid use in Appalachian Pennsylvania: cross-cutting social and community-level factors. Int J Drug Policy. 2020;78:102706.
12. Roberson PNE, Cortez G, Trull LH, Lenger K. In their own words: how opioids have impacted the lives of "Everyday" people living in Appalachia. J Appalach Health. 2020;2(4):26–36.
13. Redican KJ, Marek LI, Brock DJ, McCance-Katz EF. Exploring the etiologic factors and dynamics of prescription drug abuse in Southwest Virginia. Health Promot Perspect. 2012;2(2):153–65.
14. Sered SS. The opioid crisis and the infrastructure of social capital. Int J Drug Policy. 2019;71:47–55.
15. George DR, Snyder B, Van Scoy LJ, Brignone E, Sinoway L, Sauder C, et al. Perceptions of diseases of despair by members of rural and urban high-prevalence communities: a qualitative study. JAMA Netw Open. 2021;4(7):e2118134.
16. Thomas N, van de Ven K, Mulrooney KJD. The impact of rurality on opioid-related harms: a systematic review of qualitative research. Int J Drug Policy. 2020;85:102607.
17. Buer LM, Leukefeld CG, Havens JR. "I'm stuck": women's navigations of social networks and prescription drug misuse in Central Appalachia. North Am Dialogue. 2016;19(2):70–84.
18. Schalkoff CA, Richard EL, Piscalko HM, Sibley AL, Brook DL, Lancaster KE, et al. "Now we are seeing the tides wash in": trauma and the opioid epidemic in rural Appalachian Ohio. Subst Use Misuse. 2021;56(5):650–9.
19. Draus PJ, Carlson RG. Needles in the haystacks: the social context of initiation to heroin injection in rural Ohio. Subst Use Misuse. 2006;41(8):1111–24.
20. Smith BD, Lewis Q, Offiong A, Willis K, Prioleau M, Powell TW. "It's on every corner": assessing risk environments in Baltimore, MD using a racialized risk environment model. J Ethn Subst Abus. 2024;23(1):95–109.
21. Guise A, Horyniak D, Melo J, McNeil R, Werb D. The experience of initiating injection drug use and its social context: a qualitative systematic review and thematic synthesis. Addiction. 2017;112(12):2098–111.
22. Trappen SL, McLean KJ. Policing pain: a qualitative study of non-criminal justice approaches to managing opioid overdose during the COVID-19 pandemic. J Prev Interv Community. 2021;49(2):136–51.
23. Bourdieu P. Distinction. In: Social theory re-wired. Routledge; 1986. p. 177–92.

24. Bourdieu P. The forms of capital. In: Cultural theory: an anthology; 1986. p. 81–93.
25. Centers for Disease Control and Prevention. Multiple cause of death data on CDC WONDER. Atlanta: Centers for Disease Control and Prevention; 2025. [cited 2025 Oct 10]. Available from: https://wonder.cdc.gov/mcd.html.
26. Leukefeld C, Walker R, Havens J, Leedham CA, Tolbert V. What does the community say: key informant perceptions of rural prescription drug use. J Drug Issues. 2007;37(3):503–24.
27. Kim H, Wildeman C, Jonson-Reid M, Drake B. Lifetime prevalence of investigating child maltreatment among US children. Am J Public Health. 2017;107(2):274–80.

Upstream Determinants of Opioid Risk: Trauma, Stigma, and Social Capital in the Risk Environment Qualitative Literature

14

Being able to feel safe with other people is probably the single most important aspect of mental health.

—Bessel van der Kolk (The Body Keeps the Score, 2014)

14.1 Introduction

This chapter builds on themes in earlier qualitative studies, drawing connections between lived experiences and broader patterns found across public health, psychology, sociology, and addiction medicine. It situates those insights within a wider body of research that seeks to understand how personal and collective adversity shape substance use trajectories and overdose risk [1]. Specifically, it examines the enduring effects of adverse childhood experiences (ACEs), historical trauma, stigma, and the erosion of social capital—factors that remain underemphasized in dominant explanations of the opioid crisis. Tracing how these forces contribute to both the onset and persistence of opioid use disorder (OUD), this chapter also uncovers the structural and psychological barriers to effective treatment and long-term recovery. In doing so, it further advances the work of reframing the crisis through a social-ecological lens, moving us closer to interventions that address not just behavior, but the broken systems and legacies of inequality that shape it.

14.2 Childhood Trauma

A substantial literature has established a relationship between childhood trauma and drug use across the life course [2–4]. Compared to other substance users, people who misuse opioids (PWMO) tend to have more extensive trauma histories as well as higher rates of post-traumatic stress disorder (PTSD), which is itself associated with interpersonal trauma [5–8]. Specific types of trauma have been linked to

L. R. Webster, S. Eichberg, *Deconstructing Toxic Narratives*,
https://doi.org/10.1007/978-3-032-23135-2_14

specific substance use behaviors; for example, initiation into injection drug use (IDU) is associated with sexual and physical abuse [9–11].

Trauma has a cumulative effect that lasts into adulthood [3, 4, 12]. The Adverse Childhood Events study examined 10 distinct categories of childhood trauma and their associations with early initiation and lifetime use of illicit drugs. It showed a strong gradient for the relationship between cumulative trauma and illicit drug use beginning in adolescence and extending into adulthood [3]. It also revealed a persistent relationship between ACEs and initiation of drug use across four successive cohorts, suggesting that the effects of ACEs may be immune to social changes, including shifts in drug supply, public sentiment on drugs, and anti-drug campaigns.

Figures 14.1 and 14.2 illustrate the effects of ACEs on deaths of despair, including drug use, as well as suicide [3, 4].

The literature on ACEs shows a strong relationship between childhood traumatic events and opioid use behaviors, such as early opioid use initiation, opioid misuse, and lifetime overdose [13–15]. This research has identified associations between various ACEs, substances, diagnoses, and intervening variables [16–18]. One investigation using large sample survey data identified associations between nine types of childhood traumas and adulthood prescription pain reliever use as well as IDU [19]. Traumas included neglect, emotional, physical, and sexual abuse, parental incarceration, parental binge drinking, witnessed violence, threatened with violence, and experienced violence. The analysis revealed a high prevalence of prescription pain reliever use within the sample, with 28% having ever used by early adulthood. This percentage was prone to increasing later in life as the impact of trauma can surface after emerging adulthood [19, 20]. A strong and consistent dose–response relationship was evident between prescription pain reliever use and cumulative trauma exposure. The odds of prescription pain reliever use rose with each additional childhood trauma experienced, increasing by 34%, 50%, 70%, 217%, and 179% for one,

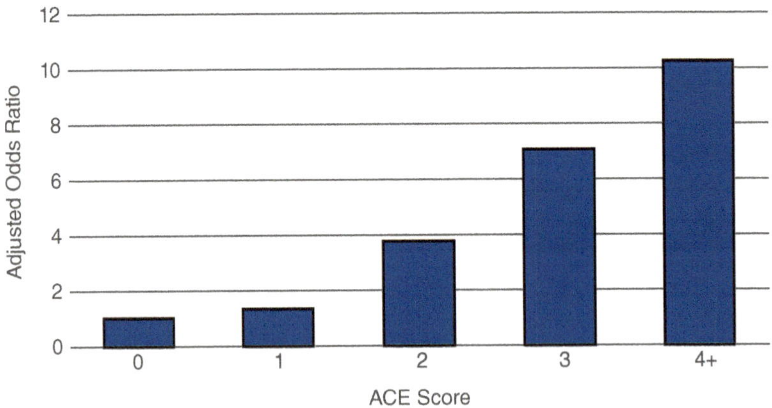

Fig. 14.1 Impact of cumulative ACE scores on the odds of intravenous drug use. Bars represent the adjusted odds ratio for scores 0 through 4+. ACEs Adverse Childhood Experiences, IV intravenous. (Source: Felitti et al. [4])

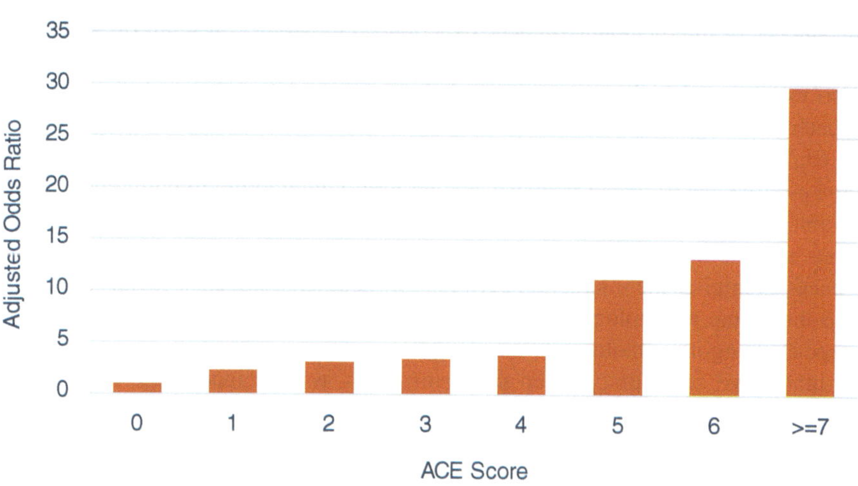

Fig. 14.2 Relationship between cumulative ACE scores and the odds of adult suicide attempts. The adjusted odds ratio indicates a sharp increase in risk as the number of adverse experiences rises, peaking at the 7 or more category. ACEs Adverse Childhood Experiences. (Source: Adapted from Dube et al. [139])

two, three, four, and five or more traumas, respectively [19]. Specific traumas—such as neglect, emotional abuse, parental incarceration, and binge drinking—were associated with a 25–55% increase in the odds of prescription pain reliever use. Notably, sexual abuse and witnessed violence were associated with almost three and five times the odds of IDU. Another investigation found that 6.7% of adolescents reported lifetime non-medical use of prescription drugs [21]. In the final multivariate model, past experiences of witnessed violence (OR = 3.76, CI = 2.65–5.33, $p < 0.001$) and lifetime PTSD (OR = 2.25, CI = 1.39–3.63, $p < 0.001$) were significantly associated with increased odds of non-medical use. Sexual and physical assault were significantly correlated with non-medical use in bivariate testing, but were no longer significant in the final multivariate model.

An analysis of 2004–2012 National Survey on Drug Use and Health data found a significant positive association between parental and adolescent non-medical prescription opioid use (adjusted OR 1.3, 95% CI, 1.09–1.56) [22]. Adolescents whose parents used prescription opioids non-medically were more likely to report their own lifetime use (13.9%) compared to those whose parents did not (8.1%). The relationship between parental and adolescent non-medical prescription opioid use varied based on the parent's sex: maternal use showed a stronger association with adolescent use (OR 1.62, 95% CI, 1.28–2.056) than paternal use. Race/ethnicity had no effect on this relationship. Other correlates of adolescent prescription opioid use included delinquency, depression, other substance use, perceived peer substance use, and parental smoking [22].

Evidence suggests that trauma, particularly interpersonal violence and child maltreatment, may be more prevalent in rural populations, especially in impoverished environments, than in non-rural areas [23–26]. A clinic-based study reported higher prevalence of interpersonal violence experienced by women in small rural (22.5%) and isolated (17.9%) areas compared to urban women (15.5%) [26]. Rural women also experienced higher severity of physical abuse than urban counterparts and greater distances from available resources.

Childhood trauma, particularly in resource-deprived or socially-isolated settings, creates a risk environment that shapes long-term vulnerability to opioid use. When trauma is compounded by geographic barriers, the structural and emotional dimensions of risk converge. Within the Risk Environment Framework (REF), these experiences exemplify the interaction between physical environments, social structures, and individual psychological outcomes—making prevention and treatment all the more challenging without systemic change.

Innovative community-based programs, such as peer recovery coach models implemented in overdose hotspots like Huntington, W.V., offer hopeful counterpoints [27]. These initiatives channel lived experience into frontline response and recovery, enhancing trust and continuity of care in structurally vulnerable areas.

14.3 Historical Trauma

Historical trauma is defined as "the traumatic experiences undergone by members or descendants of national, religious, or racial/ethnic groups, historically or at present times, as a result of colonization, war, genocide, or other forms of social, political, and cultural subjugation" [28]. Originally conceived to describe the experience of children of Holocaust survivors, the concept has since expanded globally to include colonized Indigenous groups, African Americans, Armenian refugees, Japanese-American survivors of internment camps, Palestinians, and other populations subjected to persecution, victimization, or mass trauma [29]. Historical trauma also applies to populations in regions with a long history of economic exploitation, such as Appalachia.

A central premise of historical trauma is that the psychological repercussions of the original trauma are transmitted to later generations through various biological, environmental, cultural, and social pathways, creating an intergenerational cycle of trauma response [30–32]. Given the established link between chronic stress/PTSD and chronic disease, it is plausible that individuals and groups exposed to historical trauma are more susceptible to poor health outcomes and higher disease prevalence [31, 33, 34]. Not surprisingly, historical trauma is associated with mental disorders (e.g., depression) and a greater likelihood of tobacco and substance use [32, 35, 36].

The empirical literature on historical trauma and substance use is heavily focused on Indigenous populations, particularly American Indians [28, 35, 37–40]. This population, on and off the reservation, reports high rates of alcohol and substance use, mental health disorders, suicide, violence, and behavior-related chronic diseases. Scholars argue that these disparities originate in the colonization experiences of Indigenous peoples and the historical trauma resulting from forced suppression of cultural beliefs and ways of life [41]. Regardless of origin, treatment facilities serving American Indians have lower utilization rates than other facilities due to limited resources within tribal and Indian Health Service-run behavioral health services as well as a shortage of qualified providers near reservations. Additionally, some community members believe that medication treatments conflict with traditional beliefs and healing practices, further hindering access and underscoring the need for culturally-responsive care components [42–44]. Culturally-adapted programs such as the Wellbriety Movement, founded by Don Coyhis and delivered by White Bison, integrate traditional Indigenous practices—like sweat lodge ceremonies, talking circles, drumming, and the Medicine Wheel-based 12-Step framework—as core components of recovery [45–47]. Program guides, such as those from Indian Health Service and White Bison, note that the Medicine Wheel and 12-Step model was developed from White Bison teachings and is widely used in tribal programs to combine spiritual, emotional, and community healing. This approach is one of culture as prevention and emphasizes reinforcement of cultural identity as essential to long-term healing.

Studies examining historical trauma and substance use within Indigenous populations commonly apply the Historical Losses Scale (HLS) and the Historical Losses Associated Symptoms Scale (HLASS) to quantify Indigenous historical trauma. The HLS contains 12 categories of historical losses and asks respondents to rate on an emotional scale "how frequently these losses come to mind" [32] (p. 123). Examples of historical loss include "loss of our land," "loss of our language," "loss of our traditional spiritual ways," and "loss of our people through early death." The HLASS, comprising 12 emotional and somatic responses, asks respondents to rate these responses on a frequency scale with the question "how often you feel [response] when you think about these losses" [32] (p. 125). Research has demonstrated a statistically significant relationship between higher HLS or HLASS scores and substance use; however, the nature of this relationship varies, with some studies indicating a direct association and others an indirect association, with Indigenous historical trauma mediating complex relationships between substance use and variables such as ethnic identity, discrimination, cultural activities, and stressful life events [28, 35, 38]. In some cases, findings have been contradictory across studies [39], so they should be considered with some caution. In addition, inconsistencies in adaptation, scoring, and interpretation of the scales across different studies pose challenges to drawing definitive conclusions about the relationships between variables.

A limited body of qualitative research on substance use and historical trauma in Indigenous populations gives direct voice to the populations affected by these concerns [48–50]. Overall, these studies illustrate how contemporary structures of inequality and racial discrimination intersect with past injustices to create ongoing experiences of social, economic, and political exclusion. Interviews conducted with 25 members of an American Indian reservation in Montana revealed that informants tied substance use—specifically, methamphetamines, alcohol, and prescription pills—to stressors arising from everyday living conditions, including poverty, unemployment, domestic violence, and child abuse [50]. However, they contextualized these concerns within the broader history of colonialism and forced assimilation that devastated traditional ways of life in their communities. As one informant put it, “Oppression is the overarching umbrella for all of sickness with drugs and alcohol” [50] (p. 1).

Another informant described a persistent sense of emptiness among reservation residents and ascribed the emotion to trauma passed down from generation to generation epigenetically. This informant also indicated that people on the reservation lacked understanding of the origin of these widespread feelings of loss and helplessness and had no clear pathway to healing [50]:

> There’s a hole in your heart that cannot be filled due to losing a loved one, due to something that happened maybe three or four generations ago with our grandparents. We carry that, but we don’t know what it is. And if we don’t know what it is, and we’re not offering things to help our children and our people understand, then how are we going to heal? So you have intergenerational trauma. You carry that, and it’s in our genetics (p. 11).

Historical trauma represents a time-extended structural determinant of opioid vulnerability, shaping risk through pathways of cultural dislocation, chronic stress, and systemic exclusion. The REF underscores the long-term transmission of harm through policies and collective memory, especially where culturally-appropriate services are absent. These multigenerational effects complicate individual healing and demand community-based interventions grounded in justice and reconciliation.

14.4 Stigma

Research on stigma within the field of addictive behaviors has grown over the past two decades, although the overall volume of studies remains limited [51]. Because the literature is cross-disciplinary, definitions and frameworks to investigate stigma are often inconsistent. This is further complicated by the culturally and historically-dependent nature of behaviors and statuses, which produces variable and complex understandings of stigma [52].

Sociologist Ervin Goffman defined stigma as the discrediting of an individual based on social identity or involvement in an undesirable social group [53]. Other researchers have observed that stigmatization occurs within the context of unequal social conditions and power relations, resulting in the “othering,” discrimination against, or ostracization of people with the stigmatized identity [54]. More recent conceptualizations of stigma posit several types of stigma operating at different levels of influence, thereby amplifying their impact and perpetuating poor health outcomes. These types include public stigma, perceived stigma, enacted stigma, and self-stigma [51]. These concepts have been applied to the misuse of opioids and other substances [55]. As discussed in this paper, stigma manifests in many ways from physicians’ pathologizing of addiction to drug users’ feelings of shame and fear in drug-ravaged communities.

Public stigma is maintained via stereotypes about PWMO [55]. In clinical settings, providers may hold negative perceptions of patients with substance use disorders (SUDs), characterizing them as violent, manipulative, or less motivated than other patient groups [56–58]. Patients with chronic pain often emphasize their own "responsible" use of pain medication as legitimate pain management, positioning it as superior to recreational consumption [59].

Enacted stigma refers to behaviors that manifest from public stigma. Within health care, this may lead to knowing or unwitting discrimination against patients with SUDs, resulting in compromised quality of care [60, 61]. For example, the stigma surrounding methadone is probably the most common and widespread stigma related to opioids, with clinicians and pharmacists expressing and acting on concerns about its suitability as a substitute for other opioids [62]. In treatment programs, strict care policies that disregard patient autonomy and impose harsh penalties, including treatment termination for policy violations such as smoking or positive toxicology results, reduce patient engagement and damage the provider–patient relationship [63–65]. The implementation of rigid, opioid-prescribing guidelines has also led to various forms of enacted stigma, such as strict dosage caps or duration limits and physician-imposed, noncollaborative tapers for long-term pain patients, which can increase the risk of adverse reactions and drive patients toward non-prescription opioids [66, 67].

Public and enacted stigma become structural when they are embedded in macro-level norms, laws, and policies. These structures reinforce differential treatment for PWMO, implicitly holding them accountable for a perceived lack of control and branding them as undeserving of support and care. This increases public support for criminalization [55]. Enacted stigma is also evident in the separation of drug treatment from other forms of care, leading to overly narrow treatment plans that fail to holistically address other substance use, mental health, and physical health conditions. Patients may encounter inadequate reimbursement for treatment, as insurance often covers only basic services like medication delivery and weekly healthcare provider encounters, neglecting the complex needs of patients who require additional counseling, pharmacologic therapy, and care management [68].

Internalized (i.e., self) stigma occurs when people with SUD/OUD take onboard or anticipate the public stigma associated with their behavior, resulting in negative health outcomes and barriers to recovery [69]. For example, in people with SUD/OUD, internalized and/or anticipated stigma has been linked with psychological distress and poor quality of life, persistent substance use, and avoidance of or diminished engagement with care and treatment [70–75]. Research also shows that when people with SUD do seek care, they frequently encounter discrimination and receive suboptimal quality of care [76].

It is crucial to recognize that opioid-related stigma manifests differently depending on type of opioid, method of acquisition, and the setting of use. For example, people who inject illicit opioids tend to be highly stigmatized, encountering more hostile public reactions and greater obstacles to accessing health services [75].

Stigma functions as a structural force that interacts with healthcare policy, social norms, and individual psychology to inhibit care-seeking and exacerbate marginalization. Within the REF, stigma bridges social and policy environments, reinforcing inequity and amplifying risk across levels. Its impact is particularly harsh in areas with limited harm reduction infrastructure or punitive drug enforcement, deepening spatial disparities and discouraging engagement with lifesaving care.

Programs like OnPoint NYC's overdose prevention centers embody resilience through harm reduction, offering non-judgmental, lifesaving care that counters stigmatizing systems and empowers individuals at risk [77].

14.5 Social Capital

As discussed previously, social capital refers to the beneficial outcomes derived from social networks, built upon shared values, obligations, and expectations. Social capital provides members of a social unit with assets such as social cohesion, trust, and fellowship, which can be mobilized to facilitate collective action and advance shared interests. For example, people may leverage social capital to obtain support with tasks such as managing illness, raising children or securing jobs, housing, or educational opportunities [78–80].

The term gained prominence following the 2000 publication of sociologist Robert Putnam's book, *Bowling Alone: The Collapse and Revival of American Community* [80]. Putnam argued that since 1950, as American society became more affluent with increases in time and work pressures and suburban sprawl, social capital declined, weakening community bonds and heightening individual feelings of anomie. Putnam demonstrated the decline in social capital through analysis of national surveys regarding membership and participation in civic organizations, labeling American's growing social and civic disengagement as "bowling alone" [79, 80]. While influential, Putnam's work was not universally praised, with some critics arguing that civic activity was not dwindling but instead assuming different forms [81].

Across academic disciplines, scholars use measures of social capital to explain variations in population outcomes. Communities and regions with higher levels of social capital tend to have healthier citizens, lower suicide rates, better educational outcomes, and reduced crime and fear of crime [80, 82–85]. In research on drug use, higher levels of social capital have been associated with decreased substance use among adolescents and young adults [86–88]. Economists have speculated that social capital may have significant explanatory power for why (or to what extent) unemployment elevates drug-related deaths.

Various academic and media sources have highlighted the role of community disengagement and social isolation as major drivers of deaths of despair and opioid overdoses, underscoring the impact of declining social capital [89–91]. The COVID-19 pandemic further illustrated where social isolation jeopardized wellbeing. Social capital possibly played a mediating role, for example, by motivating people to follow social distancing protocols. A study examining the effects of social capital on health outcomes during European pandemic lockdowns, conducted from mid-March until end of June 2020, found that a one-standard-deviation increase in social capital resulted in between 14% and 34% fewer COVID-19 cases per capita and between 6% and 35% fewer excess deaths per capita [92]. Investigators applied a within-county-across-counties research design to account for regional differences among countries. Similarly, another study found that shifting a county from the 25th to the 75th percentile social capital distribution (using various measures of social capital) resulted in an 18% decrease in cumulative COVID-19 infections and 5.7% decrease in deaths, reflecting less spread of the disease [93].

The significant geographic variation in opioid overdose death concentrations suggests the presence of unidentified variables that either protect against or increase vulnerability to overdoses, with social capital being a potential contributor [94]. Notably, there are considerable disparities in social capital levels across rural communities, with Midwestern counties exhibiting higher levels than other rural regions [95].

Several studies have directly explored the relationship between drug use and social capital, finding a link between the two. Ford, Sacra, and Yohros examined the effects of neighborhood characteristics such as social capital and social disorganization on adolescent prescription drug-related behaviors, revealing a significant inverse relationship between social capital and prescription drug use generally and opioid use specifically [96]. Zoorob and Salemi investigated the relationship between drug overdose mortality and social capital and observed a statistically significant inverse relationship between social capital and county-level drug overdose mortality rates [94]. Their analysis found that counties at the highest social capital quintile were 83% less likely to be in the "high-overdose" category (>16 deaths per 100,000) and 75% less likely to be in the "moderate-overdose" category (4–16 deaths), suggesting a protective effect against drug use initiation, as well as support for recovery or addiction treatment seeking.

Yang, Kim, and Matthews evaluated the thesis behind Case's and Deaton's "deaths of despair" by examining the relationship between high unemployment and opioid-related mortality rates [97]. Their analysis compared counties in states where opioid-related mortality rates had rapidly increased since 2013 to counties in states where rates had not. While they did not detect a direct association between high unemployment and opioid-related mortality rates, they did discover that high unemployment rates were negatively associated with social capital, and low social capital levels affected high opioid-related mortality.

The tie between social capital and individual and group resilience is an area of research that has been well explored in disaster research but less so in drug addiction [98]. Social capital facilitates personal and community adaptation and recovery after traumatic events, such as earthquakes, hurricanes, or disease epidemics, helping to mobilize resources and to build capacity to prepare and withstand against future catastrophe [99, 100]. Applying a resiliency framework to the study of drug use and addiction in large and small communities promises a means to create interventions that orient individuals toward the future by maximizing determination, agency, and social cooperation.

Recovery community centers like Anchor in Rhode Island demonstrate how rebuilding social capital through peer engagement and wraparound services can restore purpose and reduce isolation in the aftermath of addiction [101].

Social capital operates as a protective or amplifying factor in the risk environment, modulating how communities absorb shocks and support recovery. When social ties are frayed—through disinvestment, isolation, or mistrust—individual resilience weakens and vulnerability increases. The REF positions social capital as a mediator that can either buffer or heighten exposure to harm depending on broader structural conditions.

14.6 Barriers to Treatment and Recovery

The previously discussed factors, such as trauma, social capital deficits, and stigma, not only contribute to the risk of OUD and opioid-related mortality but also impede access to and success within addiction treatment and recovery.

Evidence-based OUD treatments, including medications for OUD (MOUD), are underused in treatment and recovery plans. In 2023, of the 48.5 (16.7%) million people aged 12 and older who reported an SUD in the past year, only 7.1 million (14.6%) received treatment and just 2.3 million (0.8%) underwent addiction treatment involving MOUD. Similarly, in 2022, only 25% of people who needed OUD treatment received MOUD [102, 103].

Compounding the problem that many people cannot—or do not—access appropriate treatment for OUD, racial and economic disparities are evident in addiction treatment, as they are in other spheres of substance misuse [104]. These disparities are rooted in a much larger system of structural racism within the American healthcare system and in an established history of medicalization that differentiates addiction treatment along racial and class lines [105].

Black, Indigenous, and People of Color (BIPOC) populations, particularly those living in poverty, face multiple challenges to OUD treatment and recovery, including barriers to health insurance, childcare, and transportation along with the broader burdens of poverty. Within the healthcare system, a legacy of institutional racism contributes to mistrust between Black patients and their white or non-Black physicians, impeding doctor–patient communication and reducing satisfaction with care [106, 107]. Medical system bias, leading to a shortage of Black and Hispanic physicians, further constrains access to culturally or linguistically sensitive or responsive treatment [108–110].

Racial and class biases influence OUD treatment outcomes. The typical reason given for why African Americans were relatively untouched by the prescription opioid epidemic is that they were "perversely protected" because of constrained access to prescription painkillers [105, 111]. This differential treatment reflects racial bias in the assessment and management of pain. Healthcare providers often undervalue or discount reports of pain from BIPOC patients, relative to white patients. As a result, Black patients are more likely to be undertreated, and when prescribed pain medications, receive lower doses [112–117]. Specifically, with prescription opioids, Black patients are less likely than white patients to receive the analgesic or to be prescribed equivalent doses across heterogeneous healthcare contexts [112]. These contexts include the following:

- End-of-life pain care [118]
- Emergency medicine [119–121] (Fig. 14.3)
- Veterans Health Administration appointments [122]
- Traumatic and surgical pain [123]
- Arthritis pain [124]
- Chronic noncancer pain [125, 126]

Treatment coverage for SUD, particularly MOUD, remains limited in many Black communities due to structural and attitudinal barriers. A review of 21 studies found that, in over 75% of cases, Black individuals had lower access to or utilization of medication-assisted treatment (MAT)/MOUD compared to white individuals (Fig. 14.4) [127]. Considered the "gold standard" of addiction care, MAT (of which MOUD is a component) involves dispensing one of three FDA-approved drugs: buprenorphine, methadone, or naltrexone in combination with counseling and behavioral therapies [128]. Methadone, a full opioid agonist, and buprenorphine, a partial opioid agonist, are associated with decreased OUD mortality [129].

Although there is abundant evidence of buprenorphine's and methadone's efficacy, the medications still face skepticism from the general public, medical and addiction treatment professionals, and law enforcement, many of whom favor medication-free approaches [128, 130]. As a result, people who receive MAT are at risk for encountering intervention stigma, which is particularly acute for those on methadone maintenance [128, 130]. Long associated with poor and BIPOC drug users, especially heroin injectors, methadone is disparaged as an inferior option to buprenorphine. Furthermore, methadone's restrictive protocols relative to buprenorphine contribute to its disfavor among patients, who sometimes label the drug "liquid shackles" [131].

Not surprisingly, when MAT is available, methadone often is the only treatment option in BIPOC communities [132, 133]. Hansen et al. compared treatment rates

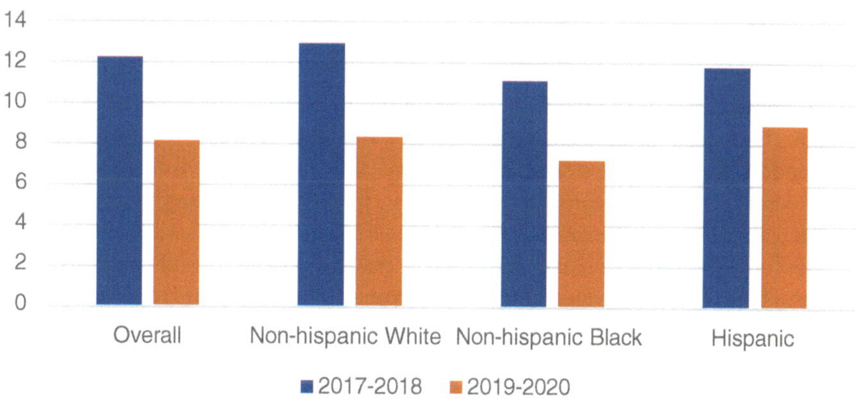

Fig. 14.3 The National The Hospital Ambulatory Medical Care Survey was discontinued in 2023, ending data collection. (Source: National Center for Health Statistics, National Hospital Ambulatory Medical Care Survey, 2017–2020)

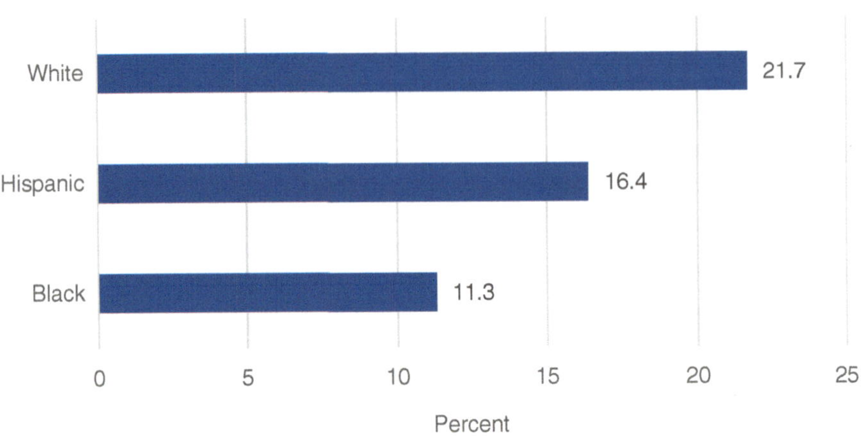

Fig. 14.4 Survey of people aged 12+ diagnosed with opioid use disorder. (Source: Substance Abuse and Mental Health Services Administration (SAMHSA), 2022 National Survey on Drug Use and Health (NSDUH))

for buprenorphine and methadone in each ZIP code in New York City (aggregated to social areas) and found that buprenorphine treatment rates were highest in areas with the greatest income and percentage of white residents, including parts of Staten Island, Queens (bordering Long Island), the North Bronx (bordering Westchester County), and lower and midtown Manhattan [132]. In contrast, methadone was concentrated in places with the greatest percentage of low-income Hispanic residents. Similar patterns of ethnic and racial treatment segregation have been seen in other studies mapping geographic distribution and spatial arrangements of treatment centers [134–136].

This differential access to buprenorphine based on race/ethnicity, income, and other factors stems from obstacles facing both patients and clinicians. Because buprenorphine is exclusively available in office settings, prescribed and dispensed by primary care physicians, patients without access to primary care, including many low-income or uninsured members of racial and ethnic minorities, are excluded. A study tracking trends in outpatient prescriptions of buprenorphine found that white patients and those using private insurance or self-pay were more likely to receive buprenorphine treatment during office visits [133]. Strikingly, for every appointment where a person of color received a prescription for buprenorphine, there were 35 such appointments for white patients.

Doctors who treat uninsured or publicly insured patients are also less likely to obtain a buprenorphine waiver due to low reimbursement rates and resource barriers that prevent them from undergoing the training required to care for buprenorphine patients [137]. Methadone is made available via federally-regulated treatment programs that are disproportionally located in low-income areas. Methadone is also a more cumbersome treatment, requiring patients to visit clinics daily (at least initially), undergo mandatory drug testing, and attend counseling [137]. Ultimately, the differences between buprenorphine and methadone treatment create a two-tiered treatment system that disadvantages BIPOC individuals with OUD.

Treatment access and recovery barriers reflect the culmination of structural harms described earlier—trauma, stigma, and low social capital—and are reinforced by policy-level inequities. As national data indicate, Black patients are significantly less likely to receive buprenorphine and more likely referred to methadone, while 92% of buprenorphine patients in national samples were white compared with just 53% of methadone recipients [137, 138]. These disparities align squarely with the policy environment dimension of the REF, showing how regulatory systems and treatment geography institutionalize risk and inequity.

14.7 Toward a Future of Equity in Care

In this chapter, we have deepened our review of the socioecological understanding of the opioid crisis by exploring key structural and psychological determinants that shape vulnerability to opioid use and overdose. Building on the qualitative accounts and the REF introduced in prior chapters, this chapter synthesizes evidence from multiple disciplines to underscore the significance of ACEs, historical trauma, stigma, and social capital. Each of these forces not only contributes to opioid use initiation and persistence but also impedes access to evidence-based treatment and long-term recovery. These determinants are often unequally distributed across communities, shaped by systemic racism, geographic disparities, and deeply rooted historical legacies.

By spotlighting these upstream drivers, we challenge prevailing narratives that blame individuals or narrowly focus on drug supply. Structural change must come by acknowledging the broader context of despair, dislocation, and disinvestment. This perspective provides a powerful counterpoint to simplistic, punitive approaches and paves the way for the next chapter, which turns toward forward-looking strategies: policies and social investments aimed at creating the conditions that reduce demand for harmful substance use. To effectively confront the crisis, we must move beyond reactive models and toward a future defined by equity, opportunity, and care. The next chapter explores transformative policy and programmatic solutions, ranging from Medicaid expansion and Housing First initiatives to harm reduction integration and culturally-grounded care models that aim to reshape the structural conditions driving opioid vulnerability.

References

1. Rhodes T. The 'risk environment': a framework for understanding and reducing drug-related harm. Int J Drug Policy. 2002;13(2):85–94.
2. Briere J, Kaltman S, Green BL. Accumulated childhood trauma and symptom complexity. J Trauma Stress. 2008;21(2):223–6.

3. Dube SR, Felitti VJ, Dong M, Chapman DP, Giles WH, Anda RF. Childhood abuse, neglect, and household dysfunction and the risk of illicit drug use: the adverse childhood experiences study. Pediatrics. 2003;111(3):564–72.
4. Felitti VJ, Anda RF, Nordenberg D, Williamson DF, Spitz AM, Edwards V, et al. Relationship of childhood abuse and household dysfunction to many of the leading causes of death in adults. The adverse childhood experiences (ACE) study. Am J Prev Med. 1998;14(4):245–58.
5. Lawson KM, Back SE, Hartwell KJ, Moran-Santa Maria M, Brady KT. A comparison of trauma profiles among individuals with prescription opioid, nicotine, or cocaine dependence. Am J Addict. 2013;22(2):127–31.
6. Mills KL, Teesson M, Ross J, Peters L. Trauma, PTSD, and substance use disorders: findings from the Australian National Survey of mental health and Well-being. Am J Psychiatry. 2006;163(4):652–8.
7. Breslau N. The epidemiology of posttraumatic stress disorder: what is the extent of the problem? J Clin Psychiatry. 2001;62(Suppl 17):16–22.
8. Norris FH. Epidemiology of trauma: frequency and impact of different potentially traumatic events on different demographic groups. J Consult Clin Psychol. 1992;60(3):409–18.
9. Ompad DC, Ikeda RM, Shah N, Fuller CM, Bailey S, Morse E, et al. Childhood sexual abuse and age at initiation of injection drug use. Am J Public Health. 2005;95(4):703–9.
10. Roy E, Haley N, Leclerc P, Cédras L, Blais L, Boivin JF. Drug injection among street youths in Montreal: predictors of initiation. J Urban Health. 2003;80(1):92–105.
11. Kerr T, Stoltz JA, Marshall BD, Lai C, Strathdee SA, Wood E. Childhood trauma and injection drug use among high-risk youth. J Adolesc Health. 2009;45(3):300–2.
12. Khoury L, Tang YL, Bradley B, Cubells JF, Ressler KJ. Substance use, childhood traumatic experience, and posttraumatic stress disorder in an urban civilian population. Depress Anxiety. 2010;27(12):1077–86.
13. Stein MD, Conti MT, Kenney S, Anderson BJ, Flori JN, Risi MM, et al. Adverse childhood experience effects on opioid use initiation, injection drug use, and overdose among persons with opioid use disorder. Drug Alcohol Depend. 2017;179:325–9.
14. Swedo EA, Sumner SA, de Fijter S, Werhan L, Norris K, Beauregard JL, et al. Adolescent opioid misuse attributable to adverse childhood experiences. J Pediatr. 2020;224:102–9.e3.
15. Afifi TO, Henriksen CA, Asmundson GJ, Sareen J. Childhood maltreatment and substance use disorders among men and women in a nationally representative sample. Can J Psychiatr. 2012;57(11):677–86.
16. Hughes K, Bellis MA, Hardcastle KA, Sethi D, Butchart A, Mikton C, et al. The effect of multiple adverse childhood experiences on health: a systematic review and meta-analysis. Lancet Public Health. 2017;2(8):e356–e66.
17. Regmi S, Kedia SK, Ahuja NA, Lee G, Entwistle C, Dillon PJ. Association between adverse childhood experiences and opioid use-related behaviors: a systematic review. Trauma Violence Abuse. 2023;25(3):2046–64.
18. Santo T Jr, Campbell G, Gisev N, Tran LT, Colledge S, Di Tanna GL, et al. Prevalence of childhood maltreatment among people with opioid use disorder: a systematic review and meta-analysis. Drug Alcohol Depend. 2021;219:108459.
19. Quinn K, Boone L, Scheidell JD, Mateu-Gelabert P, McGorray SP, Beharie N, et al. The relationships of childhood trauma and adulthood prescription pain reliever misuse and injection drug use. Drug Alcohol Depend. 2016;169:190–8.
20. Widom CS, Weiler BL, Cottler LB. Childhood victimization and drug abuse: a comparison of prospective and retrospective findings. J Consult Clin Psychol. 1999;67(6):867–80.
21. McCauley JL, Danielson CK, Amstadter AB, Ruggiero KJ, Resnick HS, Hanson RF, et al. The role of traumatic event history in non-medical use of prescription drugs among a nationally representative sample of US adolescents. J Child Psychol Psychiatry. 2010;51(1):84–93.
22. Griesler PC, Hu MC, Wall MM, Kandel DB. Nonmedical prescription opioid use by parents and adolescents in the US. Pediatrics. 2019;143(3)

23. Hink AB, Toschlog E, Waibel B, Bard M. Risks go beyond the violence: association between intimate partner violence, mental illness, and substance abuse among females admitted to a rural level I trauma center. J Trauma Acute Care Surg. 2015;79(5):709–14; discussion 15-6.
24. Martz DM, Jameson JP, Page AD. Psychological health and academic success in rural Appalachian adolescents exposed to physical and sexual interpersonal violence. Am J Orthopsychiatry. 2016;86(5):594–601.
25. Orsi R, Yuma-Guerrero P, Sergi K, Pena AA, Shillington AM. Drug overdose and child maltreatment across the United States' rural-urban continuum. Child Abuse Negl. 2018;86:358–67.
26. Peek-Asa C, Wallis A, Harland K, Beyer K, Dickey P, Saftlas A. Rural disparity in domestic violence prevalence and access to resources. J Womens Health (Larchmt). 2011;20(11):1743–9.
27. Sisk T. West Virginia City once battered by opioid overdoses confronts 'Fourth Wave' [Internet]. KFF Health News; 2024 Mar 13 [cited 2025 Aug 7]. Available from: https://kffhealthnews.org/news/article/west-virginia-opioid-overdoses-fourth-wave/.
28. Pokhrel P, Herzog TA. Historical trauma and substance use among native Hawaiian college students. Am J Health Behav. 2014;38(3):420–9.
29. Mohatt NV, Thompson AB, Thai ND, Tebes JK. Historical trauma as public narrative: a conceptual review of how history impacts present-day health. Soc Sci Med. 2014;106:128–36.
30. Kellermann NP. Transmission of holocaust trauma—an integrative view. Psychiatry. 2001;64(3):256–67.
31. Sotero M. A conceptual model of historical trauma: implications for public health practice and research. J Health Disparities Res Pract. 2006;1(1):93–108. Available from: https://ssrn.com/abstract=1350062, https://ssrn.com/abstract=1350062.
32. Whitbeck LB, Adams GW, Hoyt DR, Chen X. Conceptualizing and measuring historical trauma among American Indian people. Am J Community Psychol. 2004;33(3–4):119–30.
33. Brunello N, Davidson JR, Deahl M, Kessler RC, Mendlewicz J, Racagni G, et al. Posttraumatic stress disorder: diagnosis and epidemiology, comorbidity and social consequences, biology and treatment. Neuropsychobiology. 2001;43(3):150–62.
34. Webb NB, editor. Mass trauma and violence: helping families and children cope. New York: The Guilford Press; 2004.
35. Ehlers CL, Gizer IR, Gilder DA, Ellingson JM, Yehuda R. Measuring historical trauma in an American Indian community sample: contributions of substance dependence, affective disorder, conduct disorder and PTSD. Drug Alcohol Depend. 2013;133(1):180–7.
36. Estrada AL. Mexican Americans and historical trauma theory: a theoretical perspective. J Ethn Subst Abus. 2009;8(3):330–40.
37. Gameon JA, Skewes MC. Historical trauma and substance use among American Indian people with current substance use problems. Psychol Addict Behav. 2021;35(3):295–309.
38. Soto C, Baezconde-Garbanati L, Schwartz SJ, Unger JB. Stressful life events, ethnic identity, historical trauma, and participation in cultural activities: associations with smoking behaviors among American Indian adolescents in California. Addict Behav. 2015;50:64–9.
39. Spence N, Wells S, George J, Graham K. An examination of marijuana use among a vulnerable population in Canada. J Racial Ethn Health Disparities. 2014;1(4):247–56.
40. Wiechelt S, Gryczynski J, Johnson J, Caldwell D. Historical trauma among urban American Indians: impact on substance abuse and family cohesion. J Loss Trauma. 2012;17(4):319–36. https://doi.org/10.1080/15325024.2011.616837.
41. Garcia JL. Historical trauma and American Indian/Alaska native youth mental health development and delinquency. New Dir Child Adolesc Dev. 2020;2020(169):41–58.
42. Rieckmann T, Moore L, Croy C, Aarons GA, Novins DK. National overview of medication-assisted treatment for American Indians and Alaska natives with substance use disorders. Psychiatr Serv. 2017;68(11):1136–43.
43. Tipps RT, Buzzard GT, McDougall JA. The opioid epidemic in Indian country. J Law Med Ethics. 2018;46(2):422–36.

44. Zeledon I, Telles V, Dickerson D, Johnson C, Schweigman K, West A, et al. Exploring culturally based treatment options for opioid use disorders among American Indian and Alaska native adults in California. J Stud Alcohol Drugs. 2022;83(4):613–20.
45. Coyhis D, Simonelli R. The native American healing experience. Subst Use Misuse. 2008;43(12–13):1927–49.
46. Rowan M, Poole N, Shea B, Gone JP, Mykota D, Farag M, et al. Cultural interventions to treat addictions in indigenous populations: findings from a scoping study. Subst Abuse Treat Prev Policy. 2014;9(1):34.
47. Buffalo-Boy D, Murray J. Native American SUD peer best practices. Portland: The Regional Facilitation Center; 2022.
48. Baldwin JA, Lowe J, Brooks J, Charbonneau-Dahlen BK, Lawrence G, Johnson-Jennings M, et al. Formative research and cultural tailoring of a substance abuse prevention program for American Indian youth: findings from the intertribal talking circle intervention. Health Promot Pract. 2021;22(6):778–85.
49. Myhra L, Wieling E, Grant H. Substance use in American Indian family relationships: linking past, present, and future. Am J Fam Ther. 2015;43(1):1–12.
50. Skewes MC, Blume AW. Understanding the link between racial trauma and substance use among American Indians. Am Psychol. 2019;74(1):88–100.
51. Kulesza M, Larimer ME, Rao D. Substance use related stigma: what we know and the way forward. J Addict Behav Ther Rehabil. 2013;2(2)
52. Schur EM. Labeling deviant behavior: its sociological implications. New York: Harper & Row; 1971.
53. Goffman E. Stigma: notes on the management of spoiled identity. New York: Simon and Schuster; 2009.
54. Link BG, Phelan JC. Conceptualizing stigma. Annu Rev Sociol. 2001;27:363–85. https://doi.org/10.1146/annurev.soc.27.1.363.
55. Tsai AC, Kiang MV, Barnett ML, Beletsky L, Keyes KM, McGinty EE, et al. Stigma as a fundamental hindrance to the United States opioid overdose crisis response. PLoS Med. 2019;16(11):e1002969.
56. Gilchrist G, Moskalewicz J, Slezakova S, Okruhlica L, Torrens M, Vajd R, et al. Staff regard towards working with substance users: a European multi-Centre study. Addiction. 2011;106(6):1114–25.
57. McLaughlin D, McKenna H, Leslie J, Moore K, Robinson J. Illicit drug users in Northern Ireland: perceptions and experiences of health and social care professionals. J Psychiatr Ment Health Nurs. 2006;13(6):682–6.
58. Rao H, Mahadevappa H, Pillay P, Sessay M, Abraham A, Luty J. A study of stigmatized attitudes towards people with mental health problems among health professionals. J Psychiatr Ment Health Nurs. 2009;16(3):279–84.
59. Antoniou T, Ala-Leppilampi K, Shearer D, Parsons JA, Tadrous M, Gomes T. "Like being put on an ice floe and shoved away": a qualitative study of the impacts of opioid-related policy changes on people who take opioids. Int J Drug Policy. 2019;66:15–22.
60. Kennedy-Hendricks A, Busch SH, McGinty EE, Bachhuber MA, Niederdeppe J, Gollust SE, et al. Primary care physicians' perspectives on the prescription opioid epidemic. Drug Alcohol Depend. 2016;165:61–70.
61. Louie DL, Assefa MT, McGovern MP. Attitudes of primary care physicians toward prescribing buprenorphine: a narrative review. BMC Fam Pract. 2019;20(1):157.
62. McCradden MD, Vasileva D, Orchanian-Cheff A, Buchman DZ. Ambiguous identities of drugs and people: a scoping review of opioid-related stigma. Int J Drug Policy. 2019;74:205–15.
63. Allen B, Harocopos A, Chernick R. Substance use stigma, primary care, and the New York state prescription drug monitoring program. Behav Med. 2020;46(1):52–62.
64. van Boekel LC, Brouwers EP, van Weeghel J, Garretsen HF. Stigma among health professionals towards patients with substance use disorders and its consequences for healthcare delivery: systematic review. Drug Alcohol Depend. 2013;131(1–2):23–35.

65. Curtis J, Harrison L. Beneath the surface: collaboration in alcohol and other drug treatment. An analysis using Foucault's three modes of objectification. J Adv Nurs. 2001;34(6):737–44.
66. Benintendi A, Kosakowski S, Lagisetty P, Larochelle M, Bohnert ASB, Bazzi AR. "I felt like I had a scarlet letter": recurring experiences of structural stigma surrounding opioid tapers among patients with chronic, non-cancer pain. Drug Alcohol Depend. 2021;222:108664.
67. Manhapra A, Sullivan MD, Ballantyne JC, MacLean RR, Becker WC. Complex persistent opioid dependence with long-term opioids: a gray area that needs definition, better understanding, treatment guidance, and policy changes. J Gen Intern Med. 2020;35(Suppl 3):964–71.
68. Olsen Y, Sharfstein JM. Confronting the stigma of opioid use disorder—and its treatment. JAMA. 2014;311(14):1393–4.
69. Crapanzano KA, Hammarlund R, Ahmad B, Hunsinger N, Kullar R. The association between perceived stigma and substance use disorder treatment outcomes: a review. Subst Abus Rehabil. 2019;10:1–12.
70. Ahern J, Stuber J, Galea S. Stigma, discrimination and the health of illicit drug users. Drug Alcohol Depend. 2007;88(2–3):188–96.
71. Earnshaw V, Smith L, Copenhaver M. Drug addiction stigma in the context of methadone maintenance therapy: an investigation into understudied sources of stigma. Int J Ment Health Addict. 2013;11(1):110–22.
72. Latkin C, Davey-Rothwell M, Yang JY, Crawford N. The relationship between drug user stigma and depression among inner-city drug users in Baltimore, MD. J Urban Health. 2013;90(1):147–56.
73. Kulesza M, Watkins KE, Ober AJ, Osilla KC, Ewing B. Internalized stigma as an independent risk factor for substance use problems among primary care patients: rationale and preliminary support. Drug Alcohol Depend. 2017;180:52–5.
74. Cunningham JA, Sobell LC, Sobell MB, Agrawal S, Toneatto T. Barriers to treatment: why alcohol and drug abusers delay or never seek treatment. Addict Behav. 1993;18(3):347–53.
75. Paquette CE, Syvertsen JL, Pollini RA. Stigma at every turn: health services experiences among people who inject drugs. Int J Drug Policy. 2018;57:104–10.
76. Miller NS, Sheppard LM, Colenda CC, Magen J. Why physicians are unprepared to treat patients who have alcohol- and drug-related disorders. Acad Med. 2001;76(5):410–8.
77. OnPoint NYC. Program. New York: OnPoint NYC; [cited 2025 Aug 7]. Available from: https://onpointnyc.org/.
78. Bankston CL III, Zhou M. Social capital as process: the meanings and problems of a theoretical metaphor. Sociol Inq. 2002;72(2):285–317. https://doi.org/10.1111/1475-682X.00017.
79. Putnam RD. Tuning in, tuning out: the strange disappearance of social capital in America. Polit Sci Polit. 1995;28(4):664–83.
80. Putnam RD. Bowling alone: the collapse and revival of American community. New York: Simon & Schuster; 2000.
81. Lemann N. Kicking in groups. Atlantica. 1996;277(4):22–6.
82. Kawachi I, Kennedy BP, Glass R. Social capital and self-rated health: a contextual analysis. Am J Public Health. 1999;89(8):1187–93.
83. Helliwell JF. Well-being and social capital: does suicide pose a puzzle? Soc Indic Res. 2007;81(3):455–96. https://doi.org/10.1007/s11205-006-0022-y.
84. Rosenfeld R, Baumer EP, Messner SF. Social capital and homicide. Soc Forces. 2001;80(1):283–310. https://doi.org/10.1353/sof.2001.0086.
85. Kruger DJ, Hutchison P, Monroe MG, Reischl T, Morrel-Samuels S. Assault injury rates, social capital, and fear of neighborhood crime. J Community Psychol. 2007;35(4):483–98. https://doi.org/10.1002/jcop.20160.
86. Awgu E, Magura S, Coryn C. Social capital, substance use disorder and depression among youths. Am J Drug Alcohol Abuse. 2016;42(2):213–21.
87. Reynoso-Vallejo H. Social capital influence in illicit drug use among racial/ethnic groups in the United States. J Ethn Subst Abus. 2011;10(2):91–111.

88. Winstanley EL, Steinwachs DM, Ensminger ME, Latkin CA, Stitzer ML, Olsen Y. The association of self-reported neighborhood disorganization and social capital with adolescent alcohol and drug use, dependence, and access to treatment. Drug Alcohol Depend. 2008;92(1–3):173–82.
89. Case A, Deaton A. Deaths of despair and the future of capitalism. Princeton: Princeton University Press; 2020.
90. McLean K. "There's nothing here": deindustrialization as risk environment for overdose. Int J Drug Policy. 2016;29:19–26.
91. Achenbach J, Keating D. Unnatural causes: sick and dying in small-town America—a new divide in American death (introduction to a series of articles). The Washington Post; 2017. Available from: https://www.washingtonpost.com/unnatural-causes/?utm_term=.8e2899a1141a.
92. Bartscher AK, Seitz S, Siegloch S, Slotwinski M, Wehrhöfer N. Social capital and the spread of covid-19: insights from european countries. J Health Econ. 2021;80:102531.
93. Makridis CA, Wu C. How social capital helps communities weather the COVID-19 pandemic. PLoS One. 2021;16(1):e0245135.
94. Zoorob MJ, Salemi JL. Bowling alone, dying together: the role of social capital in mitigating the drug overdose epidemic in the United States. Drug Alcohol Depend. 2017;173:1–9.
95. Rupasingha A, Goetz SJ, Freshwater D. The production of social capital in US counties. J Socio-Econ. 2006;35(1):83–101.
96. Ford JA, Sacra SA, Yohros A. Neighborhood characteristics and prescription drug misuse among adolescents: the importance of social disorganization and social capital. Int J Drug Policy. 2017;46:47–53.
97. Yang TC, Kim S, Matthews SA. Unemployment and opioid-related mortality rates in U.S. counties: investigating social capital and social isolation–smoking pathways. Soc Probl. 2023;70(2):533–53. https://doi.org/10.1093/socpro/spab053.
98. Rudzinski K, Strike C. Resilience in the face of victimization: a Bourdieusian analysis of dealing with harms and hurts among street-involved individuals who smoke crack cocaine. Contemporary Drug Prob. 2020;47(1):3–28.
99. Aldrich DP, Meyer MA. Social capital and community resilience. Am Behav Sci. 2014;59(2):254–69.
100. Dynes RR. Community social capital as the primary basis for resilience. Newark: University of Delaware, Disaster Research Center; 2005.
101. Anchor Recovery Center: A Program of the Providence Center; 2023. [cited 2025 Aug 7]. Available from: https://anchorrecovery.providencecenter.org/.
102. Dowell D, Brown S, Gyawali S, Hoenig J, Ko J, Mikosz C, et al. Treatment for opioid use disorder: population estimates - United States, 2022. MMWR Morb Mortal Wkly Rep. 2024;73(25):567–74.
103. Substance Abuse and Mental Health Services Administration. 2023 National Survey on drug use and health (NSDUH) releases [internet]. Rockville: Substance Abuse and Mental Health Services Administration; 2023 [cited 2025 Oct 10]. Available from: https://www.samhsa.gov/data/data-we-collect/nsduh-national-survey-drug-use-and-health/national-releases/2023#highlighted-population-slides.
104. Nguemeni Tiako MJ. Addressing racial & socioeconomic disparities in access to medications for opioid use disorder amid COVID-19. J Subst Abus Treat. 2021;122:108214.
105. Substance Abuse and Mental Health Services Administration. The opioid crisis and the black/African American population: an urgent issue. Rockville: Substance Abuse and Mental Health Services Administration; 2020. Publication No. PEP20-05-02-001. Available from: https://library.samhsa.gov/product/opioid-crisis-and-blackafrican-american-population-urgent-issue/pep20-05-02-001.
106. Cooper LA, Roter DL, Johnson RL, Ford DE, Steinwachs DM, Powe NR. Patient-centered communication, ratings of care, and concordance of patient and physician race. Ann Intern Med. 2003;139(11):907–15.

107. Saha S, Komaromy M, Koepsell TD, Bindman AB. Patient-physician racial concordance and the perceived quality and use of health care. Arch Intern Med. 1999;159(9):997–1004.
108. Kennedy BR, Mathis CC, Woods AK. African Americans and their distrust of the health care system: healthcare for diverse populations. J Cult Divers. 2007;14(2):56–60.
109. Lin LA, Knudsen HK. Comparing buprenorphine-prescribing physicians across nonmetropolitan and metropolitan areas in the United States. Ann Fam Med. 2019;17(3):212–20.
110. Xierali IM, Nivet MA. The racial and ethnic composition and distribution of primary care physicians. J Health Care Poor Underserved. 2018;29(1):556–70.
111. Santoro TN, Santoro JD. Racial bias in the US opioid epidemic: a review of the history of systemic bias and implications for care. Cureus. 2018;10(12):e3733.
112. Anderson KO, Green CR, Payne R. Racial and ethnic disparities in pain: causes and consequences of unequal care. J Pain. 2009;10(12):1187–204.
113. Bonham VL. Race, ethnicity, and pain treatment: striving to understand the causes and solutions to the disparities in pain treatment. J Law Med Ethics. 2001;29(1):52–68.
114. Cintron A, Morrison RS. Pain and ethnicity in the United States: a systematic review. J Palliat Med. 2006;9(6):1454–73.
115. Freeman HP, Payne R. Racial injustice in health care. N Engl J Med. 2000;342(14):1045–7.
116. Goyal MK, Kuppermann N, Cleary SD, Teach SJ, Chamberlain JM. Racial disparities in pain management of children with appendicitis in emergency departments. JAMA Pediatr. 2015;169(11):996–1002.
117. Institute of Medicine Committee on U, Eliminating R, Ethnic Disparities in Health C. In: Smedley BD, Stith AY, Nelson AR, editors. Unequal treatment: confronting racial and ethnic disparities in health care. Washington (DC): National Academies Press (US) Copyright 2002 by the National Academy of Sciences. All rights reserved; 2003.
118. Enzinger AC, Ghosh K, Keating NL, Cutler DM, Clark CR, Florez N, et al. Racial and ethnic disparities in opioid access and urine drug screening among older patients with poor-prognosis cancer near the end of life. J Clin Oncol. 2023;41(14):2511–22.
119. Pletcher MJ, Kertesz SG, Kohn MA, Gonzales R. Trends in opioid prescribing by race/ethnicity for patients seeking care in US emergency departments. JAMA. 2008;299(1):70–8.
120. Tamayo-Sarver JH, Hinze SW, Cydulka RK, Baker DW. Racial and ethnic disparities in emergency department analgesic prescription. Am J Public Health. 2003;93(12):2067–73.
121. Todd KH, Samaroo N, Hoffman JR. Ethnicity as a risk factor for inadequate emergency department analgesia. JAMA. 1993;269(12):1537–9.
122. Saha S, Freeman M, Toure J, Tippens KM, Weeks C, Ibrahim S. Racial and ethnic disparities in the VA health care system: a systematic review. J Gen Intern Med. 2008;23(5):654–71.
123. Meghani SH, Byun E, Gallagher RM. Time to take stock: a meta-analysis and systematic review of analgesic treatment disparities for pain in the United States. Pain Med. 2012;13(2):150–74.
124. Dominick KL, Bosworth HB, Dudley TK, Waters SJ, Campbell LC, Keefe FJ. Patterns of opioid analgesic prescription among patients with osteoarthritis. J Pain Palliat Care Pharmacother. 2004;18(1):31–46.
125. Chen I, Kurz J, Pasanen M, Faselis C, Panda M, Staton LJ, et al. Racial differences in opioid use for chronic nonmalignant pain. J Gen Intern Med. 2005;20(7):593–8.
126. Burgess DJ, Nelson DB, Gravely AA, Bair MJ, Kerns RD, Higgins DM, et al. Racial differences in prescription of opioid analgesics for chronic noncancer pain in a national sample of veterans. J Pain. 2014;15(4):447–55.
127. Mark TL, Goode SA, McMurtrie G, Weinstein L, Perry RJ. Improving research on racial disparities in access to medications to treat opioid use disorders. J Addict Med. 2023;17(3):249–57.
128. Madden EF. Intervention stigma: how medication-assisted treatment marginalizes patients and providers. Soc Sci Med. 2019;232:324–31.
129. Wakeman SE, Larochelle MR, Ameli O, Chaisson CE, McPheeters JT, Crown WH, et al. Comparative effectiveness of different treatment pathways for opioid use disorder. JAMA Netw Open. 2020;3(2):e1920622.

130. Madden EF, Prevedel S, Light T, Sulzer SH. Intervention stigma toward medications for opioid use disorder: a systematic review. Subst Use Misuse. 2021;56(14):2181–201.
131. Harris S. To be free and normal: addiction, governance, and the therapeutics of buprenorphine. Med Anthropol Q. 2015;29(4):512–30.
132. Hansen HB, Siegel CE, Case BG, Bertollo DN, DiRocco D, Galanter M. Variation in use of buprenorphine and methadone treatment by racial, ethnic, and income characteristics of residential social areas in New York City. J Behav Health Serv Res. 2013;40(3):367–77.
133. Lagisetty PA, Ross R, Bohnert A, Clay M, Maust DT. Buprenorphine treatment divide by race/ethnicity and payment. JAMA Psychiatry. 2019;76(9):979–81.
134. Baxter JD, Clark RE, Samnaliev M, Leung GY, Hashemi L. Factors associated with Medicaid patients' access to buprenorphine treatment. J Subst Abus Treat. 2011;41(1):88–96.
135. Knudsen HK, Ducharme LJ, Roman PM. Early adoption of buprenorphine in substance abuse treatment centers: data from the private and public sectors. J Subst Abus Treat. 2006;30(4):363–73.
136. Schuler MS, Dick AW, Stein BD. Growing racial/ethnic disparities in buprenorphine distribution in the United States, 2007-2017. Drug Alcohol Depend. 2021;223:108710.
137. Hansen H, Siegel C, Wanderling J, DiRocco D. Buprenorphine and methadone treatment for opioid dependence by income, ethnicity and race of neighborhoods in new York City. Drug Alcohol Depend. 2016;164:14–21.
138. Goedel WC, Shapiro A, Cerdá M, Tsai JW, Hadland SE, Marshall BDL. Association of racial/ethnic segregation with treatment capacity for opioid use disorder in counties in the United States. JAMA Netw Open. 2020;3(4):e203711.
139. Dube, et al. Childhood abuse, household dysfunction, and the risk of attempted suicide throughout the life span: findings from the Adverse Childhood Experiences Study. JAMA. 2001;286(24):3089–96.

Transformational Solutions and Global Lessons 15

A paradigm shift begins with the imagination of a different kind of world.

—Donella H. Meadows (Leverage Points: Places to Intervene in a System. The Sustainability Institute, 1999)

15.1 Introduction

This chapter explores transformative solutions to the opioid crisis, building on an analysis of its social and economic determinants. Its central thesis is that meaningful change requires institutional reform informed by global successes and failures, not symbolic gestures or narrow biomedical fixes. The conventional narrative oversimplifies a complex reality by ignoring historical context, root-cause inequities, and voices of people with lived experience. Effective responses must embed racial equity, reduce stigma, and address the conditions under which addiction takes root.

We first examine prevention frameworks, expanding beyond the classical models to include primordial prevention, which targets social and environmental determinants such as poverty, trauma, and whole-system racism. Next, we turn to global lessons. Portugal's decriminalization of all drugs is highlighted as a comprehensive public health experiment that paired reform with treatment access, harm reduction, and social reintegration. In contrast, Oregon's Measure 110 demonstrates the challenges of partial reform when care systems and cultural buy-in are absent. Additional lessons from Canada, the United Kingdom, and Australia show how integrating methadone into primary care reduces stigma and expands access. Finally, we propose two key policy shifts, namely the deregulation of methadone and the over-the-counter (OTC) availability of low-dose buprenorphine. The central lesson is this: For prevention and reform efforts to endure, they should be structural, equity-focused, and whole-system.

L. R. Webster, S. Eichberg, *Deconstructing Toxic Narratives*,
https://doi.org/10.1007/978-3-032-23135-2_15

15.2 Opioid Use Disorder and Models of Prevention

Substance abuse prevention aims to avert, delay, or limit drug misuse and its associated negative health and social consequences [1–3]. Best solutions are equity--driven, targeting populations and communities disproportionately affected by opioid use disorder (OUD) or overdose, especially those previously excluded from prevention, treatment, and recovery efforts.

To guide intervention strategies, various conceptual frameworks exist within the field of addiction. The classical public health prevention framework, which categorizes preventive activities into primary, secondary, and tertiary stages to reflect the natural history of a disease, has been widely used for the past 50 years [4–8]. Originally designed for physical diseases, this framework has been adapted over time to address mental health concerns, including substance use disorders (SUDs), and, more recently, OUD [9–11].

The classical prevention model traditionally defines its levels as follows:

- Primary prevention focuses on preventing the onset of disease by halting or minimizing exposures to risks that cause disease or injury or by modifying risky behaviors that can lead to disease or injury [12].
- Secondary prevention emphasizes early disease identification and intervention to stop or slow down progression. Some of the strategies aim to restore people to health and prevent long-term problems or recurrence.
- Tertiary prevention strives to mitigate the downstream consequences of disease to improve functionality, life expectancy, and quality of life for people managing chronic or complex health problems.

However, a major limitation of the classical prevention model is its neglect of root-cause conditions contributing to health or disease, being confined as it is to a strict clinical or biomedical context [13, 14]. This involves a mechanistic understanding of addiction that typically yields clinical and pharmacological interventions.

To address this gap, the primordial stage was later added to attend to the social and environmental determinants of risk as root causes of health problems and to encourage large-scale structural changes (Fig. 15.1) [8, 15–18]. Unfortunately, primordial prevention has often been disregarded in SUD/OUD interventions, in part because the field was (re)framed in the 1980s as a scientific and clinical enterprise to enhance professional legitimacy. To rectify this omission, the American College of Preventive Medicine (ACPM) proposed a multilevel prevention framework for OUD that incorporates the primordial stage as the earliest point of intervention. This framework explicitly encourages efforts to address social determinants and root-cause inequities that drive the unequal distribution of risk for onset of OUD and overdose [18–21].

Discussing solutions for the opioid crisis, several authors have concluded that the only way to create enduring change is to tear out the deep roots of structural inequality causing and sustaining the overdose crisis. This would involve a radical overhaul

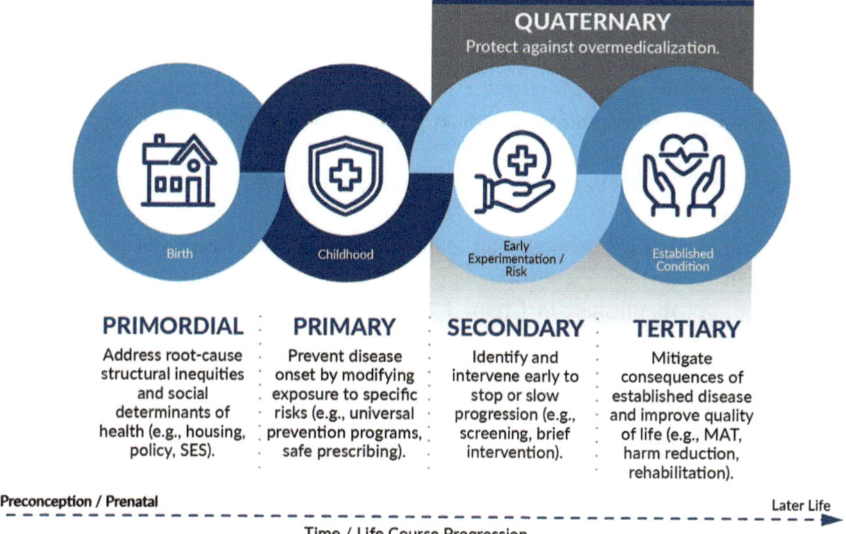

Fig. 15.1 Primordial Prevention: Incorporates efforts to address social and structural inequities to prevent the root causes of opioid use disorder (OUD) and overdose. Primary Prevention: Aims to prevent disease before it starts. Secondary Prevention: Focuses on early detection to stop or slow disease progression. Tertiary Prevention: Manages existing disease to reduce complications and improve quality of life. Quaternary Prevention: Aims to protect patients at increased risk for harm from over-testing and overmedicalization. (Source: Original figure created from concepts in Leavell and Clark [8])

of the healthcare system, the criminal justice system, and other political and economic systems. Rivera and Friedman write [19]:

> We…argue that the United States political, economic, and public health systems have helped create this crisis and, unfortunately, continue to heighten it. These same systems suggest that proposals to expand harm reduction and drug treatment capacity, to decriminalize or legalize drugs, or to reindustrialize the country sufficiently to reduce 'communities of despair' will not be enacted at a scale sufficient to end the overdose crisis. We thus suggest that in the United States at least, serious improvements in overdose rates and related policies and structures require massive social movements with a broad social change agenda (p. 1).

While primary prevention involves activities to mitigate or eliminate risk factors for onset of a medical problem, many studies in this area are designed to treat early indicators of disease rather than to prevent its onset. The focus of this prevention level is on modifying risk and protective factors directly linked to activating or impeding OUD and overdose deaths. Its orientation has shifted over time, influenced by political and social contexts. For example, in the 1960s, primary prevention was associated with community mental health and concerned with improving population health by changing social and economic conditions.

A fifth level, quaternary prevention, was proposed in 1986. It is aimed at protecting patients at an increased risk of being harmed by over-testing and overmedicalization. The Wonca International Dictionary for General/Family Practice reads: *Action taken to identify a patient at risk of overmedicalization, to protect him from new medical invasion, and to suggest to him interventions, which are ethically acceptable* [22].

Table 15.1 provides examples of relevant policies and practices at each stage of the ACPM model.

Latimore et al. have proposed an alternative preventive paradigm for OUD that integrates the socioecological framework with the classical public health prevention model [13]. As mentioned in Chap. 1, the socioecological framework highlights levels of influence on health, from the micro (individual) to the macro (societal, structural), to reveal the risk and protective factors that emerge from the synergistic interplay between people and their environments [23].

By merging these frameworks, Latimore et al. underscore the complex interactions among the three prevention levels and the socioecological levels of influence,

Table 15.1 American College of Preventive Medicine Prevention framework

Prevention level	Definition	Strategies
Primordial	Targeting the underlying social and environmental conditions that promote the onset of disease	ACE prevention and mitigation Address food insecurity Address structural racism Restructure criminal justice system
Primary	Mitigating risk factors and preventing disease from developing	Expand evidence-based prevention programs Improve access to counseling/ mental health care Promote parental and intergenerational health
Secondary	Identifying disease early and providing appropriate treatment/services to halt or slow down its progression	Improve screening and diagnosis of OUD and linkage with effective treatment Initiate and continue MOUD in carceral settings Expand access to MOUD treatment/ programs Peer recovery support
Tertiary	Managing disease to reduce negative consequences	Syringe services programs Safe use programs Community distribution of naloxone Case management for SDoH Housing for people who use drugs

Source: Adapted from Livingston et al. [18]; some strategies from Latimore et al. [56]

creating a dynamic system where factors at one level shape or are shaped by factors at other levels. This intricate approach aids the design of holistic interventions that target both the immediate downstream consequences and their upstream causes [24]. It also emphasizes the importance of social context in various settings across the prevention continuum [25].

For clarity, this chapter will employ the ACPM's multi-tiered prevention model, which emphasizes root-cause determinants at the primordial level. However, it should be recognized that structural forces and social determinants operate beyond the primordial stage, affecting prevention efforts at all stages. The four categories of prevention activities in the ACPM framework have somewhat blurred boundaries. Thus, when relevant, the chapter will discuss connections among the different levels of prevention and their implications for solutions. Expanding on the model, the chapter will further review the global evidence for frameworks that have worked and failed. It will also consider how solutions depend on different social and relational contexts amid the populations and communities who are targeted for change. Proposed solutions by category are shown in Table 15.2.

The opioid crisis has often been described in terms of its tragic outcome—overdose deaths, addictions, fractured families, and strained health systems. But such a lens focuses narrowly on symptoms, not the institutional conditions that produce them. The four approaches, primordial, primary, secondary, and tertiary, are conventional concepts that have merit, but still are limited in their reach to the broader systemic factors that need to be addressed for long-term solutions. A sustainable and ethical response to this crisis can do more than mitigate harm—it can change the conditions under which harm becomes inevitable.

The following builds on the four-level framework by ACPM, illustrated by the accompanying infographics (Fig. 15.2a, b) [26–28]. It represents a novel synthesis of global evidence and US institutional context. It offers not only a roadmap for what can be done but redefinition of what "prevention" is best in an age of compound despair, collective trauma, and economic abandonment.

The evolution of prevention—from primordial to quaternary—underscores that solutions should advance toward clinical interventions to address institutional inequities. To set the stage for more ambitious reforms, several actionable directions emerge in rethinking prevention:

- Embed primordial prevention in US drug policy by addressing poverty, racism, trauma, and social dislocation as root causes
- Recast prevention not only as risk mitigation but as reshaping social environments (housing, education, and employment)
- Apply quaternary prevention principles to guard against over-medicalization, stigma, and punitive surveillance

To determine the best solutions to prevent SUD, it is imperative to study and understand approaches that have had both positive and negative impacts internationally. The following is anchored in evidence-based international successes.

Table 15.2 American College of Preventive Medicine categories of prevention efforts

Category	Intervention
Primordial	Universal health care, Medicaid expansion in all states Legal protections for people with OUD: e.g., eliminate the illegal or current use exception to the Americans with Disabilities Act (ADA) (42 U.S.C.A. § 12,114[b]), which denies protection to anyone "currently engaging in the illegal use of drugs" Extend free healthy meals (breakfast and lunch) in all public schools Decriminalize illegal drugs Universal childcare (or increased subsidies) Housing assistance programs/tax credits Change requirements for disability benefits (no need to show prior medication use) Criminal legal reform/restructuring
Primary	Data sharing (interoperability): implement systems across health and social services/behavioral and nonbehavioral health to enhance/integrate treatment, target gaps in prevention/treatment and track outcomes for policy and planning; improve public health data sharing at state and national levels ACE prevention interventions Peer support interventions to increase self-worth, emotional support, and social capital/community building Involve individuals with shared experience in substance use and recovery to support patients in treatment Community-based research and intervention design: Engage specific populations and communities in designing, carrying out, and analyzing studies and implementing solutions (to build capacity, resilience, and social bonds and create programs that meet local needs) Increase physician/provider cultural competency training for people with low--income, mental illness and addiction, among others Training for health professionals in evidence-based pain management Training for health professionals on the needs and care of people with OUD (reduce stigma)
Secondary	Initiation and continuation of MOUD in carceral settings and upon release Education campaign: changing narrative about opioids, especially among over-burdened subpopulations, to reduce stigma Peer support (for recovery) Care coordination; Integrate primary care and mental health and treatment for OUD Revise federal law to allow methadone to be prescribed for OUD in primary care Regulatory change/alter Drug Enforcement Administration waiver framework to broaden professionals authorized to deliver MOUD Broaden access to MOUD through telemedicine by providing MOUD in community programs remotely connecting patients with physicians; ensure adequate reimbursement for tele-visits Hub-and-spoke systems of care: Vermont's hub-and-spoke model provides central, specialized substance-abuse treatment programs to stabilize patients using MOUD before referring them to local "spokes," such as community health centers or private practitioners Expand coverage for MOUD (e.g., methadone or buprenorphine as a mandated benefit) and implement other regulatory mandates for insurance to fully cover OUD treatment
Tertiary	Syringe programs Safe use facilities Expand naloxone availability/community distribution of/public access naloxone kits (e.g., on college campuses)

a

Transformational Solutions:
Synthesizing Global Evidence
Portugal
Decriminalization + Harm Reduction
Combining decriminalized drug possession with robust treatment, support, and social reintegration
Canada, UK, Australia
Methadone in Pharmacies
Expanding office-based access to methadone and integrating treatment into primary care
Prevention 2.0
Addressing Root Causes
Targeting the social determinants of health to prevent substance use

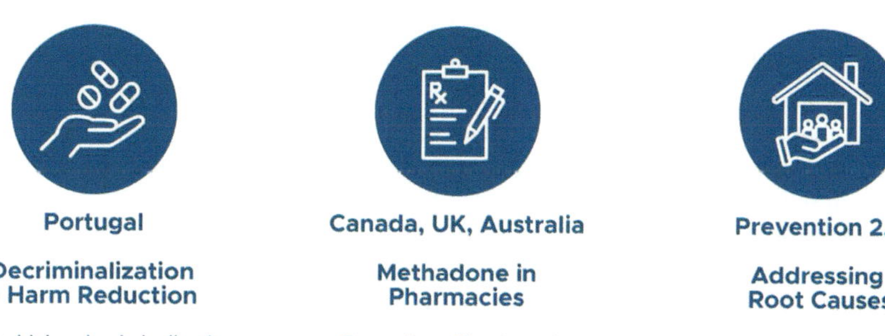

b

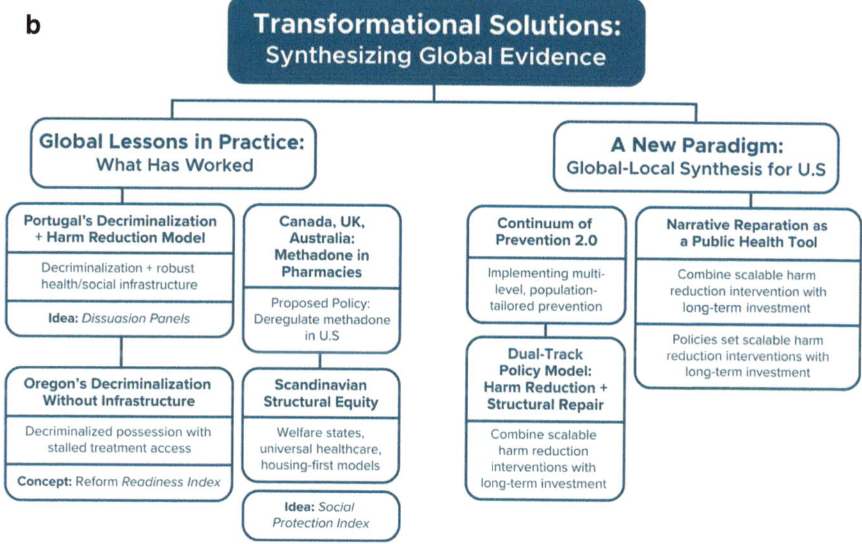

Fig. 15.2 (**a**) This figure illustrates three international models that inform systemic responses to the opioid crisis. Portugal demonstrates the effectiveness of combining drug decriminalization with treatment, harm reduction, and social reintegration. Canada, the United Kingdom, and Australia have expanded access to methadone by integrating treatment into pharmacies and primary care settings. Prevention 2.0 emphasizes targeting the social determinants of health—such as poverty, housing, and systemic inequities—to address the root causes of substance use. Together, these examples highlight the need for comprehensive, structural reforms rather than symbolic policy shifts. (**b**) This figure adapts international drug policy models, highlighting successful approaches like Portugal's decriminalization, Canada/UK/Australia's pharmacy-based methadone access, and Scandinavia's focus on structural equity. It contrasts these with the US approach and proposes new paradigms, including Prevention 2.0, that emphasize systemic, scalable reforms and dual-track models linking harm reduction with structural repair. (Source: Author's adaptation based on international drug policy research, public health prevention frameworks, and health equity scholarship, including Hughes and Stevens [26], Knutagård and Kristiansen, [27], Laqueur [28])

15.3 Portugal's Paradigm Shift: Lessons from a Bold Public Health Experiment

Portugal's turnaround from one of Europe's most severe drug crises in the 1990s to having among the lowest rates of drug-related harm today is widely recognized as a public health success. What sets Portugal apart is not simply the decriminalization of drugs, but the broader architecture of care, dignity, and social support that accompanied it. This stands in stark contrast to the punitive and fragmented systems still dominant in the United States.

At the height of Portugal's crisis, nearly 1% of its population was estimated to be addicted to heroin. Overdose deaths, HIV transmission through shared needles, and social marginalization of people who use drugs were rampant. In response, rather than escalating the War on Drugs, Portugal reframed drug use as a public health issue. In 2001, it decriminalized the personal possession and use of all drugs—not just cannabis, but heroin, cocaine, and others—pivoting from criminal punishment to public health intervention. However, this legal reform was only one pillar of a broader national strategy.

Importantly, Portugal did not legalize drugs; trafficking and large-scale possession remain criminal offenses [29]. Individuals found with small amounts (defined as a 10-day personal supply) are no longer arrested or incarcerated and are referred to a "Dissuasion Commission" (Comissões para a Dissuasão da Toxicodependência), a regional panel composed of a social worker, a legal expert, and a medical professional, offering a holistic assessment that centers dignity and support [26]. These panels assess whether the individual has an SUD and can issue administrative sanctions (e.g., fines, community service), but more importantly, they refer people to voluntary treatment and social services.

Decriminalization was just one pillar of a broader strategy. It was paired with significant investment in evidence-based treatment, including medication for opioid use disorder (MOUD), detox services, and long-term residential care. Harm reduction strategies—such as needle exchange programs, supervised consumption sites, and outreach to people who inject drugs—were central to reducing immediate risks and building trust.

Just as important was its emphasis on the social determinants of drug use: housing, employment, education, and social connection. Programs aimed to reintegrate users into society, not simply to get them to abstain from use. People could access support in the form of employment initiatives, transitional housing, and stigma reduction campaigns, which helped reduce relapse and marginalization [28].

The strategy was designed by the Portuguese Committee on Drugs under the leadership of psychiatrist João Goulão, who emphasized a non-moralistic, science-based approach. Importantly, the plan was not derailed by political changes. Instead, it maintained cross-party support and long-term funding commitments, ensuring stability and continuity.

In the two decades since, Portugal has witnessed dramatic declines in overdose deaths, new HIV infections, and incarceration for drug-related offenses. For example, between 2001 and 2012, drug-related deaths dropped by over 80%, and HIV infection rates among people who inject drugs plummeted [30, 31].

15.4 What Portugal Did That the United States Has Not Done

Portugal had a national, coordinated response with centralized oversight and evaluation. In contrast, the US response is fragmented across federal, state, and local levels, often with conflicting policies and inconsistent funding streams. The United States has pursued a punitive approach, still criminalizing drug possession in most states, particularly for Black, Indigenous, and People of Color.

US policies often neglect the root causes of substance use: poverty, housing insecurity, trauma, and lack of access to care. Portugal's model tackled these head-on. By embedding drug policy within a broader welfare system, Portugal acknowledged that addiction cannot be separated from social conditions.

Portugal intentionally used language and practices that respected the humanity of people who use drugs. This cultural shift reduced stigma and improved engagement with services. US public discourse and media coverage often perpetuate stigma, undermining efforts to treat addiction as a medical issue.

Finally, Portuguese police were trained to see users as patients, not criminals. In the United States, law enforcement remains a frontline responder to drug use, often with devastating consequences, particularly in communities that are already over-policed.

Adapting Portugal's Dissuasion Commission model for application at the US county level offers a promising pathway to redirect individuals away from jails and into care. For successful replication, however, several conditions should be met:

- Local investment in treatment capacity, housing, and case management
- Training for panelists and law enforcement to ensure a therapeutic, not punitive, ethos
- Oversight mechanisms to prevent coercive or inequitable application
- Community engagement and stigma reduction to build trust among affected populations

Portugal's experience underscores the importance of evidence over ideology. Effective drug policy is not about leniency or permissiveness; it is about realism, compassion, and social investment. Portugal's integrated public health framework offers a roadmap for reform—but only if adopted with political will and governance-level support. Without investment in care and housing, decriminalization risks repeating US policy failures (Table 15.3).

Table 15.3 Comparing global decriminalization efforts

Challenge	Oregon's approach	Portugal's model
Care infrastructure	Launched without a functioning treatment system; funds delayed nearly a year	Built treatment, housing, and reintegration supports before decriminalization
Access to services	Severe workforce shortages; over half of counties lacked behavioral health providers	Centralized system ensured access across regions
Referral mechanism	Civil citations with optional health screening—Ignored by over 95%	Mandatory appearance before a dissuasion panel with immediate voluntary care engagement
Implementation	Fragmented across counties and agencies; minimal oversight	National plan with centralized coordination and technical support
Cultural framing	Launched amid polarization and mistrust; lacking public education	Supported by a cultural shift recognizing addiction as a health issue

Portugal's paradigm shift illustrates that drug policy succeeds only when law reform is paired with health infrastructure, cultural change, and social reintegration. For the United States, the key takeaways are clear:

Lessons from Portugal

- Pair decriminalization with mandatory referral pathways (e.g., county-level dissuasion panels)
- Guarantee investment in treatment infrastructure and workforce capacity before reform
- Anchor reforms in a national strategy with bipartisan support for stability across administrations
- Launch stigma reduction campaigns that reframe drug use as a health issue, not a crime

15.5 Mainstreaming Opioid Use Disorder Treatment Through Methadone Dispensing

While Portugal's decriminalization model offers a powerful paradigm shift in how societies approach drug use, additional lessons come from high-income nations that have successfully integrated OUD treatment, specifically methadone, into mainstream health care. Canada, the United Kingdom, and Australia all provide instructive examples of how to advance away from siloed, stigmatized treatment and toward accessible, community-based models. These countries treat methadone as a core element of primary care rather than an exceptional and tightly-regulated substance.

15.5.1 Canada: National Expansion Through Primary Care and Pharmacy

Canada has implemented a decentralized model in which methadone can be prescribed by trained general practitioners and dispensed through community pharmacies. By 2020, nearly 60% of methadone patients in Canada received their medication from a pharmacy [32]. The integration of methadone into everyday healthcare settings has expanded access, especially in rural areas, and reduced stigma associated with addiction treatment. British Columbia's province-wide response to its overdose crisis includes a publicly-funded safer-supply program and integration of OUD care into primary care and harm reduction services. Despite challenges with uptake and provider training, this approach has been credited with stabilizing care continuity and reducing overdose deaths in pilot regions [33].

15.5.2 United Kingdom: Methadone in Primary Care

The United Kingdom has long operated a system where methadone is available via both specialized drug clinics and general practitioners working in collaboration with pharmacists. Community pharmacies have played a critical role: by 2018, over 1200 UK pharmacies were engaged in supervised methadone dispensing [34]. This accessibility has been credited with helping to sustain engagement in treatment and reduce illicit opioid use.

The British model emphasizes harm reduction through continuity of care. People receiving methadone are monitored for therapeutic response but without the punitive or surveillance-heavy framework seen in the United States. This has made the UK a global leader in methadone retention rates and treatment continuity [35].

15.5.3 Australia: Community-Based Accessibility

Australia's National Opioid Pharmacotherapy Strategy promotes broad access to methadone and buprenorphine through both public and private clinics as well as community pharmacies. As of 2021, approximately 70% of patients received their doses from community pharmacies [36]. This model reduces geographic and economic barriers, particularly in rural areas [36, 37].

Evidence from New South Wales showed that the integration of pharmacy-based methadone increased treatment capacity while decreasing waiting times and drop-out rates [38]. Moreover, pharmacy-based access has improved patient autonomy by facilitating flexible, consistent, and stigma-free engagement with care.

Lessons from Canada, the UK, and Australia in Methadone Mainstreaming

- Deregulate methadone prescribing for primary care physicians and nurse practitioners
- Expand community pharmacy dispensing to reduce travel burdens and stigma
- Use opioid settlement funds to build rural access, telehealth delivery, and pharmacist training
- Provide federal support for pharmacist training and telehealth models
- Position methadone as an essential medicine within primary care, not a highly restricted treatment of last resort

15.5.4 Implications for US Policy

In contrast to global best practices, US methadone regulation remains rigid and outdated. Methadone for OUD can only be dispensed through federally-certified opioid treatment programs (OTPs), often requiring daily attendance and intensive monitoring. This structure has been heavily criticized for its logistical burden and its exclusionary impact on rural and underserved communities [39].

During the COVID-19 pandemic, temporary regulatory flexibilities allowed take-home methadone doses and telehealth evaluations. Early evaluations indicated that these changes did not increase overdose rates and may have improved treatment retention [40, 41]. Yet, the United States has been slow to make these changes permanent.

Such a shift would make methadone treatment more patient-centered, scalable, and equitable, aligned with both public health logic and global best practices. There is a caveat, however: half measures and fragmented execution will not serve the purpose, as lessons from Oregon attest.

Global best practices show that methadone can be safely integrated into everyday health care. The United States should consider steps that move methadone from a siloed, stigmatized system into accessible community care.

15.6 Oregon and the Pitfalls of Partial Reform

In November 2020, Oregon made history by becoming the first US state to decriminalize the possession of small amounts of all drugs, including heroin, methamphetamine, and fentanyl. The initiative, Measure 110, promised a transformative public health approach, reallocating marijuana tax revenues to fund addiction treatment, peer support, and harm reduction services. However, just three years later, Oregon reversed course, partially recriminalizing drug possession in 2024 after public backlash over visible drug use, rising homelessness, and untreated addiction.

Table 15.4 Lessons from failure of partial reform: How could Oregon have more closely aligned with Portugal's model?

Element	Portugal	Oregon
Referral system	Mandatory appearance before dissuasion panel	Optional phone line on ticket
Treatment access	Nationally funded, coordinated services	Delayed funding, underbuilt system
Social supports	Employment, housing, integration programs	Minimal reintegration focus
National strategy	Centralized, depoliticized implementation	Fragmented, local-only execution

Why did Oregon's decriminalization falter? The measure echoed aspects of Portugal's reforms but remained piecemeal and underfunded. Oregon removed penalties but did not meaningfully replace them with a functioning system of care. The failure of Oregon's effort does not reflect the futility of decriminalization per se, but rather the dangers of implementing such a policy without the macro-level support that made Portugal's model successful. Several key missteps illustrate how partial reform can lead to political and social backlash (Table 15.4).

While Portugal spent years building a nationally-coordinated network of treatment facilities, housing supports, and social reintegration programs before decriminalization, Oregon launched its policy in the absence of a well-funded, fully-staffed addiction treatment system. Measure 110 funds were not distributed until nearly a year after the law went into effect. At the same time, Oregon faced a severe shortage of behavioral health workers. According to the Oregon Health Authority, more than half of counties lacked sufficient providers for people with SUDs [42].

Portugal's model mandates appearance before a Dissuasion Panel, which engages the person immediately, assesses their needs, and offers a path to voluntary treatment [43, 44]. Oregon, by contrast, offered neither legal obligation nor proactive outreach. Oregon relied on a non-binding citation system: tickets with an optional health assessment line, which over 95% of recipients ignored. Citations were civil violations with minimal consequences, and most people simply discarded them. A 2023 review found that only 1% of cited individuals called the health screening number printed on their ticket [45]. The citation system not only lacked enforcement but failed to divert people into care.

Furthermore, Portugal's strategy was embedded in a national plan with centralized oversight and standardization. Oregon's implementation was fragmented across counties and state agencies, with little coordination and inadequate technical assistance. Counties were given flexibility without sufficient oversight or readiness. Accountability metrics were poorly defined and inconsistently reported.

Portugal's approach also was rooted in a cultural shift that reframed addiction as a health issue rather than a criminal one. In Oregon, decriminalization occurred in the context of deep political polarization, media sensationalism, and widespread mistrust of government. Public concerns about visible drug use, especially in Portland, were amplified by a lack of shelter beds, housing-first policies, and mental health supports. Law enforcement opposition and negative media framing further undermined public confidence [46].

The US barriers to success are daunting. Ongoing political fragmentation means US drug policy remains highly decentralized, making it difficult to implement cohesive, long-term strategies. Local opposition, inconsistent leadership, and the politicization of harm reduction all undercut public health implementation. Investments are necessary, but political will is often underdeveloped. Decriminalization only succeeds when coupled with treatment, housing, and social supports. In the United States, all of these face chronic underfunding, exacerbated by workforce shortages, Medicaid barriers, and low reimbursement rates.

Oregon's Measure 110 demonstrates how partial reform can unravel when institutional support is absent. In the absence of visible improvements, decriminalization efforts are easily blamed in the media and public perception for social disorder. Without early wins or clear narratives, policies risk reversal, as happened with Oregon's 2024 recriminalization.

Oregon shows that decriminalization alone cannot solve the problem. While frameworks for engagement need improvement, Portugal's model uses mandatory appearances to create a structured opportunity for care, not punishment. The US models often swing between harsh criminalization and underpowered volunteerism, failing to build a middle ground rooted in therapeutic engagement. Policy shifts must be systemic, not symbolic, if the United States hopes to pursue durable reform.

Oregon's Lessons on Partial Reform

- Pair decriminalization with immediate treatment access and mandatory engagement mechanisms
- Build housing, employment, and reintegration services alongside legal reform
- Ensure centralized oversight and consistent implementation across counties and states
- Launch public education campaigns early to secure cultural buy-in and reduce backlash

15.7 Over-the-Counter Low-Dose Buprenorphine

A paradigm shift would be to permit low-dose buprenorphine to be available as OTC medication. Buprenorphine has a well-documented safety profile, and, at low doses, it is not more rewarding than substances already legal and widely available, such as alcohol or marijuana. Making low-dose buprenorphine OTC would serve as a meaningful harm reduction strategy, helping individuals with opioid use patterns who want to avoid more dangerous heroin or fentanyl opioids. This policy could be particularly valuable for those unwilling (e.g., due to stigma) or unable (e.g., due to cost) to access formal treatment programs, offering an early-intervention tool to reduce overdose risk and disrupt progression to more SUDs.

Low-dose buprenorphine presents a transformative opportunity for early harm reduction, but it requires safeguards and a clear vision of how it would function in practice.

OTC Buprenorphine Strategies

- Make low-dose buprenorphine available OTC as a harm reduction strategy
- Introduce packaging safeguards, pharmacist consultation models, and dosing limits to mitigate risks
- Target populations facing stigma or structural barriers (e.g., uninsured, rural, or marginalized groups)
- Use OTC access to interrupt transitions to fentanyl/heroin and reduce overdose mortality

15.8 Equity-Driven Prevention as Public Health Strategy

Effective prevention is an essential component of a public health strategy addressing substance use. The throughline across global lessons is that institutional inequities determine outcomes at every stage of prevention and reform. Any durable solution must be equity-focused: A meaningful response to the opioid crisis—at national, state, or local levels—requires confronting the institutional racism that shapes access to prevention, treatment, and recovery services. Discriminatory policies have systematically marginalized communities of color, increasing their exposure to risk, surveillance, criminalization, and limited access to evidence-based care [47–51]. These disparities are reinforced by factors like residential segregation, neighborhood disinvestment, underinsurance, and underfunded healthcare systems that repeatedly fail vulnerable populations [52, 53].

Addressing these profound inequities requires embedding racial equity throughout drug policy and programs—from inclusive research and fair funding to culturally responsive care and public health policies reflecting the lived experiences of people with SUDs. Without this coordinated, equity-driven overhaul, disparities will persist, undermining both effectiveness and fairness in substance use policy in the United States [54, 55].

Embedding Equity in All Reforms

- Require racial equity assessments in all drug policy initiatives
- Eliminate discriminatory exclusions from the Americans with Disabilities Act and related protections
- Fund culturally-responsive care models designed by and for communities of color and people with lived experience
- Expand Medicaid and move toward universal health care to dismantle structural barriers to treatment access

This chapter has outlined the evolution of prevention frameworks and discusses how they have been modified over time. Additionally, it analyzes various international prevention initiatives, including a comparative discussion of Portugal's decriminalization model and Oregon's Measure 110. This overview underscores the critical role of integrating decriminalization within a comprehensive public health approach that employs an integrative perspective. Building on these global lessons and the necessity of equity, the final chapter will outline a new framework for prevention focused on long-term healing and collective support.

References

1. Cowen EL. Changing concepts of prevention in mental health. J Ment Health. 1998;7(5):451–61.
2. Radden J. Public mental health and prevention. Public Health Ethics. 2018;11(2):126–38.
3. National Research Council (US) and Institute of Medicine (US). Committee on the prevention of mental disorders and substance abuse among children, youth, and young adults: research advances and promising interventions. In: O'Connell ME, Boat T, Warner KE, editors. Preventing mental, emotional, and Behavioral disorders among young people: progress and possibilities. Washington, DC: National Academies Press (US); 2009. https://doi.org/10.17226/12480.
4. Gordon R. An operational classification of disease prevention. In: Steinberg JA, Silverman MM, editors. Preventing mental disorders: a research perspective. National Institute of Mental Health; 1987. p. 20–6.
5. AbdulRaheem Y. Unveiling the significance and challenges of integrating prevention levels in healthcare practice. J Prim Care Community Health. 2023;14:21501319231186500.
6. Caplan G. Principles of preventive psychiatry. London: Basic Books; 1964.
7. Commission on Chronic Illness. Chronic illness in the United States, vol. 1. Cambridge, MA: Harvard University Press; 1957.
8. Leavell HR, Clark EG. Preventive medicine for the doctor in his community. 3rd ed. New York: McGraw-Hill; 1965.
9. Nelson LF, Weitzman ER, Levy S. Prevention of substance use disorders. Med Clin North Am. 2022;106(1):153–68.
10. Daniels-Witt Q, Thompson A, Glassman T, Federman S, Bott K. The case for implementing the levels of prevention model: opiate abuse on American college campuses. J Am Coll Heal. 2017;65(7):518–24.
11. Davenport TE, DeVoght AC, Sisneros H, Bezruchka S. Navigating the intersection between persistent pain and the opioid crisis: population health perspectives for physical therapy. Phys Ther. 2020;100(6):995–1007.

12. Papworth MA, Milne DL. Qualitative systematic review: an example from primary prevention in adult mental health. J Community Appl Soc Psychol. 2001;11(3):193–210.
13. Latimore AD, Salisbury-Afshar E, Duff N, Freiling E, Kellett B, Sullenger RD, et al. Primary, secondary, and tertiary prevention of substance use disorders through socioecological strategies. NAM Perspect. 2023;2023 https://doi.org/10.31478/202309b.
14. Rappaport J. The dilemma of primary prevention in mental health services: rationalize the status quo or bite the hand that feeds you. J Community Appl Soc Psychol. 1992;2(2):95–9.
15. Strasser T. Reflections on cardiovascular diseases. Interdiscip Sci Rev. 1978;3(3):225–30.
16. Jamoulle M. Information et informatisation en médecine générale. Dans: Berleur J, Lobet-Maris Cl, Poswick RF, et al., éditeurs. Les informa-G-iciens. Les professionnels de l'informatique dans leurs rapports avec les utilisateurs: Actes des III°Journées de Réflexion sur l'Informatique (3°J.R.I.); 28 et 29 novembre 1986; Namur, Belgique. 1986.
17. Kisling LA, Das JM. Prevention strategies. In: StatPearls [Internet]. Treasure Island (FL): StatPearls Publishing; 2025.
18. Livingston CJ, Berenji M, Titus TM, Caplan LS, Freeman RJ, Sherin KM, et al. American College of Preventive Medicine: addressing the opioid epidemic through a prevention framework. Am J Prev Med. 2022;63(3):454–65.
19. Rivera BD, Friedman SR. What would it really take to solve the overdose epidemic in the United States? Int J Drug Policy. 2024;128:104435.
20. Blanco C, Wiley TRA, Lloyd JJ, Lopez MF, Volkow ND. America's opioid crisis: the need for an integrated public health approach. Transl Psychiatry. 2020;10(1):167.
21. Werb D. Post-war prevention: emerging frameworks to prevent drug use after the War on Drugs. Int J Drug Policy. 2018;51:160–4.
22. Martins C, Godycki-Cwirko M, Heleno B, Brodersen J. Quaternary prevention: reviewing the concept. Eur J Gen Pract. 2018;24(1):106–11.
23. McCormick KA, Samora J, Claborn KR, Steiker LKH, DiNitto DM. A systematic review of macro-, meso, and micro-level harm reduction interventions addressing the U.S. opioid overdose epidemic. Drugs (Abingdon Engl). 2025;32(1):1–14.
24. Brady BR, Taj EA, Cameron E, Yoder AM, De La Rosa JS. A diagram of the social-ecological conditions of opioid misuse and overdose. Int J Environ Res Public Health. 2023;20(20):6950.
25. Riemer M, Reich SM, Evans SD, Nelson G, Prilleltensky I, editors. Community psychology: in pursuit of liberation and well-being. 3rd ed. Bloomsbury Academic; 2020.
26. Hughes CE, Stevens A. What can we learn from the Portuguese decriminalization of illicit drugs? Br J Criminol. 2010;50(6):999–1022.
27. Knutagård M, Kristiansen A. Not by the book: the emergence and translation of housing first in Sweden. Eur J Homelessness. 2013;7(1):93–115.
28. Laqueur H. Uses and abuses of drug decriminalization in Portugal. Law Soc Inq. 2015;40(3):746–81.
29. Greenwald GG. Drug decriminalization in Portugal: lessons for creating fair and successful drug policies. Washington, DC: Cato Institute; 2009.
30. EUDA. Portugal: country drug report 2015. Lisbon: European Union Drugs Agency; 2015.
31. Domosławski A. Drug policy in Portugal: the benefits of decriminalizing drug use. Warsaw: Open Society Foundations; 2011.
32. Gomes T, Kitchen SA, Murray R. Measuring the burden of opioid-related mortality in Ontario, Canada, during the COVID-19 pandemic. JAMA Netw Open. 2021;4(5):e2112865.
33. Irvine MA, Kuo M, Buxton JA, Balshaw R, Otterstatter M, Macdougall L, et al. Modelling the combined impact of interventions in averting deaths during a synthetic-opioid overdose epidemic. Addiction. 2019;114(9):1602–13.
34. Strang J, McDonald R, Campbell G, Degenhardt L, Nielsen S, Ritter A, et al. Take-home naloxone for the emergency interim management of opioid overdose: the public health application of an emergency medicine. Drugs. 2019;79(13):1395–418.
35. National Institute for Health and Care Excellence (NICE). Methadone and buprenorphine for the management of opioid dependence, Technology appraisal guidance; no. TA114. London: NICE; 2007.

36. Pew Charitable Trusts. In Australia, primary care and pharmacies deliver methadone. Washington, DC: Pew Charitable Trusts; 2023.
37. Cheetham A, Morgan K, Jackson J, Lord S, Nielsen S. Informing a collaborative-care model for delivering medication assisted treatment for opioid dependence (MATOD): an analysis of pharmacist, prescriber and patient perceptions. Res Soc Adm Pharm. 2023;19(3):526–34.
38. Calcaterra SL, Bach P, Chadi A, Chadi N, Kimmel SD, Morford KL, et al. Methadone matters: what the United States can learn from the global effort to treat opioid addiction. J Gen Intern Med. 2019;34(6):1039–42.
39. National Academies of Sciences, Engineering, and Medicine. Medications for opioid use disorder save lives. Washington, DC: The National Academies Press; 2019.
40. NIDA. Overdose deaths involving buprenorphine did not proportionally increase with new flexibilities in prescribing. National Institute on Drug Abuse website [Internet]; 2023. [cited 2025 Aug 30].
41. Chan B, Cook R, Levander X, Wiest K, Hoffman K, Pertl K, et al. Buprenorphine discontinuation in telehealth-only treatment for opioid use disorder: a longitudinal cohort analysis. J Subst Use Addict Treat. 2024;167:209511.
42. Zhu JM, Howington D, Hallett E, Simeon E, Amba V, Deshmukh A, et al. Behavioral health workforce: report to the Oregon health authority and state legislature, Final Report. Portland: Center for Health Systems Effectiveness, Oregon Health & Science University; 2022.
43. Drug Policy Alliance. Drug decriminalization in Portugal: learning from a health and human-centered approach. New York: Drug Policy Alliance; 2018.
44. Robinson R. In Portugal, drug decriminalization is not depenalization. Institute of Current World Affairs website [Internet]; 2024. [cited 2025 Sep 2].
45. Oregon Secretary of State. Measure 110 implementation audit. Salem: Oregon Secretary of State; 2023.
46. Bolstad E. Drug decriminalization stumbled in Oregon. Other states are taking note. Stateline; 2023.
47. Hansen H, Netherland J. Is the prescription opioid epidemic a white problem? Am J Public Health. 2016;106(12):2127–9.
48. Pamplin JR 2nd, Rouhani S, Davis CS, King C, Townsend TN. Persistent criminalization and structural racism in US drug policy: the case of overdose good Samaritan Laws. Am J Public Health. 2023;113(S1):S43–8.
49. Santoro TN, Santoro JD. Racial bias in the US opioid epidemic: a review of the history of systemic bias and implications for care. Cureus. 2018;10(12):e3733.
50. Jegede O, Bellamy C, Jordan A. Systemic racism as a determinant of health inequities for people with substance use disorder. JAMA Psychiatry. 2024;81(3):225–6.
51. Cook BL, Alegría M. Racial-ethnic disparities in substance abuse treatment: the role of criminal history and socioeconomic status. Psychiatr Serv. 2011;62(11):1273–81.
52. Tsai AC, Kiang MV, Barnett ML, Beletsky L, Keyes KM, McGinty EE, et al. Stigma as a fundamental hindrance to the United States opioid overdose crisis response. PLoS Med. 2019;16(11):e1002969.
53. Dickman SL, Himmelstein DU, Woolhandler S. Inequality and the health-care system in the USA. Lancet. 2017;389(10077):1431–41.
54. Kunins HV. Structural racism and the opioid overdose epidemic: the need for antiracist public health practice. J Public Health Manag Pract. 2020;26(3):201–5.
55. Jordan A, Martinez CP, Isom J. Incorporating a race equity framework into opioid use disorder treatment. In: Treating opioid use disorder in general medical settings. Cham: Springer International Publishing; 2021. p. 189–202.
56. Latimore AD, Salisbury-Afshar E, Duff N, Freiling E, Kellett B, Sullenger R, Salman A, and the Prevention, Treatment, and Recovery Services Working Group of the National Academy of Medicine's Action Collaborative on Countering the U.S. Opioid Epidemic. Primary, secondary, and tertiary prevention of opioid use disorder through socioecological strategies, NAM perspectives. Discussion paper. Washington, DC: National Academy of Medicine; 2023. Concepts in NAM paper used with permission from The American Institutes for Research® (AIR®).

Evolving Toward a Structural Paradigm: Prevention 2.0

16

It is not enough to know that upstream causes exist. If we want to improve outcomes, we must redesign the river.

—Sandro Galea (Well: What We Need to Talk About When We Talk About Health, 2017, p. 48)

16.1 Introduction

Substance use prevention in the United States will remain inadequate until health, labor, and justice systems are rebuilt into a single continuum of resilience. Health systems in the United States are grappling with a profound shift in addressing substance use, moving away from individual-level interventions toward a foundational "Prevention 2.0" paradigm. Rooted in social-ecological theory and social determinants of health (SDoH), this new approach recognizes that substance use is shaped by a complex interplay of socioeconomic factors, trauma, and institutional inequities.

This chapter examines this evolution, contrasting the ineffective, fear-based Prevention 1.0 with the evidence-based, wellbeing-centered Prevention 2.0 framework. We explore global lessons from nations like Portugal and Australia that have successfully implemented integrated, public health-oriented models. Finally, we propose a national wage subsidy program to bridge the community-correctional divide and address the political and fiscal barriers—such as recent federal budget cuts and administrative changes—that threaten to undermine progress. By shifting from reactive measures to proactive institutional investments, the United States can move from managing crises to transforming the systems that create them.

L. R. Webster, S. Eichberg, *Deconstructing Toxic Narratives*,
https://doi.org/10.1007/978-3-032-23135-2_16

16.2 An Evolution: From Prevention 1.0 to Prevention 2.0

Substance use prevention in the United States is evolving from a focus on individual behavior and deterrence to one that considers the broader social and ecological contexts in which substance use arises. This evolution is embodied in the transition from what is now termed Prevention 1.0 to a more nuanced and evidence-based framework: Prevention 2.0.

Prevention 1.0 emerged in the late-twentieth century as a response to rising public concern about adolescent drug use. Shaped by the political and cultural influence of the War on Drugs, it focused on deterring the initiation of substance use, particularly among youth. Its strategies centered on mass education and behavioral interventions—exemplified by campaigns like "Just Say No" and programs like D.A.R.E.—which relied on fear appeals, drug facts, and zero-tolerance messaging.

These programs assumed that drug use resulted primarily from individual moral failure or ignorance, and that increasing awareness or instilling fear would suffice to prevent initiation. Policy mechanisms reinforced this approach through criminalization, restricted access, and punitive consequences for even minor drug-related infractions.

However, despite their popularity and political appeal, these approaches failed to demonstrate meaningful long-term effectiveness. Meta-analyses of D.A.R.E., for instance, revealed no significant impact on reducing drug use among participants [1, 2]. The fundamental flaw of Prevention 1.0 was its reductionist focus on individual behavior, neglecting the more complex psychosocial and structural embedded drivers of substance use. Moreover, this model often reinforced stigma and shame, making it harder for people to seek help and further marginalizing those already vulnerable. It underestimated the powerful influence of trauma, poverty, housing insecurity, mental illness, and community disinvestment—factors now widely recognized as core contributors to substance use disorders (SUDs).

Prompted by the limitations of previous methods, researchers and public health experts developed a new approach—Prevention 2.0—grounded in social-ecological theory and supported by decades of evidence about the SDoH [3, 4]. Prevention 2.0 represents a paradigmatic shift from a narrow focus on preventing drug use to fostering wellbeing, resilience, and opportunity, particularly in structurally-disadvantaged communities. Prevention is not framed as a matter of individual virtue, but as a consequence of living conditions and whether or not those conditions support stable housing, safe relationships, economic security, and mental health [5, 6].

Programs under the Prevention 2.0 umbrella emphasize early childhood support, trauma-informed care, school–community partnerships, restorative practices, and culturally-responsive prevention efforts. Evidence shows that building self-regulation skills in childhood, ensuring access to safe environments, and mitigating toxic stress are better predictors of long-term health and behavioral outcomes than simple exposure to drug education [7, 8].

Figure 16.1 describes the evolution from Prevention 1.0 to 2.0. Crucially, Prevention 2.0 redefines success. The goal is no longer merely to prevent first use but to change the structural conditions that make harmful substance use likely. This approach aims to reduce adverse childhood experiences (ACEs), promote

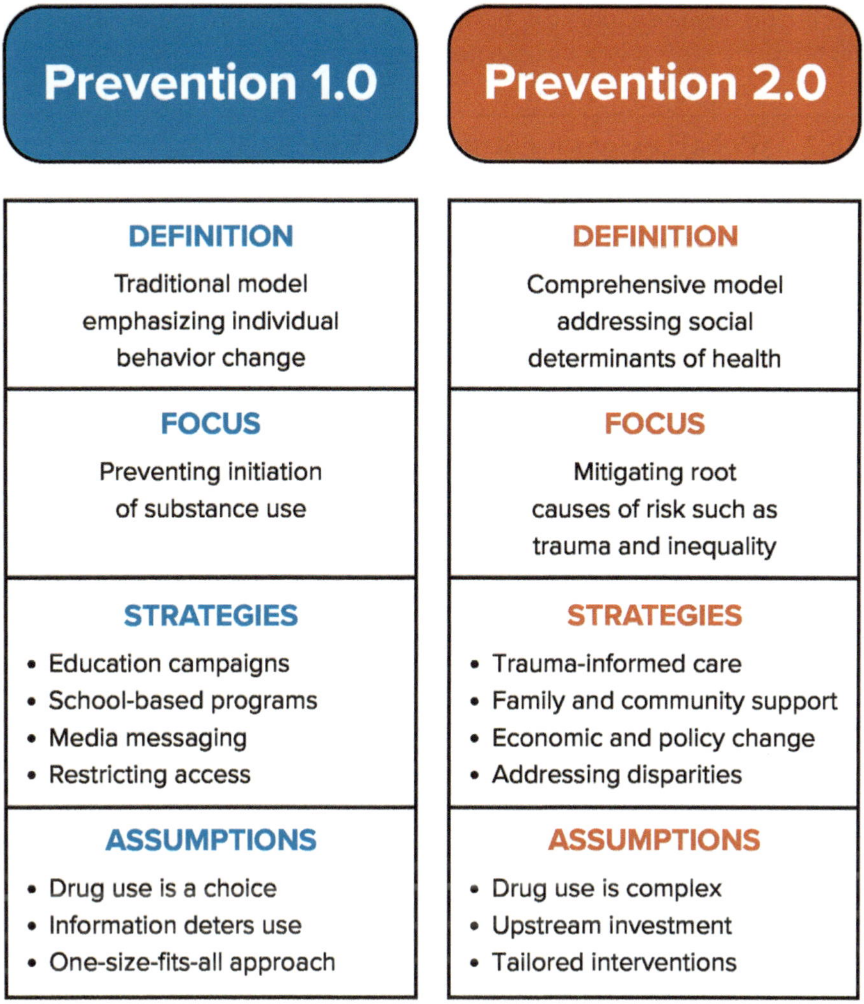

Prevention 1.0	Prevention 2.0
DEFINITION Traditional model emphasizing individual behavior change	**DEFINITION** Comprehensive model addressing social determinants of health
FOCUS Preventing initiation of substance use	**FOCUS** Mitigating root causes of risk such as trauma and inequality
STRATEGIES • Education campaigns • School-based programs • Media messaging • Restricting access	**STRATEGIES** • Trauma-informed care • Family and community support • Economic and policy change • Addressing disparities
ASSUMPTIONS • Drug use is a choice • Information deters use • One-size-fits-all approach	**ASSUMPTIONS** • Drug use is complex • Upstream investment • Tailored interventions

Fig. 16.1 Prevention 1.0 (Deterrence): Focused on fear-based messaging and punitive measures ("Just Say No," D.A.R.E.). Prevention 2.0 (Wellbeing): Emphasizes social determinants of health, trauma-informed care, and culturally-responsive strategies. Success is measured by wellbeing, not just the absence of drug use. (Source: Author's analysis, based on evidence summarized in Ennett et al. [1], West and O'Neal [2], Braveman and Gottlieb [5], and National Academies of Sciences [4, 8])

mental health, and provide pathways to meaningful education, employment, and social connection. This reflects a broader cultural and scientific recognition: that you cannot scare or punish your way out of a public health crisis rooted in inequality and despair. It challenges policymakers to exert the political will necessary to move away from reactive measures and invest long term in an equitable and responsive public health infrastructure. The new (and true) measure of success is not just the absence of drug use, but the presence of opportunity, connection, and meaning.

16.3 Global Lessons for Structural Change

As we synthesize the global lessons previously reviewed from Portugal's integrated decriminalization model, Canada's pharmacy-based methadone systems, and the emergent Prevention 2.0 framework, one theme stands out: to restructure the environment of risk itself to a deeper, upstream form of prevention. This is a new concept because it is a systems-level public health framing that has not been typical of US federal or state strategies, most of which stop at behavior-level interventions and overwhelmingly focus on treatment access, prescribing practices, and supply-side control. To meaningfully reduce substance-related harm, we must shift from managing individuals in crisis to transforming the systems that manufacture crisis.

Table 16.1 serves as a roadmap for structural change, demonstrating a new approach to substance use prevention and overdose prevention. Learning from effective global models and avoiding past mistakes (such as those in Oregon), the United States can forge a new path that combines scientific rigor, justice-based frameworks, and social investment.

Portugal's national strategy exemplifies this shift. While often lauded for decriminalizing drug possession as described in a previous chapter, Portugal's true innovation was the infrastructure that followed: investment in housing, employment services, mental health care, and non-stigmatizing support systems [9]. Similarly, Canada, the United Kingdom, and Australia have shown that integrating methadone

Table 16.1 Four categories of novel concepts to guide structural change

#	Concept	What's novel	Strategic implication
1	Shifting from managing symptoms to changing root conditions	Moves from crisis-focused treatment to addressing upstream social determinants (e.g., poverty, trauma, and housing)	Policy must invest in structural drivers of health, not just addiction services
2	Integrating global lessons for US transformation	Replaces American exceptionalism with openness to proven international models (e.g., Portugal and Canada)	Adapt successful foreign approaches (e.g., dissuasion panels, methadone in pharmacies) to fit US systems
3	Providing multilevel, multigenerational, and trauma-responsive prevention	Expands beyond youth-focused, one-time interventions to lifelong, family-based, trauma-informed strategies	Design cross-sector, upstream prevention systems that start early and span generations
4	Combining short-term survival with long-term healing	Integrates emergency response (e.g., naloxone, MOUD) with long-term supports (e.g., jobs, housing, and social connections)	Create recovery ecosystems that stabilize individuals and foster lasting wellbeing

MOUD Medications for opioid use disorder

treatment into community pharmacies and primary care, rather than isolating it in punitive, siloed systems, leads to better access and outcomes [10, 11].

These models reflect a key insight: addiction is not merely a problem of drug exposure, but of social exposure—to trauma, neglect, abandonment, and economic precarity. When people are disconnected from social connection and social supports, substances often become a substitute for what society has failed to provide [8]. The logic underlying Prevention 2.0 is a public health strategy that emphasizes trauma-informed care, early childhood support, social capital development, and housing-first policies. It is built on the understanding that wellbeing must be cultivated, not simply restored after a crisis [6].

Global models demonstrate that prevention, health, and reintegration must function as a single continuum of care. By embedding substance use policy within broader systems of housing, labor, and justice, these nations show what it means to treat addiction not as an isolated disorder, but as a societal condition [9, 11].

What these examples demand of the United States is humility. Learning from abroad requires us to abandon the myth of American exceptionalism and embrace a global evidence base for prevention and recovery. Integrating global lessons is, in itself, a new concept in the United States, which has approached national drug policy reform as an exceptional domestic problem, one requiring uniquely American solutions. This insularity is not accidental. US drug policy has been deeply rooted in moral narratives, racialized enforcement, and political posturing, making it resistant to outside influence or evidence-based recalibration [12]. As a result, the United States has remained committed to prohibitionist frameworks long after many peer nations have adopted public health-oriented, harm-reduction models.

Despite the Portugal model's demonstrated success in reducing overdose deaths, HIV transmission, and incarceration, the United States has been slow to adopt even localized analogues [13, 14]. Similarly, integration of methadone dispensing into pharmacies and primary care, designed to normalize and expand access to opioid agonist therapy, has no parallel in most of the United States, where federal restrictions still silo methadone within tightly controlled clinics [4, 10].

The global record also illustrates that transformation is not achieved in a single reform, but through sequencing: beginning with survival interventions, embedding them in health systems, and then extending outward to employment, housing, and reintegration. The United States must learn not only what to do, but in what order to do it.

The novelty of integrating global lessons into the US context acknowledges that other nations have succeeded not because they are softer on drugs, but because they have taken addiction seriously as a matter of public health, human rights, and social investment [15]. The effectiveness of universal healthcare and social safety nets depends not merely on their presence but on their strength, accessibility, and integration. The opioid crisis did not emerge simply from supply but from a toxic synergy between availability and vulnerability.

Integrating global models is especially urgent given the US polycrisis of synthetic opioids, housing instability, and mental health deterioration, contributing to over 80,000 annual drug overdose deaths [16]. Learning from other nations is not only pragmatic but also evidence-based, ethically sound, and long overdue. The United States must join other nations that recognize addiction as a social condition, treatable through evidence, dignity, and institutional change.

16.4 Multigenerational and Trauma-Informed Care

Another new, more sophisticated approach to substance use prevention is emerging: a multilevel, multigenerational, and trauma-responsive model. This is a significant shift from older models that viewed prevention as a set of discrete interventions targeting specific age groups, behaviors, and individual risk factors.

Traditionally, prevention efforts in the United States were built around a three-tiered public health model: universal prevention (for all), selective prevention (for high-risk groups), and indicated prevention (for individuals already showing signs of substance misuse) [3]. While this framework remains foundational, it is incomplete on its own. It often fails to recognize that the roots of substance use behaviors span generations and that trauma exposure in one life stage or family member can profoundly affect outcomes across time and relational networks.

A truly transformational model expands prevention in two critical ways. First, it becomes multigenerational, acknowledging that the conditions leading to substance use often originate before birth and persist across the lifespan and family lineage. ACEs, for instance, have been shown to increase the risk of early substance use, school failure, and chronic disease, while also shaping parenting behaviors in the next generation [17, 18]. Embedding support into family systems—not just individual children or teens—breaks intergenerational cycles of trauma and addiction [19].

Second, the model becomes explicitly trauma-responsive, not only recognizing the pervasive impact of trauma but designing interventions that account for it in structure, delivery, and content. Trauma-responsive prevention emphasizes safety, trust, peer support, collaboration, empowerment, and cultural relevance—key principles for reaching individuals whose substance use may be rooted in chronic adversity [20].

For example, home-visiting programs for new parents, like Nurse-Family Partnership, provide universal and selective prevention by offering parenting support, mental health screening, and substance use education in a non-stigmatizing way [21]. These programs reduce later substance use among both parents and children by promoting secure attachment, responsive caregiving, and stable home environments [22]. Similarly, early childhood trauma screening in pediatric settings—paired with supportive services—can flag risk early and offer healing before substance use begins.

Another example is *Familias Unidas*, a culturally tailored, family-centered prevention program for Hispanic parents and at-risk adolescents [23]. It strengthens parental support networks, builds parent–school partnerships, offers supervised family activities, and provides parenting classes to promote safe, stable home environments. Grounded in trauma-informed care, the program fosters healing and empowers families through culturally responsive strategies. What makes this approach new is not just its content, but its integration and scope. It links systems, including education, health care, housing, and justice, and synchronizes them across generations. It is built on the understanding that trauma in one domain (e.g., foster care) can manifest in another (e.g., juvenile detention or addiction treatment) unless there is a coordinated prevention net. It is also informed by neurodevelopmental science, which shows that brain plasticity, especially in childhood and adolescence, provides a window of opportunity to build resilience and emotional regulation [24].

Ultimately, this prevention approach is not simply an event or a curriculum but a lifelong, interwoven practice of creating safe, supportive, and equitable conditions for individuals, families, and communities. It asks not only, "How do we stop substance use?" but, more importantly, "How do we build lives where it is less necessary?"

16.5 Recovery as a Continuum of Care

Another new concept integrates short-term survival strategies with long-term healing approaches in substance use policy and practice. Administering naloxone or initiating medications for opioid use disorder (MOUD) is only the beginning of recovery, not its end. Without addressing the long-term social and system-embedded conditions that fuel addiction, such as housing insecurity, economic marginalization, and social fragmentation, many individuals remain caught in cycles of relapse, disconnection, and precarity [4].

The new paradigm recognizes that recovery is not a moment of intervention but a continuum of care and opportunity, extending well beyond clinical encounters. This model posits that the effectiveness of emergency interventions is magnified when they are embedded in a recovery ecology, a network of support that includes safe housing, meaningful employment, social connection, and community belonging [25, 26].

For example, programs that pair MOUD with supportive housing have shown significantly higher rates of treatment retention and reduced criminal justice involvement [27, 28]. Employment initiatives for people in recovery, especially when tied to peer support and job coaching, improve not just sobriety outcomes but also self-esteem and long-term stability [29]. Similarly, community reentry programs that integrate health care, vocational training, and trauma support reduce recidivism and promote continuity of care [30].

What's novel here is not the tools themselves but the intentional combination of emergency interventions with upstream determinants of wellbeing. It transcends the dichotomy of "harm reduction vs. abstinence" and instead supports multiple recovery pathways rooted in dignity, equity, and choice [26]. This model also elevates social cohesion, which is the relational fabric of communities, as a core component of recovery. Studies show that people who report stronger social bonds and a sense of belonging are more likely to sustain recovery and less likely to return to substance use in moments of stress or instability [31].

Integrating short-term survival and long-term healing acknowledges that recovery is not merely an individual accomplishment but a collective infrastructure. It requires that we build systems that don't just keep people alive but help them create lives worth living.

16.6 Bridging the Community–Correctional Divide

16.6.1 Breaking the Cycle: The Role of Employment in Correctional Health and Reentry

The proposed prevention paradigm is compelling and transformative. However, it must extend beyond community-based settings to prioritize correctional health, which is long overlooked and chronically underfunded. A comprehensive drug policy would connect community-based prevention strategies with reimagined correctional practices to disrupt the entrenched cycle of deep-seated disadvantage, substance use, and incarceration.

For decades, punitive drug laws have disproportionately targeted marginalized communities, including people living in poverty, people of color, and those with mental health conditions, transforming jails and prisons into de facto addiction management centers. Yet, these institutions lack the medical infrastructure or supportive services needed to address root causes or prepare individuals for reentry. Attempts to retrofit these facilities for therapeutic purposes have consistently fallen short, hindered by staffing shortages, inadequate healthcare infrastructure, and custodial priorities that place surveillance and control above evidence-based, trauma-informed care [32–34].

These institutional failures reflect a discriminatory social order that criminalizes poverty, race, and addiction simultaneously [12, 35]. The widespread denial of proven treatments—such as MOUD—within correctional settings exemplifies policy neglect [36].

Many incarcerated individuals enter prison with extensive trauma histories, only to face further harms unique to correctional environments: overcrowding, stigma, inadequate medical and behavioral health care, violence, hostile staff interactions, and institutional cultures prioritizing penalty over therapeutic support [37]. Under such conditions, substance use often becomes both a coping mechanism for deep emotional pain—rooted in societal disadvantage—and a survival strategy in an environment where legitimate economic opportunities are absent. Beyond re-traumatizing individuals, the correctional system further undermines recovery efforts (Fig. 16.2) [38].

Beyond these internal challenges, inadequate support service upon release—such as jobs and skills training, mental and behavioral health care, and housing assistance —undermines successful reintegration, fueling relapse and recidivism. One of the most significant barriers is the lack of stable employment, despite convincing evidence that work is a strong predictor of both sustained recovery and desistance. Stable employment provides income, structure, purpose, and social

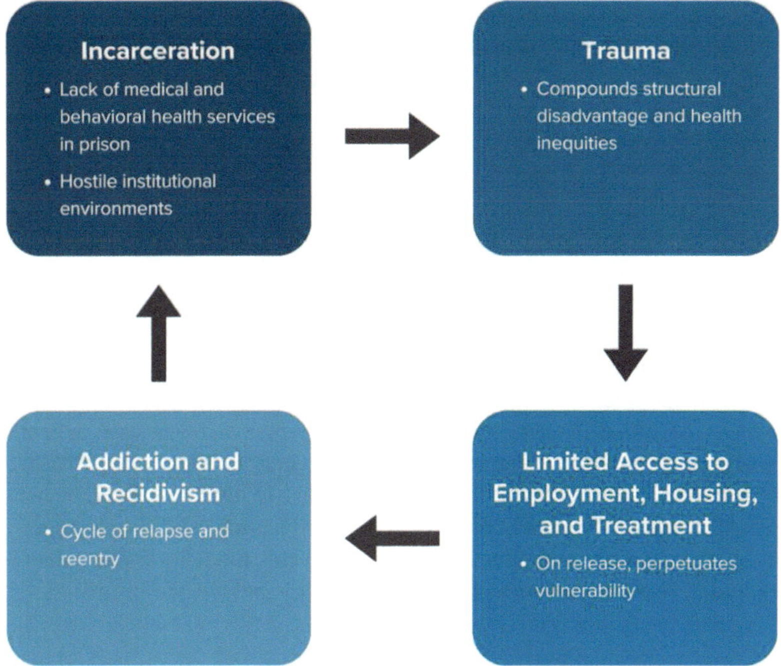

Fig. 16.2 The diagram illustrates how incarceration, trauma, limited access to employment, housing, and treatment, and cycles of addiction and recidivism are interconnected in perpetuating substance use vulnerability. Arrows indicate a cyclical relationship between structural disadvantage, health inequities, and reentry into the criminal legal system. (Source: Concepts adapted from Cloud et al. [38])

connections. Rigorous trials have shown that it reduces recidivism by roughly 16–22% [39–41].

Wage subsidy programs represent a promising labor market reentry strategy. They incentivize employers to hire individuals facing major employment barriers—including formerly incarcerated people—by reducing financial risk through partial wage subsidies or tax credits. These incentives are intended to improve employee retention, boost morale, and free resources for innovation.

Many of these programs, especially large scale, have been rigorously assessed for outcomes among diverse groups—with mixed results. For example, the Transitional Jobs Reentry Demonstration, funded by the U.S. Department of Labor, showed increased earnings for individuals during participation, but effects disappeared once subsidies ended, with little long-term impact on recidivism [42, 43]. In contrast, New York City's Center for Employment Opportunities, which couples wage subsidies with individualized support, cognitive-behavioral interventions, and job coaching, achieved a 16–22% reduction in recidivism among high-risk participants (e.g., co-occurring disorders and lengthy incarceration records) within three years post-release [42, 44].

Federal programs such as the Work Opportunity Tax Credit (WOTC) and the Federal Bonding Program offer limited incentives for hiring individuals with criminal records [45, 46]. However, the WOTC's complex paperwork and delayed tax benefits can reduce its appeal to employers, and neither program provides upfront cash flow to offset employer risk, making participation a daunting prospect.

International models offer valuable lessons on job reentry for disadvantaged workers. Portugal's decriminalization strategy, for example, prioritized rehabilitation and societal reintegration through employment programs that support recovery from substance use and help individuals secure stable work. Australia's Restart Program, also a national strategy, subsidizes employers who hire mature-age workers who have improved employment retention and reduced welfare reliance, especially when combined with tailored supports [47].

Research and international experience show that wage subsidies are most effective when embedded in comprehensive strategies that combine employment with tailored reentry programs. Transforming the carceral system demands a decisive shift from reactive, punishment-focused approaches to proactive, coordinated strategies that invest in evidence-based treatment, education, and employment pathways—before, during, and after incarceration. In this model, job placement is not the endpoint, but a milestone on the path to stability and long-term success.

16.6.2 Courts as Prevention Infrastructure: Reinterpreting Law for Prevention 2.0

US courts are not merely venues for adjudicating individual cases; they are high-leverage systems that can either entrench risk or catalyze prevention. For decades, legal interpretations have treated drug use among people with addiction as willful, illegal "choices," reinforcing punitive responses and abstinence-only conditions that conflict with medical evidence. Prevention 2.0 requires a jurisprudence that distinguishes status from conduct, recognizes relapse as part of a chronic condition, and ensures access to MOUD as standard of care [48]. Supreme Court doctrine already draws a line against punishing status (e.g., addiction) even as it permits regulation of conduct [49–51]; contemporary courts can honor that principle while applying today's science to sentencing, diversion, and problem-solving courts. Practically, this means adopting trauma-informed judicial practices; prohibiting blanket bans on MOUD; limiting carceral sanctions for clinical relapse; and using pre-plea diversion and civil "health docket" models that connect people to care, housing, and employment [11, 40, 48, 52–54]. In short, courts must move from managing noncompliance to engineering conditions for success. When courts align remedies with evidence and equity, they become upstream institutions—converting legal leverage into health, stability, and belonging.

16.6.3 From Incarceration to Integration: A National Wage Subsidy Program

A national wage subsidy program for reintegration of previously incarcerated individuals would pair financial incentives with proven system-wide support to promote sustained outcomes. Unlike short-term hiring bonuses or small tax credits, the program would treat wage subsidies as strategic investments in long-term stability and recovery. It also would target high-needs populations who have been shown to benefit more than lower-risk populations from wage subsidy initiatives. We propose that the federal government subsidize up to 50% of wages for employers who hire individuals with low-level, nonviolent drug offenses—specifically users, not distributors—who are actively enrolled in certified treatment programs lasting 12–24 months.

Employers participating in the program would be required to collaborate with local reentry programs or partner with community organizations to ensure a comprehensive continuum of care. The proposed program's targeted outcomes would be: increased hiring rates and sustained employment among individuals with SUDs and criminal records; lower rates of recidivism and relapse; enhanced health and social outcomes for participants; greater employer capacity; and reduced stigma toward employing this population.

Key elements include the following:

1. Targeting populations with elevated risk factors or complex needs, including those with multiple convictions, lengthy incarceration records, or co-occurring disorders
2. Pairing subsidies with integrated services, including case management, cognitive-behavioral therapy, clinics with MOUD, skills training, and peer recovery services
3. Integrating the WOTC and the Federal Bonding with the proposed program to develop a unified enrollment process that utilizes existing programs
4. Providing retention bonuses to employers who keep staff for 12 months after the subsidy ends
5. Providing technical assistance to employers to reduce upfront costs, administrative burden, and stigma

The deep-rooted challenges facing correctional health and substance use prevention demand a bold, integrated approach that bridges community and carceral systems. Simply expanding community programs without reforming correctional settings leaves critical gaps that perpetuate cycles of addiction, incarceration, and social inequity. By investing in comprehensive wage subsidy programs embedded in a lasting continuum of care, and by prioritizing correctional health as an essential part of public health, policymakers can disrupt these cycles and create pathways toward stability, dignity, and opportunity for all populations.

16.7 Political and Fiscal Barriers to Prevention Goals

America's public health infrastructure stands at a critical crossroads. Progress achieved over decades in combating SUDs is in danger of unraveling amid unprecedented federal budget cuts and administrative upheaval. While a vision for a transformative prevention strategy is inspiring, realizing it in today's politically charged and fiscally constrained environment is forbidding.

In early 2025, the newly created Department of Government Efficiency (DOGE) initiated sweeping administrative consolidations across federal agencies, targeting vital public health institutions, including the Centers for Disease Control and Prevention, SAMHSA, and other divisions within Health and Human Services. Key divisions were dismantled or merged, critical programs were scaled back, survey databases were eliminated, and experienced staff were dismissed, further eroding the nation's fragile public health infrastructure [55, 56].

While these administrative restructurings dealt a significant blow, legislation quickly followed. On July 4, 2025, Congress passed, and the President signed, H.R. 1—the One Big Beautiful Bill Act (OBBB)—a budget reconciliation law [57]. According to a Kaiser Family Foundation analysis of the Congressional Budget Office report, the law is estimated to reduce federal Medicaid spending by about $911 billion between 2025 and 2034 [58]. This is largely due to a national 80-hour-per-month work requirement for adults on the Affordable Care Act (ACA) expansion, more frequent eligibility checks, limitations on provider taxes, and caps on state-directed payments.

As a result, these changes are projected to increase the number of uninsured people by several million by 2034 [59]. The law disproportionately affects states that have expanded Medicaid, with more than half of the total federal funding cuts—an estimated $526 billion—falling on these states due to new provisions targeting adults in the Medicaid expansion program [60]. The law also does not extend enhanced ACA premium tax credits. Additionally, it makes those who lose Medicaid due to the new work requirements ineligible for Marketplace subsidies [58], which will further increase the uninsured rate. Given that Medicaid is the nation's single largest payer of behavioral health/SUDs services, reductions of this magnitude threaten the capacity and continuity central to Prevention 2.0 [61].

Under these conditions, states now face a stark choice: raise taxes, cut essential services, or reduce Medicaid enrollment. Projections indicate that 1.6 million Medicaid enrollees with SUDs could lose their coverage—a change that would devastate access to prevention, treatment, and recovery services nationwide [62].

Beyond the direct impact on coverage, the economic fallout is also projected to be substantial. Forecasts indicate over one million job losses nationwide and an estimated $154–183 billion decline in US economic output between 2029 and 2034 [63, 64].

Although only time will tell the full impact of these changes, one prediction is certain: these financial strains will not affect all populations equally. Marginalized groups, such as people with disabilities, those living in poverty, and individuals reentering society after incarceration, face the greatest risk of coverage loss, further entrenching service gaps and reinforcing cycles of disadvantage and instability [65–69].

Vital community services—including clinics offering MOUD and behavioral health treatment, housing assistance, and workforce training—are often the first to be cut in times of fiscal pressure. Under the OBBB, rural and underserved areas will be especially vulnerable to reductions, where hospital closures and funding shortfalls will leave the most vulnerable communities without essential care. Collectively, these findings underscore the profound human and economic costs of large-scale Medicaid cuts.

16.8 Strategies for Resilience and Sustained Momentum

Fiscal austerity and government priority realignments threaten to undermine the nation's capacity to address substance use through a public health approach. Future policy must confront ideological barriers and system-wide weaknesses, especially in underserved areas. While the broader fiscal and political environment may not yet allow for transformative change, it does not preclude action, particularly at the local level. Relevant stakeholders can deploy targeted strategies that preserve hard-won knowledge and programmatic gains, protect vulnerable populations, and maintain the existing infrastructure for an integrated public health response. Success will depend on leveraging shared assets, safeguarding critical infrastructure, and acting decisively to protect those most at risk. Equally essential is cultivating a resilient mindset—persevering with flexibility and commitment—so that when the first real opportunity for societal transformation arrives, stakeholders are ready to act.

The following approaches, grounded in real-world practice, offer a blueprint for sustaining momentum until larger foundational opportunities emerge. Systems-level change models are designed to address complex social and public health challenges by targeting the root causes rather than surface symptoms. These models aim to shift both the form and function of systems—altering policies, redistributing resources, restructuring relationships, and rebalancing power—to produce more equitable, sustainable outcomes. Systems change frameworks are well suited to facilitate institutional transformation in drug prevention, treatment, and recovery because they recognize that addiction and SUDs are complex, multifaceted issues influenced by a wide range of social, economic, cultural, and institutional factors. The following sections draw upon the Whole of Society, Collective Impact, and Health in All Policies models [70–73].

16.8.1 Foster Cross-Sector Collaboration

In today's political and economic climate, collaboration is not optional—it is essential. Strong cross-sectoral partnerships can clarify shared missions, boost morale, sustain trust, and keep grassroots engagement active. For example:

- Forming interagency task forces or committees—such as those implemented across sectors for vulnerable children—allows for joint decision-making and shared responsibility for administrative and operational responsibilities [74].
- Pooling resources and expertise—as emphasized in the Public Health 3.0 framework—enables more efficient allocation, coordinated service delivery, and the creation of policies that reflect local realities [75].
- In the absence of strong federal leadership, partnerships among states, municipalities, and civil society—exemplified by state-level cross-agency COVID-19 collaborations—can fill critical gaps, sustain continuity, and keep innovation alive [76].

16.8.2 Leverage Local Action and Pilot Programs

Conducting research and developing action plans at the municipal and county levels—when federal or state avenues are blocked—helps build the evidence base and draw attention to comprehensive, integrated public health approaches. This can include piloting programs that deliver visible, short-term wins while generating evidence sufficient to scale up.

16.8.3 Protect and Diversify Funding Streams

Programs that depend heavily on federal funding are especially vulnerable to sudden cuts, which can also restrict the use of state resources—as seen with the passage of the OBBB. Blended funding—through pooled philanthropy, private foundations, community benefit agreements—can stabilize services during downturns.

- Leverage local public health budgets, opioid settlement funds, and philanthropic investments
- Integrate substance use services into sectors like housing, workforce development, and education to reduce their risk of being cut
- Closely monitor opioid settlement funds to prevent diversion to unrelated priorities

16.8.4 Reframe the Public Narrative

Reframing the public narrative is not an effort to install a single, fixed story; it is a commitment to a patient-first, evidence-responsive framework that evolves along with science and lived experience. No single authority decides the "proper" narrative. It must be co-produced with people in pain, people with OUD, their families, clinicians, harm-reduction leaders, and communities. The aim is a narrative that advances population health while protecting individualized care—especially for those who benefit from analgesics or face the greatest risks from untreated pain or substance use.

An honest narrative begins with intellectual humility. It names uncertainty, separates what we know from what we infer, and promises revision when the evidence changes. Claims should be plain-language and testable so they can be checked against data and corrected without stigma or blame. That humility also demands precision: we must not conflate use with misuse, physiological dependence with addiction, or reductions in prescribing with improvements in public health. The narrative must hold two truths at once: prevention and harm reduction are essential public health aims, and so is preserving access to clinically-indicated pain care. Policy and communication should reflect both mandates rather than allow one to eclipse the other.

A science-based narrative recognizes heterogeneity. Risks and benefits vary by diagnosis, age, disability, race, class, and geography. Communication that pretends otherwise invites error and injustice. By naming who is most affected and why, we can design messages and policies that match real contexts: overdose prevention where fentanyl dominates; continuity and destigmatization of pain care where barriers are greatest; and recovery supports embedded across health, housing, and employment systems where social determinants drive risk.

This is the central project of *Deconstructing Toxic Narratives*: not to replace one orthodoxy with another but to strip away distortions, surface the truth, and rebuild a public story that is more accurate, modest, and humane. Done this way, reframing becomes a practice rather than a slogan—rooted in ongoing dialogue with patients, transparent sharing of data, and routine updates that incorporate new trials, real-world evidence, and community feedback. It reduces stigma, counters misinformation, and builds public trust while safeguarding room for individualized clinical judgment, ensuring that policies remain both humane and scientifically current.

16.8.5 Safeguard and Share Data

Threats to national data systems, such as SAMHSA's National Survey of Drug Use and Health, highlight the need for ongoing state and local research and evaluation in drug use and mental health [77]. Accessible, reliable data let stakeholders track trends, identify gaps, and measure impact. Effective data sharing supports evidence-based policies and collaboration helps safeguard vital information in limited-resource environments.

Actions to support include the following:

- Invest in or connect with local and state-level data infrastructure
- Intensify efforts to disseminate data in academic journals, articles, social media, and forums
- Leverage data sharing to enable rapid, coordinated responses to public health threats

16.8.6 Embrace Scientific Innovation

The new paradigm must also embrace cutting-edge pharmacology, requiring long-term commitment. Notably GLP-1 receptor agonists (GLP-1s), medications primarily developed for obesity and diabetes, have rapidly emerged as a promising new class for SUDs [78, 79]. Correlational analyses from large real-world cohorts showed patients with OUD taking GLP-1 drugs had a 40% lower overdose risk, and those with alcohol use disorder (AUD) had a roughly 50% reduction in alcohol intoxication events [78]. Another large analysis focusing specifically on patients with both OUD and type 2 diabetes reported the risk of hospitalization for overdose was cut by 40–70% when taking semaglutide compared to older diabetes medications [79]. Preclinical studies suggest that these agents may work by attenuating reward-driven cravings and compulsive behaviors [80]. Crucially, these medications are adjuncts, not a technological panacea, and should be embedded within comprehensive systems that address the structural drivers of addiction, including pain, poverty, racism, trauma, and social disconnection [81]. Rigorous clinical trials should follow, and if evidence supports their use, these agents should be made accessible and affordable.

16.9 Policy and Practice for a New Era

The future of substance use prevention will not be written by fear or punishment, but by our collective choices to invest in each other's humanity. When we dare to imagine a world where everyone deserves safety, purpose, and belonging, prevention becomes not just possible but inevitable.

The intertwined crises of substance use, structural inequity, and social disconnection demand more than incremental fixes—they require a fundamental shift in vision and practice. The evidence is unmistakable: punitive, fragmented approaches have failed [12, 35]. In contrast, integrated, trauma-informed, and equity-centered strategies offer the greatest promise for building a society grounded in collective courage, compassion, and fairness.

Political and fiscal realities will shape the path forward. In the near term, resilience, cross-sector collaboration, and targeted local action are essential to preserve critical infrastructure and protect progress. Over the long term, policymakers must be prepared to reimagine prevention, treatment, and reintegration as core pillars of a transformative public health strategy (Table 16.2).

16.9.1 A Phased Approach to Transformation

Transformation demands sustained investment, political will, and the courage to dismantle macro-level barriers that perpetuate harm. The United States can learn from international models that have shifted drug policy toward public health with measurable, ethical, and sustainable results [9, 13, 86, 87].

Table 16.2 Policy recommendations and recovery impact

Policy recommendation	Time horizon	Who should act/ Mechanism	First step	Evidence of impact
Expand MOUD access in prisons and jails	Immediate (1–2 years)	State departments of corrections should require all prisons/jails >500 inmates to provide at least one MOUD; CMS should approve Medicaid waivers for pre-release coverage	Governors issue directives to pilot MOUD programs in state prisons; states file Section 1115 waivers to cover reentry treatment	Continuation of MOUD during incarceration improves treatment retention and reduces post-release overdose deaths [82]
Enhance Medicaid coverage and continuity post-incarceration	Immediate (1–2 years)	CMS should mandate suspension (not termination) of Medicaid during incarceration and provide matching funds for states ensuring MOUD initiation within 30 days of release	States file Section 1115 waivers or SPAs to guarantee coverage at reentry	Medicaid continuity reduces emergency health utilization and supports recovery [30, 82]
Invest in trauma-informed reentry programs	Medium-term (3–7 years)	State reentry councils and DOC contracting offices should require trauma-informed training and earmark 20% of reentry budgets for counseling, peer support, and family integration	Add trauma-informed care as a scoring criterion in RFPs for reentry services	Trauma-informed reentry programs reduce re-incarceration and improve psychosocial outcomes [20, 83]
Subsidize employment for individuals in recovery	Medium-term (3–7 years)	Congress should pilot a federal wage subsidy program covering up to 50% of wages for 12 months; states can replicate using opioid settlement funds	Department of Labor convenes working group to design wage subsidy pilot; states earmark settlement funds for subsidized employment	Subsidized employment is associated with lower relapse and recidivism [39, 42, 43]

(continued)

Table 16.2 (continued)

Policy recommendation	Time horizon	Who should act/ Mechanism	First step	Evidence of impact
Implement structural racism audits in health and justice systems	Long-term (7–10+ years)	Congresss should require annual equity audits of federal health and justice funding streams, tied to corrective action plans from SAMHSA and DOJ	Commission GAO to conduct a baseline racial equity audit of SUD-related federal programs	Structural racism audits improve transparency and support equitable outcomes [84]
Modernize courts for prevention 2.0	Immediate–medium (0–3 years)	State supreme courts; legislatures; court administrators; problem-solving court networks	Issue administrative orders banning MOUD exclusions; launch mandatory judicial CLE on addiction science/ADA; pilot pre-plea diversion and civil "health dockets"	NJC MOUD bench cards and All Rise Best Practice Standards recommend MOUD access; DOJ ADA guidance prohibits discrimination against people using MOUD; studies document court barriers and improved outcomes when MOUD is available [40, 48, 52, 53, 85]
Prioritize research and access to novel therapeutics (e.g., GLP-1s)	Long-term (7–10+ years)	NIH/NIDA/ NIAAA should fund rigorous clinical trials for GLP-1s in SUDs; CMS should mandate coverage for evidence-based addiction treatment	NIH funds large-scale RCTs to confirm efficacy for OUD and AUD; states use Section 1115 waivers to explore coverage pathways	Correlational data suggest: A 40% lower overdose risk in OUD and a 50% reduction in intoxication events in AUD when prescribed for other conditions [78] A 40–70% risk of hospitalization for overdose in OUD/ T2D patients with semaglutide compared to older diabetes medications [79]

MOUD medications for opioid use disorder, *CMS* Centers for Medicare & Medicaid Services, *DOC* departments of corrections, *SPAs* State Plan Amendments, *RFPs* requests for proposals, *SAMHSA* Substance Abuse and Mental Health Services Administration, *DOJ* Department of Justice, *GAO* Government Accountability Office, *SUDs* substance use disorders, *ADA* Americans with Disabilities Act, *NJC* National Judicial College, *CLE* continuing legal education, *AUD* alcohol use disorder, *GLP-1s* GLP-1 receptor agonists, *NIH* National Institutes of Health, *NIDA* National Institute on Drug Abuse, *NIAAA* National Institute on Alcohol Abuse and Alcoholism, *T2D* type 2 diabetes

Change will unfold across horizons:

- *Some steps are immediate*: expanding access to MOUD in jails and prisons, safeguarding Medicaid continuity at reentry, and protecting public health data [30, 82]. These actions are feasible within the current political climate and will save lives today.
- *Other reforms require medium-term coordination and investment*: scaling trauma-informed reentry programs, piloting wage subsidies for people in recovery, and embedding recovery supports across health, housing, and employment systems. These steps are achievable within this decade and will stabilize families, reduce recidivism, and create pathways to dignity [42, 43, 83].
- *Durable transformation will require long-term structural change*: institutionalizing racial equity audits, embedding prevention into every policy domain, and creating a national wage subsidy program that recognizes employment as public health infrastructure. These goals will take sustained political will, but they hold the power to reorient the nation's response to substance use toward fairness, resilience, and belonging [84, 86].

Federal and state leaders must embrace this paradigm. Practitioners, advocates, and researchers must work across systems to align care, education, housing, and justice under a shared vision of dignity and resilience. Communities must shape solutions rooted in lived experience. Together, we must act decisively. If we do, we can transform a crisis of despair into a culture of possibility—where prevention is not merely a strategy, but a social contract.

References

1. Ennett ST, Tobler NS, Ringwalt CL, Flewelling RL. How effective is drug abuse resistance education? A meta-analysis of project DARE outcome evaluations. Am J Public Health. 1994;84(9):1394–401.
2. West SL, O'Neal KK. Project D.A.R.E. Outcome effectiveness revisited. Am J Public Health. 2004;94(6):1027–9.
3. National Research Council (US) and Institute of Medicine (US). Committee on the prevention of mental disorders and substance abuse among children, youth, and young adults: research advances and promising interventions. In: O'Connell ME, Boat T, Warner KE, editors. Preventing mental, emotional, and Behavioral disorders among young people: Progress and possibilities. Washington, DC: National Academies Press (US); 2009. Available from: https://www.ncbi.nlm.nih.gov/books/NBK32775/, https://doi.org/10.17226/12480.
4. National Academies of Sciences, Engineering, and Medicine. Medications for opioid use disorder save lives. Washington, DC: The National Academies Press; 2019. Available from: https://nap.nationalacademies.org/catalog/25310/medications-for-opioid-use-disorder-save-lives.
5. Braveman P, Gottlieb L. The social determinants of health: it's time to consider the causes of the causes. Public Health Rep. 2014;129(1_suppl2):19–31.
6. Substance Abuse and Mental Health Services Administration. A guide to SAMHSA's strategic prevention framework. Center for Substance Abuse Prevention, Substance Abuse and Mental Health Services Administration: Rockville; 2019.

7. Moffitt TE, Arseneault L, Belsky D, Dickson N, Hancox RJ, Harrington H, et al. A gradient of childhood self-control predicts health, wealth, and public safety. Proc Natl Acad Sci. 2011;108(7):2693–8.
8. National Academies of Sciences, Engineering, and Medicine. Fostering healthy mental, emotional, and behavioral development in children and youth: a national agenda. Washington, DC: The National Academies Press; 2019. https://doi.org/10.17226/25201.
9. Hughes CE, Stevens A. What can we learn from the Portuguese decriminalization of illicit drugs? Br J Criminol. 2010;50(6):999–1022.
10. Gomes T, Kitchen SA, Murray R. Measuring the burden of opioid-related mortality in Ontario, Canada, during the COVID-19 pandemic. JAMA Netw Open. 2021;4(5):e2112865.
11. Strang J, McDonald R, Campbell G, Degenhardt L, Nielsen S, Ritter A, et al. Take-home naloxone for the emergency interim management of opioid overdose: the public health application of an emergency medicine. Drugs. 2019;79(13):1395–418.
12. Alexander M. The new Jim crow: mass incarceration in the age of colorblindness. Revised ed. New York: The New Press; 2012.
13. Laqueur H. Uses and abuses of drug decriminalization in Portugal. Law Soc Inq. 2015;40(3):746–81.
14. Domosławski A. Drug policy in Portugal: the benefits of decriminalizing drug use. Warsaw: Open Society Foundations; 2011.
15. Room R, Reuter P. How well do international drug conventions protect public health? Lancet. 2012;379(9810):84–91.
16. U.S. Overdose Deaths Decrease Almost 27% in 2024. Atlanta: Centers for Disease Control and Prevention, National Center for Health Statistics; 2025. [cited 2025 Aug 15]. Available from: https://www.cdc.gov/nchs/pressroom/nchs_press_releases/2025/20250514.htm.
17. Felitti VJ, Anda RF, Nordenberg D, Williamson DF, Spitz AM, Edwards V, et al. Relationship of childhood abuse and household dysfunction to many of the leading causes of death in adults. The Adverse Childhood Experiences (ACE) Study. Am J Prev Med. 1998;14(4):245–58.
18. Anda RF, Felitti VJ, Bremner JD, Walker JD, Whitfield C, Perry BD, et al. The enduring effects of abuse and related adverse experiences in childhood. Eur Arch Psychiatry Clin Neurosci. 2006;256(3):174–86.
19. Yoshikawa H, Aber JL, Beardslee WR. The effects of poverty on the mental, emotional, and behavioral health of children and youth: implications for prevention. Am Psychol. 2012;67(4):272–84.
20. Substance Abuse and Mental Health Services Administration. SAMHSA's concept of trauma and guidance for a trauma-informed approach. Rockville: Substance Abuse and Mental Health Services Administration; 2014. [cited 2025 Aug 15]. Report No.: (SMA) 14-4884. Available from: https://store.samhsa.gov/sites/default/files/d7/priv/sma14-4884.pdf.
21. Changent. Nurse-Family Partnership. Changent; 2024. [cited 2025 Aug 15]. Available from: https://changent.org/what-we-do/nurse-family-partnership/.
22. Olds DL, Kitzman H, Hanks C, Cole R, Anson E, Sidora-Arcoleo K, et al. Effects of nurse home visiting on maternal and child functioning: age-9 follow-up of a randomized trial. Pediatrics. 2007;120(4):e832–45.
23. Familias Unidas programs. In: Familias Unidas. [cited 2025 Aug 14]. Available from: https://www.familias-unidas.org/.
24. Shonkoff JP, Garner AS, The Committee On Psychosocial Aspects Of C, Family Health COECA, Dependent C, Section On D, et al. The lifelong effects of early childhood adversity and toxic stress. Pediatrics. 2012;129(1):e232–e46.
25. Bassuk EL, Hanson J, Greene RN, Richard M, Laudet A. Peer-delivered recovery support Services for Addictions in the United States: a systematic review. J Subst Abus Treat. 2016;63:1–9.
26. White WL. Recovery management and recovery-oriented systems of care: scientific rationale and promising practices. Philadelphia: Great Lakes Addiction Technology Transfer Center, Northeast Addiction Technology Transfer Center, Philadelphia Department of Behavioral Health/Mental Retardation Services; 2008.

27. Tsemberis S. Housing first: the pathways model to end homelessness for people with mental illness and addiction manual. Sam Tsemberis; 2011.
28. Larimer ME, Malone DK, Garner MD, Atkins DC, Burlingham B, Lonczak HS, et al. Health care and public service use and costs before and after provision of housing for chronically homeless persons with severe alcohol problems. JAMA. 2009;301(13):1349–57.
29. Substance Abuse and Mental Health Services Administration. Treatment of stimulant use disorders, Report no.: PEP20-06-01-001. Rockville: SAMHSA; 2020.
30. Morrissey JP, Domino ME, Cuddeback GS. Expedited Medicaid Enrollment, mental health service use, and criminal recidivism among released prisoners with severe mental illness. Psychiatr Serv. 2016;67(8):842–9.
31. Kelly JF, Greene MC, Bergman BG. Beyond abstinence: changes in indices of quality of life with time in recovery in a nationally representative sample of U.S. Adults. Alcohol Clin Exp Res. 2018;42(4):770–80.
32. Binswanger IA, Nowels C, Corsi KF, Glanz J, Long J, Booth RE, et al. Return to drug use and overdose after release from prison: a qualitative study of risk and protective factors. Addict Sci Clin Pract. 2012;7(1):3.
33. Widra E. Addicted to punishment: jails and prisons punish drug use far more than they treat it. Prison Policy Initiative; 2024. [cited 2025 Jul 15]. Available from: https://www.prisonpolicy.org/blog/2024/01/30/punishing-drug-use/.
34. Russ EN, Puglisi L, Eber GB, Morse DS, Taxman FS, Dupuis MF, et al. Prison and jail reentry and health. Health Aff. 2021. [cited 2025 Aug 15]. Available from: https://www.healthaffairs.org/content/briefs/prison-and-jail-reentry-and-health.
35. Hansen H, Netherland J, Herzberg D. Whiteout: how racial capitalism changed the color of opioids in America. Oakland: University of California Press; 2023.
36. Rich JD, McKenzie M, Larney S, Wong JB, Tran L, Clarke J, et al. Methadone continuation versus forced withdrawal on incarceration in a combined US prison and jail: a randomised, open-label trial. Lancet. 2015;386(9991):350–9.
37. James DJ, Glaze LE. Mental health problems of prison and jail inmates. Washington, DC: U.S. Department of Justice, Office of Justice Programs, Bureau of Justice Statistics; 2006. [cited 2025 Aug 18]. Available from: https://bjs.ojp.gov/content/pub/pdf/mhppji.pdf.
38. Cloud DH, Parsons J, Delany-Brumsey A. Addressing mass incarceration: a clarion call for public health. Am J Public Health. 2014;104(3):389–91.
39. Laudet AB, Savage R, Mahmood D. Pathways to long-term recovery: a preliminary investigation. J Psychoactive Drugs. 2002;34(3):305–11.
40. Matusow H, Dickman SL, Rich JD, Fong C, Dumont DM, Hardin C, et al. Medication assisted treatment in US drug courts: results from a nationwide survey of availability, barriers and attitudes. J Subst Abus Treat. 2013;44(5):473–80.
41. Uggen C. Work as a turning point in the life course of criminals: a duration model of age, employment, and recidivism. Am Sociol Rev. 2000;65(4):529–46.
42. Bloom D. Employment-focused programs for ex-prisoners: what have we learned, what are we learning, and where should we go from here? New York: MDRC; 2006. [cited 2025 Aug 18]. Available from: https://www.mdrc.org/work/publications/employment-focused-programs-ex-prisoners.
43. Jacobs E. Returning to work after prison: final results from the transitional jobs reentry demonstration. New York: MDRC; 2012.
44. Redcross S, Millenky M, Rudd TR, Levshin V. More than a job: final results from the evaluation of the Center for Employment Opportunities (CEO) Transitional Jobs Program, OPRE report 2011–18. Washington, DC: Office of Planning, Research and Evaluation, Administration for Children and Families, U.S. Department of Health and Human Services; 2012.
45. Internal Revenue Service. Work opportunity tax credit. Washington, DC: U.S. Department of the Treasury; [Updated 2025 Aug 18; cited 2025 Aug 18]. Available from: https://www.irs.gov/businesses/small-businesses-self-employed/work-opportunity-tax-credit.
46. Union Insurance Group. About the FBP. Federal Bonding Program; 2022. [cited 2025 Aug 18]. Available from: https://bonds4jobs.com/about-us.

47. Department of the Prime Minister and Cabinet. Transcript of the Hon Tony Abbott MP, Prime Minister. Subject: more support for mature age job seekers. Canberra: Department of the Prime Minister and Cabinet; 2014. Available from: https://pmtranscripts.pmc.gov.au/release/transcript-23637.
48. Marlowe DB, Theiss DS, Ostlie EM, Carnevale J. Drug court utilization of medications for opioid use disorder in high opioid mortality communities. J Subst Abus Treat. 2022;141:108850.
49. City of Grants Pass v. Johnson, 603 U.S. – (2024). Available from: https://www.supremecourt.gov/opinions/23pdf/23-175_19m2.pdf.
50. POWELL v. TEXAS, 392 U.S. 514 (1968). Available from: https://tile.loc.gov/storage-services/service/ll/usrep/usrep392/usrep392514/usrep392514.pdf.
51. ROBINSON v. CALIFORNIA, 370 U.S. 660 (1962). Available from: https://tile.loc.gov/storage-services/service/ll/usrep/usrep370/usrep370660/usrep370660.pdf.
52. National Judicial College. Medication for opioid use disorder (bench card). Reno: National Judicial College; 2022. Available from: https://www.judges.org/wp-content/uploads/2022/10/Final-NJC-Benchcard-on-MOUD.pdf.
53. All Rise. Adult treatment court Best practice standards. Reno: All Rise; 2023. Available from: https://allrise.org/publications/standards/.
54. European Monitoring Centre for Drugs and Drug Addiction. Drug policy profiles: Portugal. Lisbon: European Monitoring Centre for Drugs and Drug Addiction; 2011. Available from: https://www.euda.europa.eu/system/files/publications/642/PolicyProfile_Portugal_WEB_Final_289201.pdf.
55. Williams DR, Cooper LA. COVID-19 and health equity—a new kind of "herd immunity". JAMA. 2020;323(24):2478–80.
56. ASPA Press Office. HHS announces transformation to make America healthy again. Washington, DC: U.S. Department of Health and Human Services; 2025. [cited 2025 Sep 4]. Available from: https://www.hhs.gov/press-room/hhs-restructuring-doge.html
57. Congress HR. 1: one big beautiful bill act, 119th Congress. Washington, DC: U.S. Government Publishing Office; 2025. [cited 2025 Sep 4]. Available from: https://www.congress.gov/bill/119th-congress/house-bill/1.
58. Hinton E, Diana A, Rudowitz R. A closer look at the work requirement provisions in the 2025 federal budget reconciliation law. Menlo Park: Kaiser Family Foundation; 2025. [cited 2025 Sep 4]. Available from: https://www.kff.org/medicaid/issue-brief/a-closer-look-at-the-work-requirement-provisions-in-the-2025-federal-budget-reconciliation-law/.
59. Burns A, Ortaliza J, Lo J, Rae M, Cox C. How will the 2025 reconciliation law affect the uninsured rate in each state? Menlo Park: Kaiser Family Foundation; 2025. [cited 2025 Sep 4]. Available from: https://www.kff.org/uninsured/how-will-the-2025-reconciliation-law-affect-the-uninsured-rate-in-each-state/.
60. Euhus R, Williams E, Burns A, Rudowitz R. Allocating CBO's estimates of Federal Medicaid spending reductions across the states: enacted reconciliation package. Menlo Park: Kaiser Family Foundation; 2025. [cited 2025 Sep 4]. Available from: https://www.kff.org/medicaid/allocating-cbos-estimates-of-federal-medicaid-spending-reductions-across-the-states-enacted-reconciliation-package/.
61. MACPAC. Behavioral health topic page. Washington, DC: Medicaid and CHIP Payment and Access Commission. [cited 2025 Sep 4]. Available from: https://www.macpac.gov/topic/behavioral-health/.
62. Natasha Murphy. How the big, 'beautiful' bill would undermine access to life-saving substance-use disorder treatment. Washington, DC: Center for American Progress; 2025. [cited 2025 Sep 4]. Available from: https://www.americanprogress.org/article/how-the-big-beautiful-bill-would-undermine-access-to-life-saving-substance-use-disorder-treatment/.
63. Ku L, Kwon KN, Krips M, Gorak T, Cordes JJ. How Medicaid and SNAP cutbacks in the "one big beautiful bill" would trigger big and bigger job losses across states. Washington, DC: Commonwealth Fund; 2025. [cited 2025 Sep 4]. Available from: https://www.commonwealthfund.org/publications/issue-briefs/2025/jun/how-medicaid-snap-cutbacks-one-big-beautiful-bill-trigger-job-losses-states.

64. Bradley J. Medicaid cuts could hurt the U.S. economy. New York: Investopedia; 2025. [cited 2025 Sep 4]. Available from: https://www.investopedia.com/medicaid-cuts-hurt-economy-11779578.
65. Albertson EM, Scannell C, Ashtari N, Barnert E. Eliminating gaps in Medicaid coverage during Reentry after incarceration. Am J Public Health. 2020;110(3):317–21.
66. Lin Y, Monnette A, Shi L. Effects of Medicaid expansion on poverty disparities in health insurance coverage. Int J Equity Health. 2021;20(1):171.
67. Goodman N, Morris M, Boston K. Financial inequality: disability, race and poverty in America. Washington, DC: National Disability Institute; 2019. [cited 2025 Sep 4]. Available from: https://www.nationaldisabilityinstitute.org/reports/financial-inequality-disability-race-and-poverty-in-america/.
68. Nishar S, Brumfield E, Mandal S, Vanjani R, Soske J. "It's a revolving door": understanding the social determinants of mental health as experienced by formerly incarcerated people. Health Justice. 2023;11(1). [cited 2025 Sep 4]. Available from: https://doi.org/10.1186/s40352-023-00227-8.
69. Creedon TB, Lamont H, Dey J, Branham DK, Sommers BD, Marton W. Health insurance coverage among working-age adults with disabilities: 2010–2018. Washington, DC: Office of the Assistant Secretary for Planning and Evaluation, U.S. Department of Health and Human Services; 2021. [cited 2025 Sep 4]. Available from: https://aspe.hhs.gov/reports/health-insurance-coverage-among-working-age-adults-disabilities-2010-2018-issue-brief.
70. Leischow SJ, Best A, Trochim WM, Clark PI, Gallagher RS, Marcus SE, et al. Systems thinking to improve the public's health. Am J Prev Med. 2008;35(2 Suppl):S196–203.
71. Ajaero Ijeoma D, Lubinga E. A whole-of-society (WoS) approach as a communication strategy towards addressing challenges and solutions to food insecurity and climate change in Nigeria as portrayed in the documentary film swallow (2018). J Afr Films Diaspora Stud. 2025;8(2):71–92.
72. Nakueira S. A whole-of-society approach to vulnerabilities: contestations and unintended effects. In: Between protection and harm. Cham: Springer International Publishing; 2024. p. 95–116.
73. Terry NP, Burris SC. A 'Whole of government' approach to reforming opioid use disorder legal and policy strategies. 2023. Available from: https://doi.org/10.2139/ssrn.4650706.
74. Silow-Carroll S, Rodin D, Pham A. Interagency, cross-sector collaboration to improve Care for Vulnerable Children: lessons for California from six state initiatives. Palo Alto: Lucile Packard Foundation for Children's Health; 2018. [cited 2025 Sep 4]. Available from: https://lpfch.org/wp-content/uploads/2024/02/hma_interagency_collaboration_ca_report_02.15.2018.pdf.
75. DeSalvo KB, Wang YC, Harris A, Auerbach J, Koo D, O'Carroll P. Public health 3.0: a call to action for public health to meet the challenges of the 21st century. Prev Chronic Dis. 2017;14:170017. [cited 2025 Sep 4]. Available from: https://doi.org/10.5888/pcd14.170017.
76. Higgins E, Cooper R. State cross-agency collaboration during the COVID-19 pandemic response. Washington, DC: National Academy for State Health Policy (NASHP); 2021. [cited 2025 Sep 4]. Available from: https://nashp.org/state-cross-agency-collaboration-during-the-covid-19-pandemic-response/.
77. Chatterjee R. They've tracked Americans' drug use for decades. Trump and RFK Jr. fired them. Washington, DC: NPR; 2025. [cited 2025 Aug 18]. Available from: https://www.npr.org/sections/shots-health-news/2025/05/29/nx-s1-5407849/samhsa-nsduh-trump-rfk-jr-hhs-cuts.
78. Qeadan F, McCunn A, Tingey B. The association between glucose-dependent insulinotropic polypeptide and/or glucagon-like peptide-1 receptor agonist prescriptions and substance-related outcomes in patients with opioid and alcohol use disorders: a real-world data analysis. Addiction. 2025;120(2):236–50.
79. Wang W, Volkow ND, Wang Q, Berger NA, Davis PB, Kaelber DC, et al. Semaglutide and opioid overdose risk in patients with type 2 diabetes and opioid use disorder. JAMA Netw Open. 2024;7(9):e2435247.
80. Jerlhag E. GLP-1 receptor agonists: promising therapeutic targets for alcohol use disorder. Endocrinology. 2025;166(4):bqaf028.

81. Szalavitz M. The breakthrough drug to conquer addiction: Ozempic? The New York Times; 2024. [cited 2025 Nov 10]. Available from: https://www.nytimes.com/2024/10/18/opinion/addiction-ozempic-glp-1.html.
82. Rich JD, Chandler R, Williams BA, Dumont D, Wang EA, Taxman FS, et al. How health care reform can transform the health of criminal justice-involved individuals. Health Aff (Millwood). 2014;33(3):462–7.
83. French MT, Zarkin GA, Hubbard RL, Rachal JV. The effects of time in drug abuse treatment and employment on posttreatment drug use and criminal activity. Am J Drug Alcohol Abuse. 1993;19(1):19–33.
84. Bailey ZD, Krieger N, Agénor M, Graves J, Linos N, Bassett MT. Structural racism and health inequities in the USA: evidence and interventions. Lancet. 2017;389(10077):1453–63.
85. U.S. Department of Justice, ADA. Opioid use disorder. Washington: U.S. Department of Justice; 2022. Available from: https://www.ada.gov/resources/opioid-use-disorder/.
86. Csete J, Kamarulzaman A, Kazatchkine M, Altice F, Balicki M, Buxton J, et al. Public health and international drug policy. Lancet. 2016;387(10026):1427–80.
87. Greenwald GG. Drug decriminalization in Portugal: lessons for creating fair and successful drug policies. Washington, DC: Cato Institute; 2009.

Appendices

Appendix A: Summary of Econometric Study Findings

L. R. Webster, S. Eichberg, *Deconstructing Toxic Narratives*,
https://doi.org/10.1007/978-3-032-23135-2

Study type	Study authors	Source	Method	Focus	Result
Unemployment	Hollingsworth et al. (2017)	Mortality data included 3138 counties over 16 years, yielding 50,148 observations	Panel study (longitudinal) with fixed effects regression	County- and state-level analysis of the relationship between local unemployment rates and opioid-related deaths and emergency department (ED) visits between 1999 and 2014	A one percentage point increase in the county unemployment rate predicted opioid fatalities by a statistically significant 0.19 per 100,000 (3.6%) Opioid-related ED visits showed strong effects for Black individuals as well as whites
	Carpenter et al. (2016)	Pooled data with 800,000 + respondents to National Surveys on Drug Use and Health (NSDUH) for 2002–2013	Quasi-experiment: fixed effects regression and difference-in-differences models	The effect of state unemployment rates on self-reported use of illicit drugs, such as analgesics, cocaine, and heroin	Ecstasy use was positively and strongly associated with unemployment rates but results for other classes of drugs were negative or inconsistent Using clinical measures for SUDs, disorders involving analgesics (both opioid and non-opioid versions) and hallucinogens were strongly related to unemployment, with the most robust effects concentrated in non-elderly adult white men with low levels of education
	Betz and Jones (2018)	Combines various sources to provide 26,337 observations on nonmetro counties and 13,649 on metro counties	Fixed-effects regression	The relationship between opioid overdose mortality and employment and earnings per worker in certain industries for 2001–2014	Job loss and wage declines in lower skilled industries are associated with higher opioid overdose mortality rates The relationship is especially strong for rural white men in goods-producing sectors as well as Black male and female workers in the services sector
	Maclean et al. (2020)	TEDS, an all-payer administrative database compiled annually by the US government and state substance abuse agencies, with 1187 observations	Fixed-effects model	The effect of business cycles, using state unemployment as a proxy, on admissions per 100,000 to specialty substance abuse treatment between 1992 and 2015	Statistically significant evidence shows that total admissions are impacted across the business cycle for all drug types For heroin, it was found that a one percentage point increase in the state unemployment rate led to a 5.9% reduction in admissions

Plant closures and trade liberalization policies	Venkataramani et al. (2020)	Included 112 manufacturing counties located in 30 commuting zones (primarily in the US South and Midwest) with at least 1 automotive assembly plant as of 1999	Quasi-experiment: Fixed-effects regression with difference-in-differences analysis	The association between automotive assembly plant closures and opioid overdose mortality rates among working-age adults from 1999 to 2016	In counties exposed to plant closures, mortality rates increased by 8.6 opioid overdose deaths per 100,000 individuals over 5 years, an 85% rise relative to the pre-closure mortality rate The greatest increases in deaths occurred among non-Hispanic white men
	Autor et al. (2013)	Data on the value of US imports and exports between 2000 and 2007. Regional economies were defined using the 772 Commuting Zones (CZs) on the mainland US	Quasi-experiment: Fixed-effects regression with difference-in-differences analysis	Relationship between declines in US manufacturing jobs brought on by import competition from China, and mortality due to opioid and alcohol overdoses	As measured over decades, the loss of manufacturing jobs negatively affected working-age males via reductions in manufacturing jobs and wage levels, and increased opioid overdose mortality
	Charles et al. (2019)	Multiple sources: supplements of the Current Population Survey (CPS; IPUMS, Census and American Community Surveys, restricted to persons aged 21–55 focusing on commuting zones	Fixed effects	The relationship between declining local manufacturing and opioid use and death from 2001 to 2016	Declining local manufacturing employment is related to rising local opioid use and deaths Manufacturing decline in a local area in the 2000s had large and persistent negative effects on local employment rates, hours worked, and wage
	Pierce and Schott (2020)	Microdata from the CDC from 2000 to 2013 and two sets of tariff rates in the US tariff schedule Counties in the sample were distributed across 741 commuting zones	Quasi-experiment: Difference-in-differences approach	Relationship between deaths of despair, including fatal drug overdoses, and changes in US trade policy, specifically the granting of Permanent Normal Trade Relations (PNTR) to China in October 2000	Counties with greater exposure to PNTR displayed relative increases in deaths of despair, including opioid fatalities Effects were mainly observed among the white working-age population Also, greater exposure to change in trade policy led to adverse changes in unemployment and labor force participation rates, a possible mechanism by which trade policy increases drug-related mortality

(continued)

Study type	Study authors	Source	Method	Focus	Result
Economic expansion/ improvement	Musse (2020)	Scanner data from more than 170 million opioid transactions and more than 1 billion sales of over-the-counter (OTC) painkillers	Quasi-experiment: difference-in-differences framework	Effects of opioid transactions and sales of over-the-counter (OTC) painkillers on the mechanisms driving demand for pain medication during employment shocks	A one percent increase in the employment-to-population ratio decreases the per capita demand for opioids by 0.20 percent, while it increases the per capita demand for OTC painkillers by 0.14% Employment expansion affects opioid use through two channels: (1) increasing physical pain from work in expanding injury-prone industries or (2) reducing mental distress that can contribute to substance abuse
	Metcalf and Wang (2019)	Dataset includes 3100 counties, with mortality data for 2000–2016 from the CDC merged with coal production data from Energy Information Administration (EIA)	Fixed-effect model	Whether greater reliance on coal mining activity in a county's economy leads to higher or lower opioid mortality	A 1% increase among the coal-producing counties in the share of coal miners in the workforce increased the opioid mortality rate by 0.192 % One possible explanation for this finding is that increasing coal mining activity results in more workplace injuries followed by more opioid prescriptions and higher opioid death rates
	Dow (2020)	Geocoded CDC Multiple Causes of Death data for 1999–2017 for adult 18–64	Quasi-experiment: Difference-in-differences models	State-level analysis of the effect of minimum wage policies on deaths of despair	No significant effects on drug or alcohol-related mortality, but significant reductions in non-drug suicides

Opioid supply	Harris et al. (2020)	Data for 10 states from the prescription drug monitoring program and (PDMP) databases as well as data from the Bureau of Labor Statistics (BLS) for 2010–2015	Fixed effects	The relationship between prescription opioids and county-level labor market outcomes, such as labor force participation rates, employment-to-population ratios, and unemployment rates	A 10% increase in opioid prescriptions leads to a 0.56% point reduction in labor force participation
	Deiana and Giua (2018)	The final sample encompassed 741 commuting zones across the US	Quasi-experiment: Fixed effects with difference-in-differences approach	The impact of five sets of opioid-related state laws on labor market conditions and illegal activities at the county level from 2000 to 2014	An improvement in labor market participation and a rise in crime after implementation of laws to limit the supply of prescription opioids
	Park and Powell (2020)	Social Security Administration (SSA) Fiscal Year Disability Claim Data, focusing on adults, aged 18–64 and Bureau of Economic Analysis (BEA) and CES data, involving a survey of places of business representing workers covered by unemployment insurance	Fixed-effects regression	State-level analysis of the effects of transition from prescription opioids to illicit opioids (after the reformulation of Oxycontin) on labor supply and disability insurance from 2001 to 2015	Disability insurance applications and enrollment significantly increased in states with higher pre-reformulation rates of OxyContin misuse while labor market engagement decreased Shifts in labor supply and disability insurance were not associated with rates of broad analgesic misuse

(continued)

Study type	Study authors	Source	Method	Focus	Result
	Laird and Nielsen (2017)	Danish administrative data to examine the full population of the 1925–1980 birth cohorts. This information was connected with an individual's prescription drug use, their primary care provider, municipality of residence, and labor market outcomes from 1995 to 2013	Fixed effects and a semi-exogenous separation of an individual from their doctor due to a cross-municipality move	The impacts of physician prescribing behaviors on patient prescription drug use and labor market outcomes for the four classes of prescription drugs used most frequently to treat musculoskeletal and mental health disorders, including opioids	A general practitioner with a 10% point higher opioid prescription rate increases the probability of an individual using prescribed opioids by a 4.5 percentage point and a 1.5 percentage point decrease in labor market participation
	Savych et al. (2018)	Data from 28 states for injuries between 2008 and 2013 in situations where workers had more than seven days of lost work time WCRI Detailed Benchmark/Evaluation Database was the source for payment information on disability claims	Fixed effects	The effects of local opioid prescriptions on the duration of temporary disability benefits among workers with work-related low back injury	Longer term opioid prescribing stretches the length of temporary disability episodes among individuals receiving Workers Compensation benefits Durations for claims of temporary disability with prescription opioids were more than triple the duration for claims without prescription opioids
	Currie et al. (2018)	Prescription data was acquired from IQVIA, a company specializing in pharmaceutical market intelligence	Fixed-effects regression	County-level analysis for 2006–2014 to determine the relationship between per capita opioid prescription rates and employment-to-population ratios	No simple causal relationship between economic conditions and the abuse of opioids The estimated effect of opioids on employment-to-population ratios was positive but modest for women, with no relationship for men. Ambiguous findings for the effects of employment-to-population ratios on opioid prescriptions

Appendix B: Geographic/Spatial Analysis Research

Study authors	Sources	Method	Focus	Result
Ghertner and Groves (2018)	Data sources:: US Census; BLS; CDC; DEA Automation of Reports and Consolidated Orders System (ARCOS) (2006–2016); CMS Prescription Drug Event File (2006–2016); CDC for drug overdose deaths (2006–2016); and HCUP State Inpatient Databases and State Emergency Department Databases (2011–2014)	Geographic analysis/linear regression models	County-level analysis of the relationship between economic opportunity, substance use, and opioid prevalence measures	On average, counties with poorer economic conditions are more likely to have higher substance misuse prevalence measures. This relationship was clustered in specific areas of the country; rural areas were most affected, including Appalachia, parts of the West, Midwest, and New England However, some high poverty areas had low rates of overdose deaths and opioid-related hospitalizations and were seemingly protected from the opioid epidemic
Wilkes et al. (2021)	Sources: Data on opioid-related hospital inpatient stays and emergency department visits from the Healthcare Cost and Utilization Project, 2010–2018 and US Census demographic data	Generalized linear mixed models	To assess the incidence of opioid use, based on geographic and population characteristics	Regions in the west of the US were most affected by the opioid epidemic across all population center sizes; alternatively, communities in the northwest coastal region were least affected. Within the northwest, the opioid epidemic appeared to improve when moving from urban population densities to more rural population densities. However, population size centers in other regions did not show any clear trends

(continued)

Study authors	Sources	Method	Focus	Result
Pear et al. (2019)	Source: community hospital discharges from Healthcare Cost and Utilization Project's State Inpatient Databases and state governments, 2002–2014 Demographic estimates came from GeoLytics, Inc., 2016 Urbanicity was measured with a modified version of the USDA's 2010 Rural-Urban Commuting Area codes	Ecological time-series study using hierarchical Bayesian Poisson space-time models	Assessed the relationship between socioeconomic indicators and prescription opioid overdose (POD) and heroin overdose (HOD) based on degree of urbanicity of ZIP codes in 17 states	Higher rates of POD were found in more economically disadvantaged ZIP codes across the urban–rural continuum Economic disadvantage (% in poverty, low educational attainment) had a greater impact on HOD in urban than rural areas, indicating that HOD rates in rural places may have different drivers
Monnat (2019)	Sources: Mortality and prescribing data from CDC and demographic and labor market information from U.S. Census Bureau for 2000–02 and 2014–16	Linear random-effects regression models	Examined relationships between white drug mortality rates and socioeconomic and opioid supply metrics over time in counties spanning the rural–urban spectrum and within various rural labor markets	Economic distress, family distress, persistent population loss, and opioid supply factors were associated with significantly higher drug mortality rates in all rural and urban contexts Effect sizes varied across the urban–rural continuum and across rural labor markets Ultimately, the highest drug mortality rates were disproportionately concentrated in counties that were economically distressed and mining and service sector dependent (and thus greater exposure to prescription opioids and fentanyl)

Monnat et al. (2019)	Sources: CDC mortality data (2002–2004 and 2014–2016) and county-level US Census data	Multivariate and multivariable regression models	Examines associations of county-level population, economic and labor market characteristics and drug mortality rates to predict probability of membership in "opioid mortality classes"	Identified six "opioid mortality classes" reflecting low-to-high mortality levels and growth rates Overall, drug mortality rates are higher in counties characterized by more economic disadvantage, more blue-collar and service employment, and higher opioid-prescribing rates High heroin and "syndemic" opioid mortality counties (high rates across all major opioid types) are more urban, have larger concentrations of professional workers, and are less economically disadvantaged
Peters et al. (2020)	Sources: CDC fatal overdose rates in 2002–04, 2008–12, and 2014–2016 and U.S. Census Bureau's American Community Survey	Latent profile analysis	Classified counties into distinct classes based on overdose rates for specific opioids	Identified three distinct epidemics (prescription opioids, heroin, and prescription-synthetic opioid mixtures) and one syndemic involving all opioids e.g., Prescription-related epidemic counties, whether rural or urban, have been "left behind" the rest of the nation. These communities are less populated and more remote, older and mostly white, have a history of drug abuse, and are former farm and factory communities that have been in decline since the 1990s
Hochstetler and Peters (2023)	Sources: CDC mortality data; US Census American Community survey and other official sources	Latent profile analysis; Multivariate general linear model	Expanded Peters et al. (2019) and Monnat et al. (2019) to categorize counties by syndemic composition and predict their location using mortality rates from 2017–19	America does not have a single drug crisis but multiple epidemics that are spatially diverse requiring different policy responses

Appendix C: Qualitative Studies on Risk Environment

Authors, Year	Participants	Location	Drugs Discussed	Economic	Physical	Social	Policy
Thomas et al. (2020)	Systematic Review			Deindustrialization, economic decline, and economic distress created an environment where individuals used opioids to manage financial stress Economic strain also led some participants to engage in riskier drug-related practices such as injecting to cut costs associated with use	Frayed or absent infrastructure; lack of recreational options; transportation barriers due to scattered populations and large geographic distances between destinations; difficulty accessing services and treatment facilities and challenges recruiting and retaining staff	Stigmatization of people who misuse opioids (PWMO); lack of anonymity in rural settings; families and social networks provide support and help with managing stigma; easy access to prescription opioids in the home or intergenerational drug use; development of risk norms	Limited coverage and accessible harm reduction and drug treatment services; high clinician caseloads
Guise et al. (2017)	Systematic Literature Review	Urban and Rural Studies				Social networks encourage injecting drugs; injecting drugs for a sense of belonging to particular social groups; socialization process that normalizes injecting drugs; injecting drugs to cope with pain and traumatic experiences	

Schalkoff et al. (2021)	34 community stakeholders (interviews)	Appalachia	Prescription opioids	Environmental/community trauma referring to the profound economic distress following deindustrialization Lack of economic opportunity linked to pervasive despair and lack of trust Fears of corruption in local government Weakened community cohesion and prevented the possibility of recovery		Sexual assault, domestic violence, and other physical and sexual trauma throughout communities Youth exposed to traumatic drug-related issues Emotional burnout among first responders	
Thompson et al. (2020)	20 key stakeholders (includes residents) (interviews)	Appalachia	Prescription opioids Heroin	Structural and social inequalities in the community Household and community economic challenges, including the absence of funding for support services, jobs and community resources Lack of community engagement Despair		Intergenerational drug use Familial stress, violence and dysfunction Drug use normalized throughout the community Difficulty asking for help (norm)	

(continued)

Authors, Year	Participants	Location	Drugs Discussed	Economic	Physical	Social	Policy
Linton et al. (2021)	22 Community Stakeholders (interviews)	Baltimore	Heroin	Economically-depressed area Housing instability	Lack of drug-related prevention and treatment services; lack of transportation; lack of payment assistance; lack of recreational opportunities	Non-medical prescription opioid (NMPO) normalized and socially acceptable Interpersonal violence and abuse Intergenerational drug use Stigma	Police brutality; zero tolerance policies; lack of integration of mental health and drug treatment; one-size-fits-all drug programs
Cloud et al. (2019)	19 male and female residents (interviews)	Appalachia	Heroin Prescription opioids Methamphetamines	Poor job market Sense of powerlessness and depression	Lack of opportunities for social activity; lack of mental health services; fear of law enforcement shaped the physical places and social environments in which people used drugs	Stigma Strong family ties (protective mechanism) Interfamilial drug use Cultural tradition of reluctance to seek help	Local political opposition to sterile needle programs
Sered (2019)	Over 60 adults (interviews) plus field research	Weymouth, MA (suburb)	Prescription opioids, later transitioning to heroin and fentanyl	Decline of blue-collar and union jobs; labor market shifts	A deteriorating sense of community Sense of betrayal by institutions Loss of social capital and cultural capital		Catholic Church abuse scandal; Educational tracking; pressure on all kids to go to college

Williams and Francis (2022)	62 Black adults and youth (11 focus groups)	Dane County, WI	Opioids (primary focus) Specific drugs mentioned: heroin, prescription drugs, promethazine, and cocaine	Low-income	Poor social infrastructure; lack of "third" (neutral) spaces to gather; social isolation		Interlocking systems of oppression/structural racism Harassment by law enforcement, hospital administrators, Child Protective Services, social workers, landlords, and school administrators
McLean (2016)	Clients of substance use treatment center (interviews)	City of McKeesport, located in the Monongahela Valley region of Pennsylvania	Heroin	Economically depressed, deindustrialized, lack of job opportunities; a growing drug market offers recreation and employment	Absence of harm reduction services; transportation barriers to overdose prevention education and free naloxone	Lack of social support	
George et al. (2021)	60 community members and coalitions (Focus groups)	Urban and rural areas in Central Pennsylvania		Financial distress	Fraying infrastructure, lack of transportation; lack of access to health care; inadequate education system	Family fragmentation; loss of community	

(continued)

Authors, Year	Participants	Location	Drugs Discussed	Economic	Physical	Social	Policy
Draus and Carlson (2006)	25 self-described injectors	Rural Ohio	Heroin	Inject heroin to save money Use drugs to escape bleak economic situation		Sexual assault	
Redican et al. (2012)	Mixed Methods: Surveys and seven focus field interviews of key community stakeholders	Southwestern Virginia	Oxycodone, hydrocodone, methadone, and morphine, fentanyl, dilaudid, barbiturates, or benzodiazepines	High rates of workplace injuries for employment in logging and coal mining leads to legitimate use of prescribed opioids for pain relief…can lead to inappropriate use Poverty/unemployment Despair and boredom		Culture of acceptance of prescription drug use—for physical and emotional pain Adolescent use by young adults Youth are exposed early and have access to these drugs through their family's medicine cabinets Lack of family cohesion—high rates of child abuse and neglect	
Leukefeld et al. (2007)	70 key Informants in four groups	Two counties in Appalachian Kentucky	Prescription drugs – oxycodone, hydrocodone, methadone; benzodiazepines	Hopelessness Lack of opportunity Disabled people with Medicaid benefits sell their prescription drugs; also, elderly sell their prescription drugs to supplement their income			Need for treatment funding

Buer et al. (2016)	16 women (interviews)	Central Appalachia	Primary drug is prescription opioids	Socioeconomic inequalities, including poverty, unemployment, and lack of affordable health care Difficult to find a secure job w/living wages if female	Geographic isolation Mental health care and substance abuse treatment are inaccessible due to waiting times, cost and transportation issues Lack of access to medication-assisted treatment Financial barriers and administrative paperwork prevent women from accessing buprenorphine and methadone at local clinics	Domestic violence Fear of leaving drug networks Economic inequalities constrain care strategies and keep women in abusive, violent relationships Family relationships/ ties one of only avenues to quit drugs	Child Protective Services (and policies targeting mothers) used as threat
Rigg and Murphy (2013)	90 users of prescription opioid (interviews)	South Florida	Prescription opioids	Housing instability	Easier to get pills than heroin Contact with the healthcare system	Family history of substance use Romantic relationships – drug centered Emotional trauma	
Roberson et al. (2020)	Online survey and 26 patients at clinics (interviews)	Central and Southern Appalachia	Opioids	Poverty Low education levels		Social networks increase resiliency	Programs and policies limit access to opioid prescriptions

(continued)

Authors, Year	Participants	Location	Drugs Discussed	Economic	Physical	Social	Policy
Walters et al. (2023)	Nineteen in-depth semi-structured interviews with PWID and 4 with key informants who professionally work with PWID	Rural southern Illinois	Opioids and methamphetamines (injected)	Poverty Lack of economic opportunity Unaffordable housing and high living expenses Healthcare costs	Drug use/risk practices and settings Sharing or reusing equipment due to lacking access to new equipment Lack of services Lack of information about latest therapies for HCV	Stigma (in healthcare and other interactions), Hard to use drugs privately	Heavy policing, discrimination from pharmacists and police
Trappen and McLean (2021)	Part of ongoing research study (see McLean 2016) Interviews with 15 residents, some but not all reported ongoing illicit drug use, knew and/or maintained relationships with people who used illicit drugs, or were receiving ongoing medical treatment for mental health and substance use issues	McKeesport, PA	Prescription opioids but increasing use of illicit/synthetic opioids	Economic deterioration, deindustrialized, low labor force participation, poverty, economic tension	Uneven spatial development (community growth in some areas but not others) Fear of crime	Social isolation exacerbated by COVID-19	Fear of police (prevents requests for services) Fear of overdose

Smith et al. (2022)	Interviews with 21 African American adults with a history of illicit drug use	Baltimore, Maryland	Illicit drug use	Economic hardship	Increased visibility of drug markets	Normalization of drug use within social networks	
Nolte et al. (2020)	Interviews with 31 Stakeholders in health care, harm reduction, addiction, public health, and law enforcement Interviews with 22 Persons who use drugs (PWUDs) Part of a larger epidemiological and policy mixed-methods study	Rural Northern New England	Syndemic focus: heroin, cocaine/crack, opiate painkillers, buprenorphine, street fentanyl, and methamphetamine	Economic distress, high unemployment, economic disparities	Drug risk practices and settings Sharing or reusing needles due to lacking access to new equipment Geospatial access issues, transportation gaps, medications for opioid use disorder (MOUD) treatment less common than other modalities Some barriers to syringe access	Stigma in healthcare settings barrier to care Also distrust or feel disrespected by doctors Normalization of drug use within family and community trauma	Monitoring and controlling supply of prescription opioids lead to use of alternative drugs like heroin Policy climate limits action

Index

L. R. Webster, S. Eichberg, *Deconstructing Toxic Narratives*,
https://doi.org/10.1007/978-3-032-23135-2

GPSR Compliance

The European Union's (EU) General Product Safety Regulation (GPSR) is a set of rules that requires consumer products to be safe and our obligations to ensure this.

If you have any concerns about our products, you can contact us on ProductSafety@springernature.com

In case Publisher is established outside the EU, the EU authorized representative is:

Springer Nature Customer Service Center GmbH
Europaplatz 3
69115 Heidelberg, Germany

Batch number: 10370736

Printed by Printforce, the Netherlands

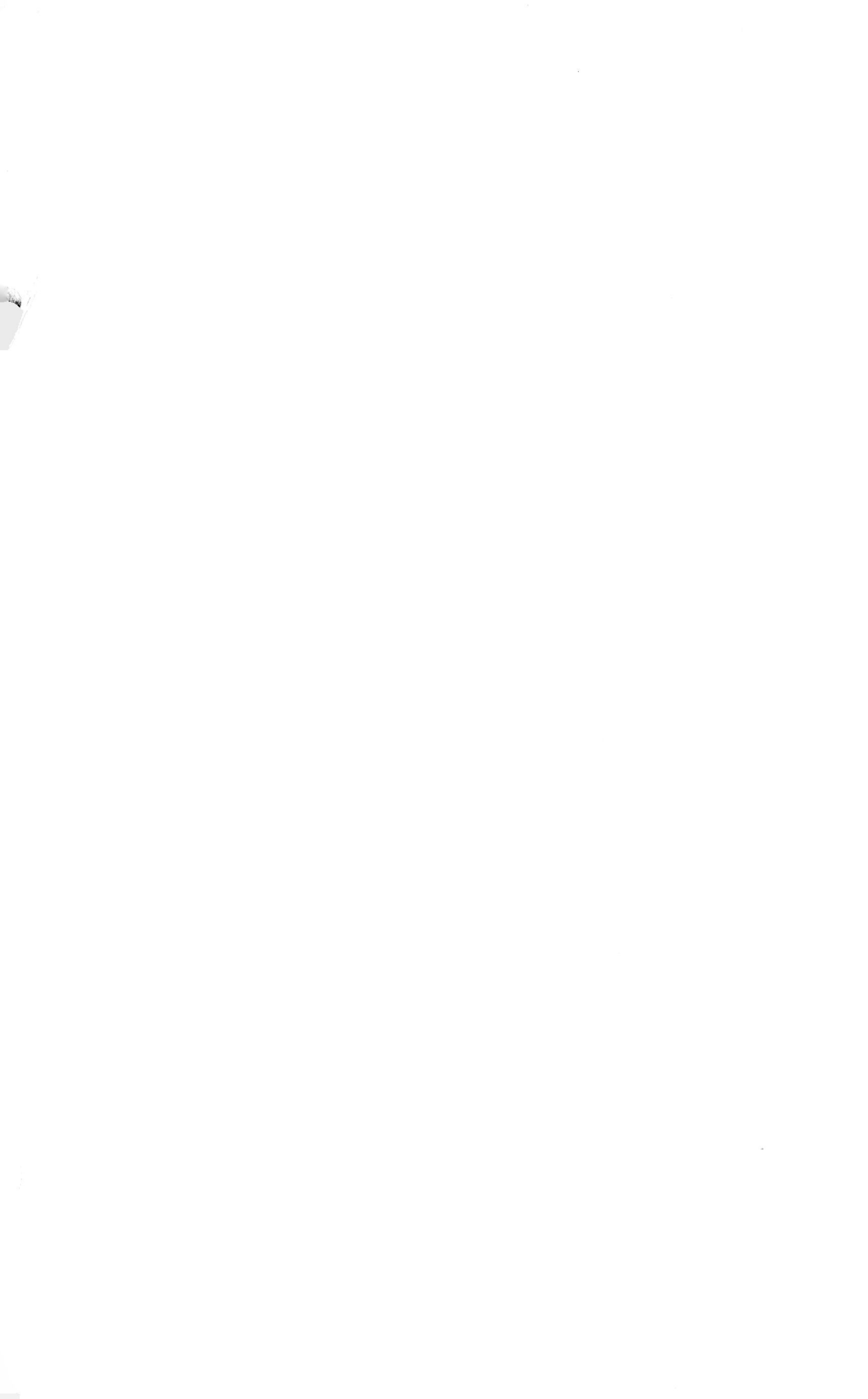